20074
.v94

Readings on the Behavior Disorders of Childhood

Edited by
James R. Frazier
Donald K. Routh
University of North Carolina

MSS Information Corporation
655 Madison Avenue, New York, N.Y. 10021

This is a custom-made book of readings prepared for the
courses taught by the editors, as well as for related courses
and for college and university libraries. For information
about our program, please write to:

MSS INFORMATION CORPORATION
655 Madison Avenue
New York, New York 10021

MSS wishes to express its appreciation to the authors of the
articles in this collection for their cooperation in making
their work available in this format.

Library of Congress Cataloging in Publication Data

Frazier, James R   comp.
    Readings on the behavior disorders of childhood.

    CONTENTS: Maturation of pattern vision in infants
during the first six months, by R. L. Fantz, J. M. Or
and M. S. Udelf.--Concept learning in discrimination
tasks, by E. C. Caldwell and V. C. Hall.--Speech perception in infants, by P. D. Eimas and others.
RJ499.F72   618.9'28'9008   72-86267
ISBN 0-8422-5005-0
ISBN 0-8422-0202-1 (pbk)

CONTENTS

SECTION V: SPECIFIC ACADEMIC DIFFICULTIES

SECTION VI: CHILD NEUROSIS

SECTION VII: CHILD PSYCHOSIS

Preface

The present collection of readings in the behavior disorders of childhood grew out of the practical demands of teaching courses in this area to graduate and advanced undergraduate courses in psychology. Most of the articles selected for inclusion in the book have appeared repeatedly on course reading lists and have continued to command the interest of students and to underscore some of the salient theoretical and practical issues in child psychopathology.

A glance at the table of contents will indicate that the editors of this collection view the field of behavior disorders in children more broadly than most. Besides articles in traditional areas such as child neurosis, psychosis, and antisocial behavior, there are others concerned with disorders of sensation and perception, with motor development and cerebral palsy, with the development and disorders of speech and language, and with academic skill deficits in children. Biological and social aspects are included to prevent a narrow psychological focus, and the laboratory approach is well represented in addition to strictly clinical studies. Finally, the infant and preschool age groups receive an emphasis equal to that given older children.

This breadth of definition of the field relates to the fact that both of the editors have worked during most of their careers in settings where more than the traditional three mental health fields (psychiatry, psychology, and social work)

were represented. We have worked alongside
pediatricians, neurologists, and pediatric
nurses; speech and hearing clinicians,
special educators, and physical and occupational therapists; and even pedodontists,
nutritionists, and biochemists. We have
learned very well that children's problems
do not neatly divide themselves along
traditional professional and scientific
boundary lines and that ignorance of the
insights of a neighboring discipline can
impoverish one's ability to see the child
whole and to plan an approach to his
problems.

SECTION I

DISORDERS OF SENSATION AND PERCEPTION IN CHILDHOOD

MATURATION OF PATTERN VISION IN INFANTS DURING THE FIRST SIX MONTHS[1]

ROBERT L. FANTZ, J. M. ORDY, AND M. S. UDELF

Western Reserve University and St. Vincent Charity Hospital, Cleveland

Studies of the vision of young infants have been confined largely to the stimulus variables of intensity, wave length, and movement. This is apparently due to two assumptions: first, that tests of pattern vision are not feasible during the early months; and second, that negative results would be obtained in any case due to the immaturity of the eye and brain, which is presumed to prevent the focusing of an image on the retina, to interfere with precise retinal reception and neural transmission, and to exclude "cortical vision" (McGraw, 1943; Pratt, 1946; Zubek & Solberg, 1954).

Both assumptions have been challenged by studies comparing the visual attention given to stimuli differing only in form or pattern. Consistent differential response to patterns was shown by infants throughout the first 6 mo. (Fantz, 1958) and as early as 1 day of age (Stirnimann, 1944). These studies, using large patterns, indicated that although pattern vision may be very poor in the early months, it is not absent. Data on visual acuity at various ages were needed to clarify the issue. The resolution of visual detail involves most of the structures and functions underlying pattern and spatial vision. Thus visual acuity can provide a behavioral measure of the maturation of the basic visual mechanism as a foundation for studying the development of adaptive responses to specific visual patterns.

A so-called acuity test described by Gesell, Ilg, and Bullis (1949) consists of placing a small sugar pellet at a certain distance in front of the infant and noting any reaction to it. A technique developed by Schwarting (1954) requires the visual pursuit of a fine wire moving across a lighted area. A more sensitive technique involving visual pursuit, often used to test the acuity of animals, con-

sists of observing the reflex eye and head movements to a large field of moving stripes and decreasing the width of stripes until this optokinetic nystagmus response is no longer present (Morgan & Stellar, 1950). Recently Gorman, Cogan, and Gellis (1957), using this technique with infants under 5 days of age found that 93 of 100 infants responded to stripes subtending a visual angle of 33.5 min., while few responded to stripes one-third as wide.

Although this result indicates a much better developed visual system in the newborn infant than had been assumed, its meaning for the maturation of pattern vision is uncertain. Structures which are important in the mediation of pattern vision—the central retina and the cerebral cortex—are not essential for the nystagmic response to patterned stimulation, at least in the adult animal (Morgan & Stellar, 1950; Walsh, 1957). Furthermore, the reflex response to a moving pattern covering most of the visual field is a very different type of visual performance from the "voluntary" attention to the pattern of localized stationary objects. The latter response, representing a closer approach to the way pattern vision functions in most adaptive behavior of the adult, formed the basis for the acuity test in the present experiments. The optokinetic technique was used for comparison with the differential fixation test in the second study.

Young infants tend to look at patterned surfaces in preference to homogeneous ones (Berlyne, 1958; Fantz, 1958; Stirnimann, 1944). If we present a graded series of patterns and find the smallest which elicits a differential ocular response, we know that visual detail at least that fine can be resolved. This method was shown to be feasible in a preliminary study (Fantz & Ordy, 1959). Infants from 2 to 5 mo. responded to stripes subtending a visual angle as small as 18 min., while younger infants did not respond consistently to the sizes of pattern used.

[1] This research was supported by Grants M-2497 and M-5284 from the National Institute of Mental Health, United States Public Health Service. It was carried out with the cooperation of DePaul Infant Home.

JOURNAL OF COMPARITIVE AND PSYCIOLOGICAL PSYCHOLOGY, 1962 Vol. 55., pp. 907-917.

Experiment 1

The main aim was to obtain more complete data on the early development of acuity by using a larger sample of infants and a wider range of pattern size. A second aim was to find the effect of testing distance on the level of acuity to provide information on the maturation of accommodation for nearby distances. A third aim was to try to separate two parts of the total visual response to pattern: reflex responses to a peripheral pattern, and maintenance of a central fixation of the pattern.

Method

Procedure. The procedure was to place an infant in a crib inside a test chamber and to expose above him a striped pattern and a plain gray comparison object for 20 sec. Ocular responses were observed through a peephole and recorded on timers and counters. A second exposure was made with reversed object positions. The initial positions were determined randomly. Stripes of varying widths were presented in this way in random order during a single test session. Within 2 weeks or less, each infant was given three such tests but with the distance of the stimulus objects changed. The order of testing at the three distances was varied systematically for all age levels.

Apparatus. The test chamber was basically a wooden box 2 ft. sq. and 30 in. high, resting on a low table. The lower half of the front side of the chamber was open so that a small hammock-type crib could be rolled underneath until the infant's head was directly under an observation hole in the center of the ceiling. The stimulus objects were attached to the ceiling to the right and left of this ¼-in. peephole. For the 5- and 10-in. distances, the objects extended down from the ceiling on dowel rods which were slanted so as to not be visible to the infant. Fine adjustments of the distance were made for each S by raising or lowering the crib.

The objects were placed in position in the chamber through rectangular openings 14 by 5 in. high along the top of the right and left sides of the chamber. These openings also gave additional space needed for the 20-in. separation of the 8-in. stimulus objects. The ceiling of the chamber extended over the side openings to prevent the infant's seeing into the room (see Fig. 1). The inside of the chamber was a nonglossy, dark saturated blue color which tended to quiet the infants and gave a contrasting background for the lighter achromatic objects.

The illumination of objects at each distance came through a horizontal slit in the back of the chamber from two 25-w. projection bulbs not visible to the infant. They were directed obliquely to the object surfaces to eliminate glare, resulting in only about 4 ft-c of light reflected from the objects according to an illumination meter. The lights were equidistant from the test and comparison objects and also from the objects at the three test distances, to equate illuminance. Background illuminance was also held constant.

The objects were hidden from view between exposures by drawing two window shades horizontally across the middle of the chamber. A 2-in. hole in the center of the closed shades served to attract the infant's gaze to the center and, at the same time, allowed E to wait until the gaze was midway between the objects before opening the shades, in order to minimize position preferences.

Stimulus objects. The test patterns were squares with vertical black and white stripes of equal width. A series of five pattern sizes was used, each presented with the same gray square, matched in luminous reflectance. All objects were nonglossy photographic prints glued to posterboard. The original striped patterns were made by a scale-making machine tool accurate to .0001 in. Stimulus objects of a different size were used for each test distance (measured from the infant's eyes to the point midway between the test and comparison objects). For the 5-in. distance, the objects were 2-in. squares placed 5 in. apart, center to center; for the 10-in. distance, 4-in. squares 10 in. apart; for the 20-in. distance, 8-in. squares 20 in. apart. This resulted in a constant visual angle of 20° subtended by each test object and a constant visual angle of 53° between the two objects presented together (see Fig. 1). The width of stripes also increased in proportion to distance, as shown in Table 1, to give a constant retinal size.

Response measure. The S's eyes were observed through the hole in the ceiling of the chamber. Tiny reflections of the stimulus objects were clearly visible on the cornea, under the given conditions of contrasting figures against a homogeneous ground. The location of one of these reflections over the pupil provided a simple criterion of fixation. If the left reflection was over the pupil, for example, the infant was looking at the object on the left. Since coordination of the two eyes was not always good in the early months, the location of a reflection over either pupil was accepted to indicate fixation as long as the reflection of the other object was not over the pupil of the other eye (which rarely occurred).

A reliability check of this criterion of fixation was made in an earlier study using photographic recordings (Fantz, 1956). Good agreement in the relative attention given to different objects was shown in independent analyses of the photographs. Direct observation of responses was used in the present experiments for greater clarity of observation and simplicity of procedure.

Fixations of the right and left objects were recorded by pressing the right or left of two telegraph-key switches. Each switch activated a Veeder counter when first pressed, to record the number of separate fixations, and also started a Thompson stop clock, to record the accumulated duration of fixations of the object during a 20-sec. exposure. Timers and counters stopped automatically at the end of the exposure.

Subjects. The Ss were 37 infants 1 to 22 weeks of age and included all infants under 6 mo. available at a foundling home at the time of the experiment excepting six who persistently cried or otherwise made testing impossible. The infants had been screened for gross abnormalities of any sort upon admittance to the

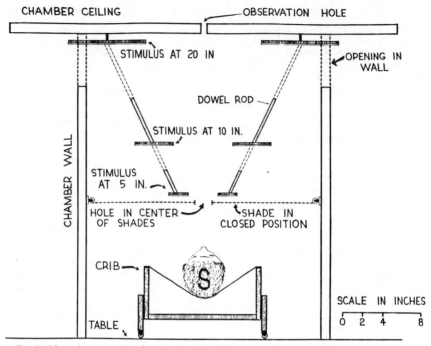

CHAMBER CEILING — OBSERVATION HOLE

STIMULUS AT 20 IN

OPENING IN WALL

DOWEL ROD

STIMULUS AT 10 IN.

STIMULUS AT 5 IN.

CHAMBER WALL

HOLE IN CENTER OF SHADES

SHADE IN CLOSED POSITION

CRIB

TABLE

SCALE IN INCHES
0   2   4   8

FIG. 1. Schematic cross section through the middle of the testing chamber, with the stimulus objects used at the three test distances superimposed on the same drawing. (The drawing is to scale except for the ¼-in. observation hole.)

home and, in addition, after the study had an ophthalmological examination which indicated no apparent ocular pathology.

In order to be able to finish a test session before the infant became fussy or fell asleep, the smaller pattern sizes were omitted for the younger infants and the largest pattern was omitted for the older ones. This selection was based on preliminary results suggesting the acuity level at each age.

Results and Discussion

The scores for the two consecutive test periods with reversed right and left positions of the striped and plain objects were combined to balance out the position preferences shown by a number of the infants. Even a consistent tendency to look more at the right or at the left object did not in most cases prevent the infant from also showing consistent differential object fixation with the position effect controlled.

The main data analysis is based on the relative fixation time for patterned and unpat-

terned objects. Table 2 gives the consistency of predominant responses to stripes for infants of all ages. At each distance the three larger pattern sizes were each significantly differentiated from gray according to one-tailed sign tests. Thus, the tendency shown in previous studies for infants to attend more to patterned objects was verified under the present conditions to provide the necessary

TABLE 1

PATTERN SIZES FOR EACH TESTING DISTANCE

Visual Angle Subtended by Stripe (min.)	Width of Stripe (in.)		
	5 in. Dist. 2 in. Sq.	10 in. Dist. 4 in. Sq.	20 in. Dist. 8 in. Sq.
5	$1\frac{1}{28}$	$\frac{1}{64}$	$\frac{1}{32}$
10	$\frac{1}{64}$	$\frac{1}{32}$	$\frac{1}{16}$
20	$\frac{1}{32}$	$\frac{1}{16}$	$\frac{1}{8}$
40	$\frac{1}{16}$	$\frac{1}{8}$	$\frac{1}{4}$
80	$\frac{1}{8}$	$\frac{1}{4}$	$\frac{1}{2}$

10

TABLE 2
VISUAL FIXATION RESPONSES TO SUCCESSIVE
PATTERN SIZES BY INFANTS OF ALL
AGES AT EACH DISTANCE

Test Dist. (in.)	No. Infants Responding More to Stripes (in minutes of visual angle) vs. No. for Gray Comparison Object (G)[a]				
	5/G	10/G	20/G	40/G	80/G
5	10/6	14/15	29/6**	27/7**	17/1**
10	6/11	16/14	28/8**	33/3**	14/5*
20	10/7	19/11	25/10*	28/8**	17/2**
Total[b]	8/9	16/14	29/8**	34/3**	18/2**

[a] Since not all pattern sizes were used at each age level, the total N varies with stimulus pair.

[b] Based on combined scores for each infant at the three distances.

* $p < .05$ level.

** $p < .001$ level.

basis for estimating how fine a pattern can be resolved.

Age. The results for the three tests at different distances were included together for the analysis of age differences. With a criterion of 75% of the tests showing longer response to the patterned than to the plain object, the minimum separable visual angle for both the first and the second month of age was 40 min.; for each of the next 2 mo., 20 min.; and over 4 mo., this criterion was almost reached (73%) for 10 min. That these data actually measure a sensory threshold was suggested by an abrupt change at the criterion point from a near-chance result (equal tests favoring stripes and gray) to a consistent choice of stripes over gray. Such a change was shown by all but the oldest group, in which case a majority of tests showed a choice of even the finest stripes presented.

The consistency of choice of the two above-threshold patterns by the youngest group is particularly noteworthy in view of the supposed absence of the ability to fixate as well as to see pattern in the neonate. The 80-min. stripes were visually selected over gray in 15 of 18 tests; the 40-min. stripes, in 13 of 17 tests; while the 20-min. stripes were selected in half the tests.

Another basis for estimating the threshold for pattern at each age level is the average strength of the response differential for each size of pattern, shown in Figure 2. Again there is a clear separation between the close-to-

chance response level (equal duration of fixation of stripes and gray) for most below-threshold results and the uniformly high differential response to above-threshold patterns. A lower threshold was suggested for the second month; otherwise there is agreement with the frequency criterion.

Distance. One possible cause of less acute vision during the first month or two than later on is inability of the optical mechanism to focus a clear retinal image of a near object. It is known from ophthalmological measurements that the young infant is hyperopic ("farsighted"), which has been attributed to the short distance between lens and retina (Mann, 1950). The hyperopic eye requires accommodation of the lens to focus at any distance and especially at a short distance. However, it is often stated that the neonatal infant has little if any power of accommodation (McGraw, 1943; Pratt, 1946). If true, this would mean a blurred retinal image, with consequent loss of acuity at short test distances. This blurring would be expected to be accentuated by the low illumination used in this study due to the resultant large pupillary opening and reduction in depth of focus.

However, test distance had no noticeable effect on the response to pattern of a given

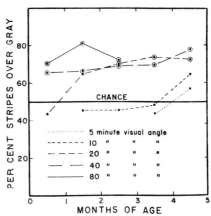

FIG. 2. Differential strength of visual fixation response to squares with varying angular fineness of pattern, averaged for tests at three distances for all infants at a given age. (Encircled points indicate that 75% of individual tests showed predominant response to pattern.)

retinal size for the range of sizes and distances used. This is shown in Table 2 for all ages combined. Likewise, the data for successive age groups did not reveal any relation between distance and visual acuity. In particular, the infants under 1 mo. of age attended equally to above-threshold patterns when placed at the three distances: stripes subtending 80 min. received an average of 70%, 73%, and 69% of the fixation time at 5, 10, and 20 in., respectively, while the corresponding figures for stripes half as wide were 63%, 65%, and 64%. Gorman et al. (1957) found a similar level of acuity in newborn infants tested at 6 in. for optokinetic nystagmus.

These results give behavioral evidence that the neonatal infant, in spite of being hyperopic, can focus sharply enough at a very short distance to resolve a near-threshold pattern, thus implying considerable power of accommodation. This is in agreement with anatomical and ophthalmological information (Mann, 1950; Pieper, 1949) suggesting that the optical system of the eye is functional at birth.

Since binocular coordination on a nearby object is not perfected for several months after birth, it is an interesting question why this would not impair visual acuity at close range. The answer may be that the doubling of the retinal image of an object due to lack of convergence need not obscure the pattern of either image provided it is superimposed on a homogeneous background.

Central fixation vs. peripheral reflex. Two other developmental factors which have been cited as causes of poor vision in the early months are the late maturation of the central retina compared with the periphery, and the supposed late appearance of nonreflex visual responses. Information on these factors was given by analyzing the fixation-time data into two component responses:

1. The *number* of separate fixations of each object during a test period, showing the number of times a stimulus falling on the peripheral retina elicits eye and head movements to bring the stimulus to the center of the visual field. The relative number of fixations of patterned and plain objects thus measures peripheral vision and reflex response tendencies.

2. The average *length* of fixation, derived by dividing the accumulated fixation time by the number of fixations, showing the length of time central fixation was maintained by interest in the object. The relative length of fixation of patterned and unpatterned objects thus measures vision in a more central area of the retina and the tendency to inhibit movements to peripheral stimuli.

Both measures indicated greater responsiveness to a visible pattern than to gray, but the differential for length of fixation was more pronounced and more consistent than for number of fixations. The relative consistency of the two measures is shown in Table 3, based only on data from the finest pattern discriminated by each age group. The frequencies for length of fixation are almost identical to those for total response time, while the differential for number of fixations is less consistent.

Figure 3 compares graphically the strength of the selectivity for a patterned object as measured by the average number of eye movements toward a peripheral stimulus and by the average duration of a central fixation. The relative responsiveness to gray and to stripes for each measure is shown by the relative distances along the scale. The areas enclosed by the two coordinates represent the resultant total response time for gray or for stripes during 40 sec. of testing. The stripes-gray differential is proportionally greater along the horizontal axis than along the vertical axis, especially for the infants under 3 mo.,

TABLE 3

Comparison of the Differential Response to a Near-Threshold Pattern Based on Three Different Measures of Visual Fixation

Age (mo.)	N	Width of Stripes (min.)	No. Infants Favoring Stripes vs. Gray for Each Measure[a]		
			No. of Fixations[b]	Mean Length of Fixation	Resultant Fixation Time
0–1	7	40	4/3	5/2	6/1
1–2	6	40	4/1	6/0	6/0
2–3	7	20	4/3	6/1	6/1
3–4	7	20	5/1	7/0	7/0
4–5	10	10	7/2	8/2	8/2
Total	37		24/10	32/5	33/4

[a] Based on total scores for each infant on three tests at different distances.
[b] Total N is lower due to three tie scores.

12

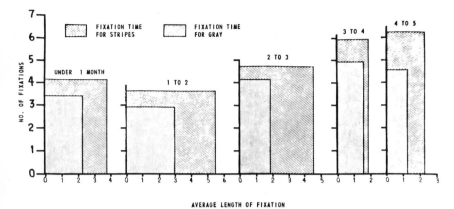

AVERAGE LENGTH OF FIXATION

Fig. 3. The relative contribution of two component responses (measured along the two coordinates) to the resultant total fixation time for patterned and for plain stimuli (area of the striped and of the gray portion) averaged for all pattern sizes and test distances.

for whom fixations were longer in general than for older infants.

These results do not prove that macular vision was more acute than peripheral vision, since the stimulus objects were so large that nonmacular parts of the retina may have contributed to the acuity shown by the central fixation component of the visual response. What these results do mean is that the overall response to fine patterns must be attributed primarily to sustained visual interest in a patterned stimulus once it falls on a broad central region of the retina, rather than to the peripheral response component. Stirnimann's results with newborns also imply sustained fixation of patterns. This central attentiveness to fine details, which might be considered the voluntary part of the fixation response, is thus present in immature form from the first month of life. Further development of this response and further maturation of the macula are undoubtedly important causes of the improvement in visual acuity during the early months.

Experiment 2

The pattern fixation test of acuity was compared with a more conventional acuity test based on the optokinetic nystagmus response to a moving striped field. It was hoped that the two different techniques would provide a check on each other and perhaps also clarify the role of various factors in the

development of acute vision. The testing was done by another investigator using mostly new Ss.

Method

Optokinetic test. The apparatus was similar to that used by Gorman et al. (1957). A roll of 16-in.-wide heavy paper had four 6-ft. sections of vertical black and white stripes alternating with 2-ft. sections of plain gray. The width of the stripes in the successive sections was $\frac{1}{8}$ in., $\frac{1}{16}$ in., $\frac{1}{32}$ in., and $\frac{1}{64}$ in., respectively. This paper was rolled from one drum to another around semicircular, 1 in.-wide strips of metal at either edge of the paper and in the middle, thus forming a half-cylinder chamber under the paper and between the drums. The hammock crib used in the first study was placed in such a position in this chamber that Ss eyes were in the center and about 10 in. from the paper all around the arc. Gray boards extended partway down from either edge of the paper to restrict the infant's view into the room and thus keep his attention on the moving stripes. The drums were turned by a hand crank so the speed could be easily varied. Fairly uniform illumination of the stripes was provided by a 25-w. incandescent bulb placed near the center of the chamber and level with the infant's head.

The procedure was to move the section of $\frac{1}{8}$-in. stripes slowly around the arc and observe the response from the front or back of the chamber. If pursuit eye and head movements in the direction of the stimulus movement were clearly present, followed by saccadic eye movements in the opposite direction, the next finer stripes were used, and so on. If the response was negative or uncertain, the same section of stripes was moved back and forth a number of times at varying speeds in the attempt to elicit a nystagmic response. When the response was in doubt, the test was repeated later. Two levels or qualities of nystagmic response were recorded: "Poor" responses were counted as

13

positive in the data analysis when there was agreement between two separate tests given before and after the pattern fixation test; a "good" response on either test was counted.

Pattern fixation test. The apparatus was the same as for Experiment 1. Only the 4-in. squares were used, at a distance of 10 in. and 10 in. apart. The largest pattern was omitted so that the same four widths of stripes were used as in the optokinetic test. For each infant the test started with the $\frac{1}{2}$-in. pattern paired with the gray comparison object; then the objects were reversed for another 20 sec. exposure. Successively smaller patterns were presented in the same manner. Only the accumulated fixation time for each object was recorded. Illumination was given by a single 25-w. incandescent bulb level with the infant's head and equidistant from the two stimuli. The amount of light reflected from the stripes was almost as much as in the optokinetic test and about the same as for the fixation test in Experiment 1.

Subjects. The Ss were 46 healthy infants 4 days to 6 mo. of age of which 10 had been used 3 mo. earlier in the first study.

Results and Discussion

The results are presented in Table 4 for each month of age and for each size of pattern. The data for the two techniques have a somewhat different meaning. For the fixation test, a close-to-equal frequency of infants responding more to stripes and more to gray indicates lack of discrimination; for the optokinetic test, a "zero" first frequency indicates lack of nystagmic response to that pattern size, while an intermediate value has no certain interpretation and could mean individual differences or fluctuations in sensory threshold or motor coordination, or errors of observation due to ambiguity of the response. However, for either technique a high percentage of response to pattern is indicative of visual resolution. A criterion of 75% was chosen to give a rough comparison of the threshold value for the two techniques. According to this criterion, the threshold differs only at two age levels—lower for the optokinetic test from 1 to 2 mo. and lower for the fixation test from 3 to 4 mo.

This close correspondence is surprising in view of the small samples and the difference in mechanism underlying the two responses. It is possible that factors which might be expected to favor better performance on the fixation test (i.e., a stationary stimulus pattern falling on the retinal area of most acute vision), were balanced by factors which might tend to result in poorer performance by young

TABLE 4

Comparison of Visual Acuity Data from Pattern Fixation (F) and Optokinetic (O) Nystagmus Tests of Same Infants

Age (mo.)	Test	No. Infants Responding to Stripes of Each Size (in min.) vs. No. Not Responding			
		5	10	20	40
0–1	F	2/3	2/3	**6/1**	**6/1**
	O	0/7	0/7	**7/0**	**7/0**
1–2	F	5/4	6/4	6/4	**10/0**
	O	0/10	6/4	**10/0**	**10/0**
2–3	F	3/4	5/3	**7/2**	**8/1**
	O	0/9	3/6	**9/0**	**9/0**
3–4	F	**6/1**	**7/1**	**8/0**	**8/0**
	O	1/7	**6/2**	**8/0**	**8/0**
4–5	F	4/3	**6/1**	**7/0**	**7/0**
	O	3/4	**7/0**	**7/0**	**7/0**
5–6	F	4/1	**5/0**	**5/0**	**5/0**
	O	**5/0**	**5/0**	**5/0**	**5/0**
All ages	F	24/16	31/12	**39/7**	**44/2**
	O	9/37	27/19	**46/0**	**46/0**

Note.—Entries in boldface indicate stripe response frequencies meeting the 75% criterion.

infants on the fixation test (i.e., a nonreflex and more variable type of response, requiring better oculomotor coordination and a greater degree of cortical involvement than does optokinetic nystagmus). Whether or not this is the correct interpretation, the agreement between the two techniques gives support for the results of the pattern fixation test.

An interesting methodological comparison was brought out in the process of recording the two different responses to pattern. Optokinetic nystagmus was often fleeting and irregular with the younger Ss and the finer stripes. Consequently, qualitative judgments were necessary, and these judgments for near-threshold patterns varied considerably in repeated observations. The expected objectivity of the optokinetic test was not apparent. In contrast, the fixation test of acuity involved a simple, unambiguous criterion of fixation at each moment, and a quantitative criterion of differential response for each test.

Table 5 combines the fixation-test results of the first two studies, using 2-mo. intervals. With this increase in sample size, the results

14

TABLE 5
Combined Fixation Acuity Data for the First and Second Studies

Age (mo.)	N^a	No. Infants Favoring Stripes vs. No. Favoring Gray (in min.)				
		5/G	10/G	20/G	40/G	80/G
0–2	30	7/7	10/11	18/12	28/2**	12/1*
2–4	31	11/10	18/12	28/3**	28/3**	6/1
4–6	22	14/8	19/3**	22/0**	22/0**	—
Total	83	32/25	47/26*	68/15**	78/5**	18/2**

a Number in each cell often is less than total N since all pattern sizes were not used at each age level in the first study and the 80-min. pattern was not used at all in the second study.

* $p < .01$ level (sign test).

** $p < .001$ level (sign test).

are very consistent. The threshold pattern size for the first 2 mo. is 40 min.; for the next 2, 20 min.; and for the last 2 mo., 10 min. of visual angle.

Experiment 3

The last study was undertaken primarily to make certain of the reliability of the differential fixation test of acuity. The visual responses of each infant were observed and recorded independently by two people. Repeatability was determined from two tests of each infant under the same conditions. A further control consisted of using two shades of gray as comparison object—one lighter and one darker than the striped patterns—instead of matching the reflectance as previously. The illumination was increased to see if the threshold would be lowered.

Method

The apparatus was the same as in Experiment 2 with these exceptions. Instead of attaching stimulus objects to the ceiling of the chamber, stripes and gray were visible through two holes in the ½-in. ceiling, each 7 by 5 in. wide, and 12 in. apart, center to center. New striped and gray stimuli were used, placed 15½ in. from the infant's eyes. They were larger than the holes and were placed directly on top of the chamber so as to cover the holes. This arrangement permitted quick changing of the objects between test periods.

Observations were made through two ½-in. holes, one adjacent to the lower edge (toward the infant's feet) of each stimulus object. The two Os, one on each side of the chamber, each recorded the fixation times by means of silent finger switches and timers out of sight of the other O. During the first series of tests, the O on the left of the chamber placed the stimulus objects in position without the other O's knowing which was the striped pattern or the width of stripes. In the repeat series of tests, the O on the right handled the

objects. The scores of the two Os were not compared until after the series of tests was completed.

Four widths of stripes (¼₄, ½₂, ½₆, and ¼ in.) were used with each infant in random sequence. Two consecutive 20 sec. periods were given with each pattern size. For the second period, the right and left positions were reversed and a different gray comparison object was used. The initial positions and the gray used first were determined randomly. One gray had a slightly higher, the other a slightly lower, luminous reflectance than the striped patterns. Both stripes and grays had a mat finish to eliminate glare.

Four 60-w. incandescent lamps with reflectors were placed in the bottom four corners of the chamber, below the infant's eyes. To give further diffusion of the light and reduce glare on the chamber walls above the lights, the walls were covered with finely knit, medium blue jersey cloth. The ceiling was a lighter blue than in the previous studies to reduce the figure-ground contrast and thus favor acute vision. The ceiling was just enough darker than the stimulus surfaces to make reflections of the latter clearly visible in the infant's eyes. The lights were connected to a Powerstat set at 90% voltage, which seemed to give about the maximum of light without discomfort to the younger infants. An illumination meter measured about 12 ft-c close to the stimulus surfaces, roughly three times as much as in the first study.

Subjects. The Ss were 23 healthy infants ranging from 7 to 29 weeks of age. (Younger infants were not available at this time.) Each was given two complete tests within 2 weeks or less, at median ages of 14 and 15 weeks.

Results and Discussion

Reliability. The differential responsiveness to stripes was remarkably consistent between the simultaneous recordings of two Os and also between repeated tests of the same infants. In terms of the frequency of choice of stripes and of gray, the three larger patterns were responded to significantly (.01 level, sign test) for all four sets of data. There was no appreciable difference in the results from Os with and without knowledge of the stimuli.

Figure 4 gives a comparison of the four sets of data in terms of average strength of responsiveness to patterned surfaces over plain. The four curves are very similar, each showing differential response for all but the finest stripes.

These results indicate reliability of the testing technique and response measurement. They further show that very similar responses were observed through different peepholes, one close to each stimulus. This is of interest because a change in O's position theoretically can displace the corneal reflection of an object relative to the pupil, which indicates whether

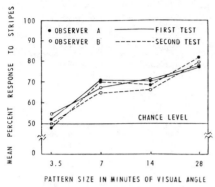

FIG. 4. Reliability of the differential fixation test of acuity as shown by similarity in results of two tests of the same infants, each recorded independently by two Os.

or not the object is fixated. When O is in line with the object and the infant, a fixated object is reflected directly over the pupil. This superposition is not always exact when O is to one side of the object, depending on the degree of curvature of the cornea and the distance between cornea and pupil for a particular S. While any resulting error should be equalized for right and left objects when O is in the center, the position of the Os in this study would accentuate any such error by increasing the left O's error for the right object and vice versa. Since the Os agreed nevertheless, the influence of this factor in the previous studies, using a center observation hole, may be dismissed.

Reflectance control. When the test periods with different comparison objects were analyzed separately, no difference was shown. About an equally low amount of visual attention was directed toward the gray with higher reflectance than the stripes (an average of 33% of the response time for all infants and tests) and toward the gray with lower reflectance than the stripes (31% of response time). In terms of the numbers of infants favoring stripes or gray, a significant response to pattern was shown both for pairings with the light gray and the dark gray. This was true in each test and for each pattern size except the smallest, which was not differentiated in the combined results. Thus, the differential response was clearly due to the presence or absence of pattern, not to a brightness difference. Similarly, Berlyne (1958) found no significant difference in the visual attention given by infants to white, gray, and black, while differences in pattern aroused differential responses.

Age and illumination. Table 6 gives an age breakdown of the results, averaged for the two Os. The frequencies are the numbers of tests favoring stripes or gray, including the two tests for each infant described above, as well as preliminary tests given to the same and to six additional infants. The larger patterns were differentiated at all age levels while the narrowest stripes, subtending only 3.5 min., elicited increasing visual response with age and passed the 75% criterion during the sixth month. If the several tests for each infant over 5 mo. are averaged and combined with the same age group in Experiment 2, 10 of 12 infants show a differential response to either 3.5- or 5-min. stripes, the finest used in the respective studies.

The threshold for pattern suggested by the data in Table 6 is lower at each age level than in the earlier experiments (Table 5). Although there were several changes in conditions, this is most likely due to better illumination of the stimuli and background, since illumination is known to affect the acuity of adults markedly.

GENERAL DISCUSSION

The results of the various acuity tests give a far different picture of the development of pattern vision than the common view that the young infant can see only vague masses of light and dark, or is lacking in pattern

TABLE 6
VISUAL FIXATION RESPONSES TO PATTERNS OF SUCCESSIVE SIZES BY INFANTS AT VARIOUS AGE LEVELS WITH INCREASED ILLUMINATION
(INCLUDES ONE TO THREE TESTS OF EACH INFANT)

Age (mo.)	N[a]	No. of Tests Favoring Stripes vs. No. Favoring Gray			
		3.5/G	7/G	14/G	28/G
2–3	14	11/11	**16/6**	**17/5**	**18/4**
3–4	12	11/7	**14/4**	**15/2**	**16/2**
4–5	10	7/4	**9/3**	**11/1**	**12/0**
5–6	8	9/3	**11/1**	**10/2**	**12/0**

NOTE.—Entries in boldface indicate stripe response frequencies meeting the 75% criterion.

[a] The total N was 28 since some infants were tested at several age levels.

vision until several months of age due to immaturity of the visual system or the need for visual experience. Instead, pattern vision becomes progressively more acute, starting with the ability of the neonate to see stripes as narrow as $\frac{1}{8}$ in. at a 10-in. distance. By 6 mo., $\frac{1}{64}$-in. stripes can be resolved at 10' or at 15 in.

These figures cannot be taken as absolute limits of visual resolution at the various age levels without knowing the optimal testing conditions, such as illumination, figure-ground contrast, type of pattern, size of field, etc., and without data from a large, representative sample of infants using a wide range of pattern sizes. Even so, these studies show much more acute vision than previous studies. At 4 mo. Chavasse (1939) found an acuity of 20/2560 in the Snellen notation, based on the reaction to a small pellet, while the present results would correspond roughly to 20 200 or better at this age. At 6 mo., Chavasse found an acuity of 20/960, and Schwarting (1954) gives the figure of 20/400 based on the pursuit of a fine line, compared with 20/100 or 20/70 according to the pattern fixation test results above.

The only comparable result was obtained by Gorman et al. (1957) based on optokinetic nystagmus to moving stripes. They found an acuity of 20/670 in newborn infants, compared with 20/400 in the present optokinetic test and 20/800 in the fixation test of infants under 1 mo. with lower illumination. When all ages are considered, the present results for the optokinetic and fixation tests are similar (Table 4).

The above comparison of present results with previous ones justifies the unconventional use of a "stimulus preference" method for determining a sensory threshold. The usual arguments against such a method are that negative results do not necessarily mean inability to discriminate, and that even if positive results are obtained they would be more variable and show lower sensitivity than methods providing better motivation, as by means of reward or instructions or by using a reflex response. However, the differential fixation test of acuity has revealed much finer visual resolution than other methods based on a "voluntary" response and about equal to those based on a reflex response. Furthermore, one could hardly ask

for less variability among Ss than shown by the visual choice of a near-threshold pattern in preference to gray by 28 of 30 infants under 2 mo. of age (Table 5); or less variability in repeated tests or between independent observations than shown by the similar curves in Figure 4. The differential fixation method thus is a sensitive and reliable test of visual acuity in spite of being based on free choice rather than forced or reinforced behavior; in fact *because* it is based on an innate and yet nonreflex response, the method gets meaningful results with Ss too immature for traditional tests of pattern vision.

The infant has the ability to see fairly fine patterns from the first month of life; to see equally well at 5, 10, and 20 in.; and to respond to patterns by continuing to gaze voluntarily at a pattern falling on the central retina as well as by reflexly turning toward a peripheral pattern or following a large moving pattern with eyes and head. These facts imply that all parts of the visual system, from the optical apparatus of the eye to the visual centers of the brain, are functional soon after birth, however structurally immature they are. This conclusion is in essential agreement with the best available anatomical, neurophysiological, ophthalmological, and behavioral information. Contrary to some reports, studies of newborn infants have shown that some degree of fixation and accommodation is present (Gesell et al., 1949; Pieper, 1949), that retinal hemorrhages are rare (Chase, Merritt, & Bellows, 1950), and that electrophysiological activity of the retina and visual cortex is elicited by visual stimulation (Ellingson, 1958; Horsten & Winkelman, 1960). The arguments purporting to prove lack of cortical vision in the young infant are inconclusive, while the present data are sufficient evidence for cortical vision, since pattern vision is completely absent in mammals from rats to humans without visual cortex (Morgan & Stellar, 1950).

The marked increase in the precision of pattern vision during the first 6 mo., from a threshold of 40 to 5 min. or less, is easily explained by the extensive maturation of the visual apparatus during this period. Probably of most importance are the increased density of macular receptors, completed myelinization of nerve fibers, maturation of the visual cortex, and improved skill in foveal fixation.

Neither visual learning nor postnatal maturation are necessary for the infant to see and respond to a patterned stimulus when the response is innate and the stimulus intrinsically interesting. Knowing this and knowing the approximate acuity at various ages should make it easier to find out how and when pattern vision comes to be used to perceive objects and space and to direct more complex behaviors.

SUMMARY

The differential fixation test of visual acuity was used to determine the ability of the young infant to resolve and attend to fine patterns. It was based on the natural tendency of infants to fixate a striped stimulus more than a gray stimulus. Each of a series of patterns with different widths of stripes was exposed to the infant in a controlled fashion to determine the finest pattern differentiated from gray according to relative duration or number of fixations.

In Experiment 1, 37 infants were tested at three distances with patterns subtending the same visual angle. No difference in acuity was shown at 5, 10, and 20 in., suggesting the ability to accommodate for near vision from early infancy. Under 1 mo. the minimum separable visual angle was 40 min. ($\frac{1}{8}$-in. stripes at 10 in.); by 5 mo. this was reduced to 10 min. The total visual response to pattern was due primarily to maintaining the central fixation of a pattern rather than to the reflex fixation of a peripherally seen pattern.

Experiment 2, using 46 infants, showed about the same level of acuity for differential fixation of patterns as for optokinetic nystagmus to a moving striped field. The fixation test supported Experiment 1 and suggested a pattern threshold of 5 min. by 6 mo. of age.

In Experiment 3, 23 infants over 2 mo. old were tested twice with responses recorded independently by two Os. The four sets of data were very similar in frequency of choice of each size of pattern and in average strength of differential responsiveness to pattern, indicating the reliability of the testing method. A lower threshold for pattern was shown than in the other studies, probably due to better illumination.

The results refute the common opinion that the young infant is lacking in pattern
vision or can see only vague masses of light and dark. The results imply that all parts of the visual mechanism, from cornea to cortex, function to some degree in the neonate, although further development of visual structures and functions during the first 6 mo. causes progressively more acute vision.

REFERENCES

BERLYNE, D. E. The influence of the albedo and complexity of stimuli on visual fixation in the human infant. *Brit. J. Psychol.*, 1958, **49**, 315–318.

CHASE, R. R., MERRITT, K. K., & BELLOWS, M. Ocular findings in the newborn. *Arch. Ophthal., Chicago*, 1950, **44**, 236–242.

CHAVASSE, F. B. *Worth's squint or the binocular reflexes and the treatment of strabismus.* (7th ed.) Philadelphia: Blakiston, 1939.

ELLINGSON, R. J. Electroencephalograms of normal, full-term newborns immediately after birth with observations on arousal and visual evoked responses. *EEG clin. Neurophysiol.*, 1958, **10**, 31–50.

FANTZ, R. L. A method for studying early visual development. *Percept. mot. Skills*, 1956, **6**, 13–15.

FANTZ, R. L. Pattern vision in young infants. *Psychol. Rec.*, 1958, **8**, 43–47.

FANTZ, R. L., & ORDY, J. M. A visual acuity test for infants under six months of age. *Psychol. Rec.*, 1959, **9**, 159–164.

GESELL, A., ILG, F. L., & BULLIS, G. E. *Vision: Its development in infant and child.* New York: Hoeber, 1949.

GORMAN, J. J., COGAN, D. G., & GELLIS, S. S. An apparatus for grading the visual acuity of infants on the basis of optokinetic nystagmus. *Pediatrics*, 1957, **19**, 1088–1092.

HORSTEN, G. P. M., & WINKELMAN, J. E. Development of the ERG in relation to the histological differentiation of the retina in man and animals. *Arch. Ophthal., Chicago*, 1960, **63**, 232–242.

McGRAW, M. B. *The neuromuscular maturation of the human infant.* New York: Columbia Univer. Press, 1943.

MANN, I. *The development of the human eye.* New York: Grune & Stratton, 1950.

MORGAN, C. T., & STELLAR, E. *Physiological psychology.* New York: McGraw-Hill, 1950.

PEIPER, A. *Die Eigenart der Kindlichen Hirntactigkeit.* Leipzig, Germany: Thieme, 1949.

PRATT, K. C. The neonate. In L. Carmichael (Ed.), *Manual of child psychology.* New York: Wiley, 1946. Pp. 190–254.

SCHWARTING, B. H. Testing infants' vision. *Amer. J. Ophthal.*, 1954, **38**, 714–715.

STIRNIMANN, F. Ueber das Farbenempfinden Neugeborener. *Ann. Paedia.*, 1944, **163**, 1–25.

WALSH, F. B. *Clinical neuro-ophthalmology.* Baltimore: Williams & Wilkins, 1957.

ZUBEK, J. P., & SOLBERG, P. A. *Human development.* New York: McGraw-Hill, 1954.

Concept Learning in Discrimination Tasks[1]

EDWARD C. CALDWELL
University of Washington

AND

VERNON C. HALL[2]
Syracuse University

The problem of false positives in psychological research has been vividly and amply demonstrated by Rosenthal (1963) in his discussion of experimenter bias. Campbell (1957) and Campbell and Stanley (1963) have discussed this problem in relation to experimental design. The present authors (Caldwell & Hall, 1969) have argued that an additional source of false positives lies in incomplete analysis of the criterion task employed (see Gagné, 1965; Gagné & Paradise, 1961; Miller, 1962). The field of computer simulation has brought this need for completeness into sharp focus.

In order to construct a preliminary model of behavior in the task, the researcher needs an idea or ideas about the behavior in the task. The idea may come from observing behavior, asking people what they are doing while performing the task, or from cogitating on what type of device would be required to perform the task. The next step is to construct a model, that is, write a program

for a computer embodying this idea. In the course of this activity, the researcher realizes the inadequacy of his original idea(s). He discovers that he needs more information. To get this information he may have to reanalyze old data or run new experiments. Thus the researcher encounters some of the advantages of computer models—the requirement for completeness and precision, etc. The only real constraint on the model builder is that his statements be unambiguous and complete (Feigenbaum & Feldman, 1963, pp. 271, 273).

It is a very simple task to test a computer model for precision and completeness. Since the model is the program, one need merely run it to check both criteria. Unfortunately, verbal models are not so readily evaluated and thus may often represent incomplete analyses of behavior that in turn generate false positives.

The present research was designed to show that the developmental curves of Gibson, Gibson, Pick, and Osser (1962) that have appeared in many prominent publications (Epstein, 1967; Gibson, 1963a, 1963b, 1965) do in fact represent false positives regarding the ability of young children to detect differences among letterlike forms. These false positives result in part from inadequate task analysis.

[1] This research was supported by Grant OEO-4120 and Contract 1620.1632 of the United States Office of Education.

[2] Requests for reprints should be sent to Vernon C. Hall, Department of Psychology, Syracuse University, 331 Huntington Hall, Syracuse, New York 13210.

DEVELOPMENTAL PSYCHOLOGY, 1970, Vol. 2., pp. 41-48

Regarding these developmental curves, Gibson et al. argued, "The improvement in such discrimination from four to eight is the result of learning to *detect* these differences and of *becoming more sensitive* to them [italics added, p. 904]." Later Gibson (1963a) argued that this learning represents "perceptual learning of the distinctive features," and this kind of learning is not "of the paired associates type. It is rather helping the child to *'pay attention to'* those features that are invariant and distinctive [italics added, p. 21]." In 1962, Gibson et al. suggested that the learning involved might well be unrelated to verbal learning:

Teachers apparently give a good deal of concentrated and highly verbal attention to reversal and rotation errors. It may be that the child learns which varying dimensions of letters are significant and which are not by simply looking repeatedly at many samples containing both varying and invariant features [p. 905].

In 1965 she had concluded "that it is perceptual learning and need not be verbalized is probable (though teachers do often call attention to contrasts between letter shapes)

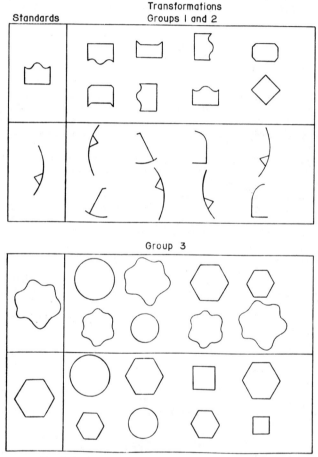

FIG. 1. Symbols used for overlay task for groups indicated.

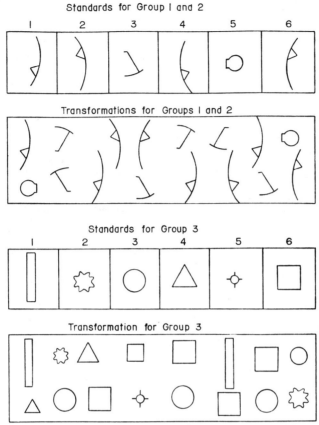

FIG. 2. Standards and transformations used for the card-selection task. (While the same set of figures, as transformations, was used for all of the standards, their orders were randomized for each standard. These standards and transformations were in the format of Davidson's Letter Perception Test.)

[p. 1068]." There seems to be little doubt that Gibson et al. perceive their study as demonstrating that 4-year-olds exhibit a perceptual deficit that is corrected through perceptual learning of a variety quite removed from verbal learning. If one were to correct for this deficit he would do so in terms of helping subjects *learn to detect, become more sensitive to and pay attention to* the stimuli, for example, Hendrickson and Muchl (1962) and Jeffrey (1966, 1968).

It is the contention of the present authors that an important element has been omitted by Gibson et al. in their analysis of the criterion task. When a child handed the experimenter a transformation, for example, a reversal, he may have done so for different reasons. First, he may have not been "able to see" the difference. Second, he may not have attended to the difference; that is, he may have been able to see the difference but did not notice it. Finally, he may have been fully aware of the difference but considered it irrelevant; that is, he may have assumed that orientation had nothing whatever to do with determining whether

TABLE 1

MFANS AND STANDARD DEVIATIONS OF
PERCENTAGE SELECTED

Group	Correct	Line to curve	Rotation and reversal	Per-spective	Break and close
Group 1					
Nursery					
M	83.6	18.6	15.8	62.6	10.2
SD	21.7	13.0	16.8	19.9	9.9
2nd grade					
M	92.8	10.9	5.3	66.4	3.4
SD	5.6	6.1	3.6	18.5	6.0
Group 2					
Nursery					
M	96.6	41.7	82.2	85.9	20.3
SD	8.4	17.6	14.1	12.5	17.2
2nd grade					
M	95.6	12.5	87.2	66.6	3.8
SD	5.9	10.1	7.1	18.5	10.2
Group 3					
Nursery					
M	91.4	30.3	42.5	70.2	15.9
SD	8.1	19.3	28.8	17.1	21.4
2nd grade					
M	90.7	5.9	10.7	39.0	2.7
SD	8.4	5.7	20.7	16.7	4.2
Group 4 (Gibson replication group)					
Nursery					
M	94.3	40.0	53.0	82.1	29.3
SD	9.4	19.9	27.1	14.1	23.1
2nd grade					
M	95.5	11.3	11.2	69.2	5.1
SD	5.2	8.0	15.3	21.9	5.3
Original Gibson study					
4 yr.	94.5	37.0	46.3	79.6	15.9
8 yr.	96.1	5.9	5.3	59.0	3.8

things are the same or different. It is this third possibility that has been overlooked by Gibson et al. as it undoubtedly has been by many other investigators. Thus, the differential performance over age groups, it is argued, is not due merely to "learning to detect," "becoming more sensitive to," or "paying attention to" the distinctive features. One may readily detect, be highly sensitive to, or pay close attention to the distinctive features in the discrimination task, but unless the subject holds the appropriate concept of same and different, that is, identical to the experimenter's relatively arbitrary concept, no amount of visual scrutiny will provide the subject with a correct response. Detection of distinctive features is no doubt a necessary but not a sufficient condition for success on the discrimination task. Likewise, while perceptual learning is necessary, it is argued that

concept learning is equally necessary and in fact largely accounts for the developmental curves beyond 4 years.

With the above viewpoint in mind, the present authors decided to test the following hypotheses:

1. When nursery school children are given warm-up and feedback on a task designed to produce a concept of same and different identical to the experimenter's concept there is no difference between nursery school children and second graders on line to curve and rotation and reversal errors.

2. When nursery school children are given warm-up and feedback that give inappropriate information regarding rotation and reversal but appropriate information regarding line to curve transformations, they make more rotation and reversal errors than second graders or nursery school children given appropriate information regarding rotations and reversals.

3. When second graders are given warm-up and feedback as in Hypothesis 2 above, they make more rotation and reversal errors than second graders and nursery school children given appropriate information.

Method

Subjects

Subjects were 72 nursery school children (38 males and 34 females) and 72 second graders (35 males and 37 females) randomly assigned by grade level to one of four treatment groups: (1) orientation relevant, (2) orientation irrelevant, (3) minimal information regarding orientation, and (4) exact replication of Gibson et al. The designation N refers to nursery school children and 2 to second graders. The younger subjects (mean age 4.35, ranging from 4.10 to 5.20) were white and randomly selected from 105 subjects attending a nursery school, supported by the National Laboratory for Early Childhood Development through the United States Office of Education, in a lower-middle to middle-class neighborhood. The second graders (mean age 8.02, ranging from 7.55 to 8.77) were white and randomly selected from 120 subjects attending one public school in the same school district. All subjects were run during the months of March and April.

Procedure

Gibson et al. presented subjects with 12 letterlike forms, each of which had 12 transformations:

The transformations chosen were as follows: three degrees of transformation of line to

TABLE 2

ANALYSES OF VARIANCE SUMMARIES

Transformation	Source	df	SS	MS	F
Correct	Treatments (A)	3	1,551	517.0	4.5[a]
	Grade level (B)	1	205	205.0	1.28
	A × B	3	568	189.3	1.68
	Error	136	15,341	112.8	
Line to curve	Treatments (A)	3	3,767	1,255.7	6.3**
	Grade level (B)	1	18,067	18,067.0	90.8**
	A × B	3	2,726	908.7	4.6**
	Error	136	27,057	198.9	
Rotation and reversal	Treatments (A)	3	111,477	37,159.0	9.5**
	Grade level (B)	1	13,964	13,964.0	37.4**
	A × B	3	11,811	3,937.0	10.5**
	Error	136	50,762	373.3	
Perspective	Treatments (A)	3	11,436	3,812.0	11.6**
	Grade level (B)	1	7,951	7,591.0	24.2**
	A × B	3	5,762	1,921.0	5.8**
	Error	136	44,738	329.0	
Break and close	Treatments (A)	3	2,153	717.7	3.4*
	Grade level (B)	1	8,289	8,289.0	39.5**
	A × B	3	1,428	476.0	2.3
	Error	136	28,528	209.8	

[a] While this was significant, the Scheffé comparison showed no differences. Groups 1-N and 2-N were most different. See Table 3.
* $p < .05$.
** $p < .01$.

curve or curve to line (1, 2, or 3); five transformations of rotation or reversal, i.e., 45° rotation, 90° rotation, 180° rotation, right-left reversal, and up-down reversal; two perspective transformations, a 45° slant left and a 45° backward tilt; and two topological transformations, a break and a close. . . . half the forms (the symmetrical ones) lacked two transformations, since either the right-left reversal or up-down reversal was identical with the standard and the 180° rotation was identical with the other. The cells in these cases were filled with the standard [pp. 897–898].

A standard form was placed on the top center row of a five-row matrix board. Each of the four rows below the standard held 13 cards (1¼-inch square on which the transformations were mounted). In each of these rows a given standard and its 12 transformations were placed in random order.

After the experimenter had put the appropriate standard in the center of the top row, the subject went through a given row searching for any form that was "exactly like the standard." When he found one he tipped it forward and continued until he had scanned the entire row. (Tipping the cards forward rather than handing the card to the experimenter represents the only procedural change in the study. This was done to facilitate assembly of materials for the next subject.)

The warm-up treatments consisted of an overlay procedure and a card-selection task. For the overlay procedure the standards in Figure 1 were reproduced on 2 × 2 inch 3M Projection Transparencies Type 127 by use of a Thermofax Copier. The standards were mounted in 2 × 2 inch Super Easymount slide holders for ease of handling. Each set of standards and transformations from Figure 1 was duplicated, cut into 1 11/16-inch squares, mounted on 7 × 14 inch pieces of red poster board in a layout similar to Figure 1 and coated with plastic. The subject was seated at a table with the board before him and instructed to find in the group of transformations those that were exactly like the standard. The experimenter said,

It's really very easy if you are careful. You take this [the plastic overlay] and line it up on this one [the standard] then you put it on top of these [the transformations]. If they line up so it looks like only one of them is there, then they are exactly the same. If some part doesn't line up, if some of the lines aren't on top of each other, then they are different.

The experimenter demonstrated with the first two figures. Note that the first figure is a rotation of the standard. For Groups 1-N and 1-2, the experimenter said, as he put the transparency on this figure,

When you put this one on top of this one you have to be careful *not* to turn it around or over like this. For some of them, like this

23

TABLE 3

SUMMARY OF SCHEFFÉ COMPARISONS OF MEANS

Groups 1-N	1-2	2-N	2-2	3-N	3-2	4-N	4-2
1-N		L-C R&R	R&R			L-C R&R	
1-2		L-C R&R	R&R	R&R		L-C R&R PER	
2-N							
2-2					L-C	L-C PER	
3-N		R&R	R&R				
3-2	R&R	L-C R&R PER	R&R PER	L-C R&R PER		L-C R&R B&C PER	PER
4-N		R&R	R&R				
4-2		L-C R&R	R&R	R&R		L-C R&R B&C	

Note.—Column heading indicates group making more selections. L-C is line to curve; R&R is rotation and reversal; B&C is break to close; PER is perspective.

one, if you did turn it around, the figures would line up, but no fair turning it around. You must compare them without turning them around or over in any way, because they are different if they have to be turned.

For Groups 2-N and 2-2, the experimenter said, as he placed the transparency on this first figure, "When you put this one on top of this you may have to turn it around or over like this to make them line up. You can turn them any way you like and as long as they line up, that means they are the same." The experimenter gave appropriate feedback to each group after each judgment and if necessary encouraged the subjects in Groups 2-N and 2-2 to rotate the standard when making a judgment. Groups 3-N and 3-2 were given instructions identical to those of Groups 1 and 2 except no mention of turning the standard was made since orientation was virtually irrelevant for their stimuli. (See Figure 1.) However, since a 25% size differential was relevant, Groups 3-N and 3-2 had to attend closely.

The card-selection task was in the format of the criterion task and employed the standards and transformations shown in Figure 2. Overlays were available for the standards and were used fre-quently to check the subject's response. Feedback appropriate for each group, as in the overlay task, was given after each decision by the subject; that is, for Groups 1-N and 1-2 orientation was relevant, for Groups 2-N and 2-2 orientation was irrelevant, and for Groups 3-N and 3-2 no specific information regarding orientation was given.

Results

The results were analyzed in terms of percentage of stimulus cards chosen in each of five categories: (a) correct, that is, identical to the standard; (b) line to curve transformations; (c) rotation and reversal transformations; (d) perspective transformations; and (e) break and close transformation. Table 1 gives the mean percentage and standard deviation in each of the eight groups for the five categories. Five 4×2 (Treatment $\times$ Grade) analyses of variance were computed, one for each category.[3] Since the nature of the treatments would tend to produce heterogeneity of variances, significance was set at the .01 level. Likewise, for comparison of means, the Scheffé test was used with the level of significance set at .01. A summary of the analyses of variances is presented in Table 2. Table 3 shows the matrix of results from the Scheffé tests with the column heading indicating the group that made more selections.

The predictions from the hypotheses were: (a) Groups 1-N and 1-2 would not differ from each other on line to curve or rotation and reversal errors. Table 3 shows that this hypothesis was confirmed. (b) Group 2-N would make more rotation and reversal errors than Groups 1-N and 1-2, and these three groups would not differ on line to curve errors. Table 2 shows that while the predicted differences occurred in the rotation and reversal errors, Group 2-N also made more line to curve errors than Groups 1-N and 1-2. (c) Group 2-2 would make more rotation and reversal errors than Groups 1-N and 1-2, and the three groups would not differ on rotation and reversal er-

[3] Five $4 \times 2 \times 2$ (Treatment $\times$ Grade $\times$ Sex) analyses were subsequently computed using the unweighted means analysis for unequal Ns (Winer, 1962) for the sex factor. No new interactions or main effects were found significant. The authors would like to acknowledge Percy N. Peckhaw for his assistance in the analysis of these data.

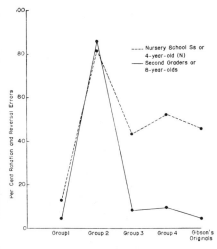

FIG. 3. Percentage of rotation and reversal errors by groups.

rors. Table 2 shows that this prediction was confirmed.

Discussion

First it should be noted from Table 1 that the nursery school children in the replication study, Group 4-N, performed very much like the 4-year-olds in the Gibson et al. study. Furthermore, Table 3 shows that Group 4-N made more break and close errors than did their second-grade counterpart. Since Gibson et al. did not obtain this result, it can be argued that the nursery school children in the present study were certainly not superior to the 4-year-olds of the Gibson et al. study at least relative to the respective 8-year-olds or second graders. Hence the superiority of Group 1-N cannot likely be attributed to population differences.

There were no differences in the number of correct responses. Hence the treatments did not merely manipulate the quantity of cards selected by the subject. The fact that there were no differences between Groups 1-N and 1-2 on any of the transformation indicates that nursery school children perform much like second graders when given a 6–10-minute warm-up designed to give them an adequate concept of same and different. Since Groups 2-N and 2-2 made more ro-

tation and reversal errors than all of the other groups, it is obvious that they quickly employed the concept that shape, regardless of orientation, was what the experimenter meant by *same*. Figure 3 clearly indicates this result of concept learning.

The unanticipated result that Group 2-N made more line to curve errors than Groups 1-N and 1-2 requires consideration. During warm-up, since orientation was irrelevant, less attention was demanded of Group 2-N for correct responses. No close inspection of the stimuli was required since those that were different were different on many dimensions. Hence their poorer performance may well have been due to a "set" of looking only for an object that had roughly the same shape. Attention, or in Gibson's terms, "learning to detect," "becoming more sensitive to distinctive features," is an important factor here.

Obviously then both attention and concept learning are important variables in this discrimination task. An attempt was made to separate the contribution of each by use of Groups 3-N and 3-2, for which attention was essential (due to the size transforma-

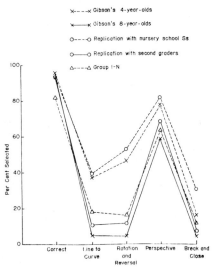

FIG. 4. Comparison of Gibson's 4-year-olds and 8-year-olds with equivalent replicated groups and Group 1-N of the present study.

tion) but for which relatively little information was available regarding orientation. Since Groups 1-N and 3-N did not differ on any transformation at the .01 level, it can be argued that there was little if any difference in the attentional requirements for the two groups. Further, the difference that was greatest between the two groups was on rotation and reversal errors. This was significant at the .05 level using the Scheffé comparison. In addition, the subjects in Group 3-2 performed significantly better than all the other second graders in perspective transformations. This discrimination requires considerable attention. A final suggestion that attention was equal for the two kinds of warm-up conditions comes from an earlier study (Caldwell & Hall, 1969) in which it was argued that analysis of irrelevant errors indicated equivalent attention.

It is tempting to view the differences observed in Figure 3 between Groups 1-N and 3-N as the effects of the orientation factor, that is, concept learning, and the difference between Groups 1-N and 4-N as a combination of orientation and attention factors.

Regardless of the relative influence of these two variables, an important and obvious conclusion is that nursery school children are able to discriminate as well as second graders when given very brief but appropriate experiences. Figure 4 demonstrates graphically the irrelevance of grade and/or age as a variable since Group 1-N, a group of nursery school children, coincide very closely with the 8-year-olds of the Gibson et al. study and the present replication group, Group 4-2. It is apparent that when tasks are more adequately analyzed into their component skills and young children are trained in these skills, they perform much more adequately than many of the normative studies indicate they are capable of. Certainly more than perceptual learning is involved here, that is, more than merely learning to pay attention to the stimuli, and verbalization it would seem is very important.

REFERENCES

CALDWELL, E. C., & HALL, V. C. The influence of concept training on letter discrimination. *Child Development*, 1969, **40**, 63–71.

CAMPBELL, D. T. Factors relevant to the validity of experiments in social settings. *Psychological Bulletin*, 1957, **54**, 297–312.

CAMPBELL, D. T., & STANLEY, J. C. Experimental and quasi-experimental designs for research on teaching. In N. L. Gage (Ed.), *Handbook of research on teaching*. Skokie, Ill.: Rand McNally, 1963.

EPSTEIN, W. *Varieties of perceptual learning*. New York: McGraw-Hill, 1967.

FEIGENBAUM, E. A., & FELDMAN, J. *Computers and thought*. New York: McGraw-Hill, 1963.

GAGNÉ, R. M. *The conditions of learning*. New York: Holt, Rinehart & Winston, 1965.

GAGNÉ, R. M., & PARADISE, N. E. Abilities and learning sets in knowledge acquisition. *Psychology*, 1961, **75** (14, Whole No. 518).

GIBSON, E. J. Development of perception: Discrimination of depth compared with discrimination of graphic symbols. *Monograph of the Society for Research in Child Development*, 1963, **28**(1, Serial No. 86). (a)

GIBSON, E. J. Perceptual development. *Yearbook of the National Society for Studies in Education*, 1963, **62**, Part I. (b)

GIBSON, E. J. Learning to read. *Science*, 1965, **148**, 1066–1072.

GIBSON, E. J., GIBSON, J. J., PICK, A. D., & OSSER, H. A developmental study of the discrimination of letter-like forms. *Journal of Comparative and Physiological Psychology*, 1962, **55**, 897–906.

HENDRICKSON, L. N., & MUEHL, S. The effect of attention and motor response pretraining on learning to discriminate B and D in kindergarten children. *Journal of Educational Psychology*, 1962, **53**, 236–241.

JEFFREY, W. E. Discrimination of oblique lines by children. *Journal of Comparative and Physiological Psychology*, 1966, **62**, 154–156.

MILLER, R. B. Task description and analysis. In R. M. Gagné (Ed.), *Psychological principles in system development*. New York: Holt, Rinehart & Winston, 1962.

ROSENTHAL, R. On the social psychology of the psychological experiment: The experimenter's hypothesis as unintended determinant of experimental results. *American Scientist*, 1963, **51**, 268–283.

WINER, B. J. *Statistical principles in experimental design*. New York: McGraw-Hill, 1962.

PETER D. EIMAS
EINAR R. SIQUELAND
PETER JUSCZYK
JAMES VIGORITO

Speech Perception in Infants

In this study of speech perception, it was found that 1- and 4-month-old infants were able to discriminate the acoustic cue underlying the adult phonemic distinction between the voiced and voiceless stop consonants /b/ and /p/. Moreover, and more important, there was a tendency in these subjects toward categorical perception: discrimination of the same physical difference was reliably better across the adult phonemic boundary than within the adult phonemic category.

Earlier research using synthetic speech sounds with adult subjects uncovered a sufficient cue for the perceived distinction in English between the voiced and voiceless forms of the stop consonants, /b-p/, /d-t/, and /g-k/, occurring in absolute initial position (1). The cue, which is illustrated in the spectrograms displayed in Fig. 1, is the onset of the first formant relative to the second and third formants. It is possible to construct a series of stimuli that vary continuously in the relative onset time of the first formant, and to investigate listeners' ability to identify and discriminate these sound patterns. An

investigation of this nature (2) revealed that the perception of this cue was very nearly categorical in the sense that listeners could discriminate continuous variations in the relative onset of the first formant very little better than they could identify the sound patterns absolutely. That is, listeners could readily discriminate between the voiced and voiceless stop consonants, just as they would differentially label them, but they were virtually unable to hear intraphonemic differences, despite the fact that the acoustic variation was the same in both conditions. The most measurable indication of this categorical perception was the occurrence of a high peak of discriminability at the boundary between the voiced and voiceless stops, and a nearly chance level of discriminability among stimuli that represented acoustic variations of the same phoneme. Such categorical perception is not found with nonspeech sounds that vary continuously along physical continua such as frequency or intensity. Typically, listeners are able to discriminate many more stimuli than they are able to identify absolutely, and the dis-

SCIENCE, 1971, Vol. 171., pp. 303-306.

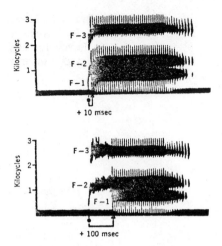

Fig. 1. Spectrograms of synthetic speech showing two conditions of voice onset time (VOT): slight voicing lag in the upper figure and long voicing lag in the lower figure. The symbols *F-1*, *F-2*, and *F-3* represent the first three formants, that is, the relatively intense bands of energy in the speech spectrum. [Courtesy of L. Lisker and A. S. Abramson]

criminability functions do not normally show the same high peaks and low troughs found in the case of the voicing distinction (3). The strong and unusual tendency for the stop consonants to be perceived in a categorical manner has been assumed to be the result of the special processing to which sounds of speech are subjected and thus to be characteristic of perception in the speech or linguistic mode (4).

Because the voicing dimension in the stop consonants is universal, or very nearly so, it may be thought to be reasonably close to the biological basis of speech and hence of special interest to students of language development. Though the distinctions made along the voicing dimension are not phonetically the same in all languages, it has been found in the cross-language research of

Lisker and Abramson (5) that the usages are not arbitrary, but rather very much constrained. In studies of the production of the voicing distinction in 11 diverse languages, these investigators found that, with only minor exceptions, the various tokens fell at three values along a single continuum. The continuum, called voice onset time (VOT), is defined as the time between the release burst and the onset of laryngeal pulsing or voicing. Had the location of the phonetic distinctions been arbitrary, then different languages might well have divided the VOT continuum in many different ways, constrained only by the necessity to space the different modal values of VOT sufficiently far apart as to avoid confusion.

Not all languages studied make use of the three modal positions. English, for example, uses only two locations, a short lag in voicing and a relatively long lag in voicing. Prevoicing or long voicing lead, found in Thai, for example, is omitted. Of interest, however, is the fact that all languages use the middle location, short voicing lag, which, given certain other necessary articulatory events, corresponds to the English voiced stop /b/, and one or both of the remaining modal values. The acoustic consequences for two modes of production are shown in Fig. 1; these correspond to short and long voicing lags, /b/ and /p/, respectively.

Given the strong evidence for universal—and presumably biologically determined—modes of production for the voicing distinction, we should suppose that there might exist complementary processes of perception (6). Hence, if we are to find evidence marking the beginnings of speech perception in a linguistic mode, it would appear reasonable to initiate our search with investigations of speech sounds differing along the voicing continuum. What was done experimentally, in essence, was to compare the discriminability of two synthetic speech sounds separated by a fixed difference in VOT under two conditions: in the first condition the two stimuli to be discriminated lay on opposite sides of the adult phonemic boundary, whereas in the second condition the two stimuli were from the same phonemic category.

The experimental methodology was a modification of the reinforcement procedure developed by Siqueland (7). After obtaining a baseline rate of high-amplitude, nonnutritive sucking for each infant, the presentation and intensity of an auditory stimulus was made contingent upon the infant's rate of high-amplitude sucking. The nipple on which the child sucked was connected to a positive pressure transducer that provided polygraphic recordings of all responses and a digital record of criterional high-amplitude sucking responses. Criterional responses activated a power supply that increased the intensity of the auditory feedback. A sucking rate of two responses per second maintained the stimulus at maximum intensity, about 75 db (13 db over the background intensity of 62 db).

The presentation of an auditory stimulus in this manner typically results in an increase in the rate of sucking compared with the baseline rate. With continued presentation of the initial stimulus, a decrement in the response rate occurs, presumably as a consequence of the lessening of the reinforcing properties of the initial stimulus. When it was apparent that attenuation of the reinforcing properties of the initial stimulus had occurred, as indicated by a decrement in the conditioned sucking rate of at least 20 percent for two consecutive minutes compared with the immediately preceding minute, a second auditory stimulus was presented without interruption and again contingent upon sucking. The second stimulus was maintained for 4 minutes after which the experiment was terminated. Control subjects were treated in a similar manner, except that after the initial decrease in response rate, that is, after habituation, no change was made in the auditory stimulus. Either an increase in response rate associated with a change in stimulation or a decrease of smaller magnitude than that shown by the control subjects is taken as inferential evidence that the infants perceived the two stimuli as different.

The stimuli were synthetic speech sounds prepared by means of a parallel resonance synthesizer at the Haskins Laboratories by Lisker and Abramson. There were three variations of the bilabial voiced stop /b/ and three variations of its voiceless counterpart /p/. The variations between all stimuli were in VOT, which for the English stops /b/ and /p/ can be realized acoustically by varying the onset of the first formant relative to the second and third formants and by having the second and third formants excited by a noise source during the interval when the first-formant is not present. Identification functions from adult listeners (8) have indicated that when the onset of the first formant leads or follows the onset of the second and third formants by less than 25 msec perception is almost invariably /b/. When voicing follows the release burst by more than 25 msec the perception is /p/. Actually the sounds are perceived as /ba/ or /pa/, since the patterns contain three steady-state formants appropriate for a vowel of the type /a/. The six stimuli had VOT values of -20, 0, $+20$, $+40$, $+60$, and $+80$

msec. The negative sign indicates that voicing occurs before the release burst. The subjects were 1- and 4-month-old infants, and within each age level half of the subjects were males and half were females.

The main experiment was begun after several preliminary studies established that both age groups were responsive to synthetic speech sounds as measured by a reliable increase in the rate of sucking with the response-contingent presentation of the first stimulus ($P < .01$). Furthermore, these studies showed that stimuli separated by differences in VOT of 100, 60, and 20 msec were discriminable when the stimuli were from different adult phonemic categories; that is, there was reliable recovery of the rate of sucking with a change in stimulation after habituation ($P < .05$). The finding that a VOT difference of 20 msec was discriminable permitted within-phonemic-category discriminations of VOT with relatively realistic variations of both phonemes.

In the main experiment, there were three variations in VOT differences at each of two age levels. In the first condition, 20D, the difference in VOT between the two stimuli to be discriminated was 20 msec and the two stimuli

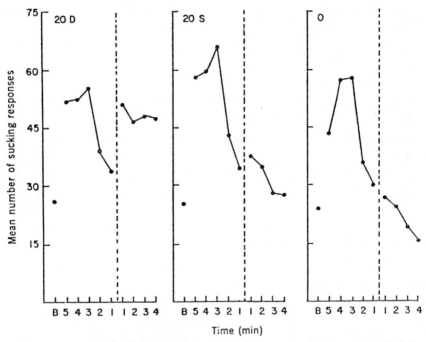

Fig. 2. Mean number of sucking responses for the 4-month-old infants, as a function of time and experimental condition. The dashed line indicates the occurrence of the stimulus shift, or in the case of the control group the time at which the shift would have occurred. The letter B stands for the baseline rate. Time is measured with reference to the moment of stimulus shift and indicates the 5 minutes prior to and the 4 minutes after shift.

were from different adult phonemic categories. The two stimuli used in condition 20D had VOT values of +20 and +40 msec. In the second condition, 20S, the VOT difference was again 20 msec, but now the two stimuli were from the same phonemic category. In this condition the stimuli had VOT values of −20 and 0 msec or +60 and +80 msec. The third condition, 0, was a control condition in which each subject was randomly assigned one of the six stimuli and treated in the same manner as the experimental subjects, except that after habituation no change in stimulation was made. The control group served to counter any argument that the increment in response rate associated with a change in stimulation was artifactual in that the infants tended to respond in a cyclical manner. Eight infants from each age level were randomly assigned to conditions 20D and 20S, and ten infants from each age level were assigned to the control condition.

Figure 2 shows the minute-by-minute response rates for the 4-month-old subjects for each of the training conditions separately. The results for the younger infants show very nearly the identical overall pattern of results seen with the older infants. In all conditions at both age levels, there were reliable conditioning effects: the response rate in the third minute prior to shift was significantly greater than the baseline rate of responding ($P < .01$). As was expected from the nature of the procedure, there were also reliable habituation effects for all subjects. The mean response rate for the final 2 minutes prior to shift was significantly lower than the response rate for the third minute before shift ($P < .01$). As is apparent from inspection of Fig. 1, the recovery data for the 4-month-old infants were differentiated by the nature

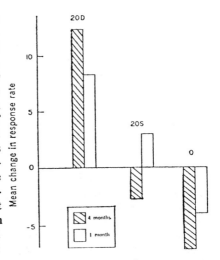

Fig. 3. The mean change in response rate as a function of experimental treatments, shown separately for the 1- and 4-month-old infants. (See text for details.)

of the shift. When the mean response rate during the 2 minutes after shift was compared with the response rate for the 2 minutes prior to shift, condition 20D showed a significant increment ($P < .05$), whereas condition 20S showed a nonsignificant decrement in responding ($P > .05$). In the control condition, there was a fairly substantial decrement in responding during the first 2 minutes of what corresponded to the shift period in the experimental conditions. However, the effect failed to reach the .05 level of significance, but there was a reliable decrement when the mean response rate for the entire 4 minutes after shift was compared with the initial 2 minutes of habituation ($P < .02$). The shift data for the younger infants were quite similar. The only appreciable difference was that in condition 20S there was a nonsignificant increment in the response rate during the first 2 minutes of shift.

In Fig. 3 the recovery data are summarized for both age groups. The mean change in response rate (that is, the mean response rate for the initial 2 minutes of shift minus the mean response rate during the final 2 minutes before shift) is displayed as a function of experimental treatments and age. Analyses of these data revealed that the magnitude of recovery for the 20D condition was reliably greater than that for the 20S condition ($P < .01$). In addition, the 20D condition showed a greater rate of responding than did the control condition ($P < .01$), while the difference between the 20S and control conditions failed to attain the .05 level of significance.

In summary, the results strongly indicate that infants as young as 1 month of age are not only responsive to speech sounds and able to make fine discriminations but are also perceiving speech sounds along the voicing continuum in a manner approximating categorical perception, the manner in which adults perceive these same sounds. Another way of stating this effect is that infants are able to sort acoustic variations of adult phonemes into categories with relatively limited exposure to speech, as well as with virtually no experience in producing these same sounds and certainly with little, if any, differential reinforcement for this form of behavior. The implication of these findings is that the means by which the categorical perception of speech, that is, perception in a linguistic mode, is accomplished may well be part of the biological makeup of the organism and, moreover, that these means must be operative at an unexpectedly early age.

References and Notes

1. A. M. Liberman, P. C. Delattre, F. S. Cooper, *Language and Speech* 1, 153 (1958); A. M. Liberman, F. Ingemann, L. Lisker, P. C. Delattre, F. S. Cooper, *J. Acoust. Soc. Amer.* 31, 1490 (1959). It should be emphasized that the cues underlying the voicing distinction as discussed in the present report apply only to sound segments in absolute initial position.
2. A. M. Liberman, K. S. Harris, H. S. Hoffman, H. Lane, *J. Exp. Psychol.* 61, 370 (1961).
3. P. D. Eimas, *Language and Speech* 6, 206 (1963); G. A. Miller, *Psychol. Rev.* 63, 81 (1956); R. S. Woodworth and H. Schlosberg, *Experimental Psychology* (Holt, New York, 1954).
4. A. M. Liberman, F. S. Cooper, D. P. Shankweiler, M. Studdert-Kennedy, *Psychol. Rev.* 74, 431 (1967); M. Studdert-Kennedy, A. M. Liberman, K. S. Harris, F. S. Cooper, *ibid.* 77, 234 (1970); M. Studdert-Kennedy and D. Shankweiler, *J. Acoust. Soc. Amer.*, in press.
5. L. Lisker and A. S. Abramson, *Word* 20, 384 (1964).
6. P. Lieberman, *Linguistic Inquiry* 1, 307 (1970).
7. E. R. Siqueland, address presented before the 29th International Congress of Psychology, London, England (August 1969); ——— and C. A. DeLucia, *Science* 165, 1144 (1969).

8. L. Lisker and A. S. Abramson, *Proc. Int. Congr. Phonet. Sci. 6th* (1970), p. 563.
9. Supported by grants HD 03386 and HD 04146 from the National Institute of Child Health and Human Development. P.J. and J.V. were supported by the NSF Undergraduate Participation Program (GY 5872). We thank Dr. F. S. Cooper for generously making available the

facilities of the Haskins Laboratories. We also thank Drs. A. M. Liberman, I. G. Mattingly, A. S. Abramson, and L. Lisker for their critical comments. Portions of this study were presented before the Eastern Psychological Association, Atlantic City (April 1970).

SECTION II

DISORDERS OF MOTOR DEVELOPMENT

The Relation of Childhood Characteristics to Outcome in Young Adults with Cerebral Palsy

Zelda S. Klapper   Herbert G. Birch

Introduction

WE have detailed knowledge of the characteristics of handicapped persons at specific points in their development, but little is known about their whole life course. This is particularly true for cerebral palsy, in which, as Crothers (1951) has pointed out, gaps in our knowledge are 'due to the fact that most of us have studied our patients as children and have not been sufficiently aware of the end-results' (p. 6). Only a longitudinal follow-up investigation of a clinically well-defined sample can provide such knowledge of the natural history of the disorder and its developmental course. Such a study also allows us to evaluate the prognostic value of our early diagnosis and the effectiveness of our management in promoting social habilitation.

Some studies (Crothers and Paine 1959, Remboldt 1959) concerned with physical status and the extent of orthopedic handicap in adult life have been conducted, and the relationship between early diagnostic category and physical status as a young adult has been explored, as have the influence of surgical intervention and physical and occupational therapy on motor functioning. However, little informa-

tion is available on how such children eventually function socially and personally as human beings.

A recent international seminar on rehabilitation (United Nations 1960) emphasised the need for such information : 'the primary objectives of rehabilitation are humanitarian and social. The handicapped person must be helped to develop his residual working capacity to the full and to occupy his rightful place in the family and the community. In a work-centred competitive society the unsuccessful are looked down upon. They feel themselves humiliated in their families and communities because of their inability to earn their living' (p. 10). The assessment of function in the handicapped young adult must extend beyond physical status to include both his personal functioning and his productive social involvement.

The available evidence on the vocational functioning of cerebral palsied adults suggests strongly that their integration into the productive life of the community is significantly limited. Reports from Israel (Kideon 1962), Denmark (Hansen 1960), Scotland (Moir 1960, Ingram 1964), England (Dunsdon 1952, Stephen 1961), and the United States (Machek and Collins

DEVELOPMENTAL MEDICINE AND CHILD NEUROLOGY, 1966, Vol. 4 pp. 645-656.

1961, Jones *et al.* 1962) all support this view. In spite of organized attempts to improve the vocational and social adjustment of the cerebral palsied children in all these countries, the findings point uniformly to significant difficulties in occupational placement in adulthood. These findings agree with those of Crothers and Paine (1959), who found that less than a quarter of their sample were suitable for non-sheltered employment as adults.

Little information is available from these studies regarding the childhood characteristics of these handicapped adults, although clinical experience suggests that there is a definite relationship between diagnostic classification, extent of physical handicap and intellectual status in early childhood and outcome in later life. Since this relation is not necessarily direct or simple it appeared desirable to carry out a follow-up study on a group of young cerebral palsied adults who were evaluated as children 14–15 years ago.

The present report derives from a follow-up study in 1962 and 1963 of a group of cerebral palsied children whose physical, psychological and social background status was carefully investigated in 1947 and 1948. The emphasis of the study was on their psychological, occupational and social outcome. This paper deals with their social and vocational outcome. The details of their psychological growth and development will be separately reported.

Subjects, Method and Procedure

A group of 155 children aged 2–16 years were studied in 1948. The age distribution of the sample at the time of the initial study is presented in Table I, which shows that there were 86 boys and 69 girls in the group, with more than 90 of the children falling in the age range of 5–10 years.

The largest initial medical diagnostic group consisted of children with spastic hemiplegia (64). Next in order, and very close together in frequency of occurrence, were spastic tetraplegia (23), spastic paraplegia (21), and athetosis (22). A few of the children were ataxic (8), and others were monoplegic (4), triplegic (4) or had a mixed form of cerebral palsy (9).

Initially, 14 children were physically untestable on standard psychological tests and the remainder had IQs up to 125 (Table II). The modal IQ score was in the low borderline normal range, and the figures reflect the usual finding that between two-thirds and three-quarters of cerebral palsied children fall in the borderline to defective groups of mental functioning.

TABLE I
Age When First Examined

Age in yr.		No. of children	
2		3	
3	}2–4	8	}27
4		16	
5		18	
6	}5–7	26	}51
7		7	
8		17	
9	}8–10	11	}42
10		14	
11		14	
12	}11–13	12	}30
13		4	
14		4	
15	}14–16	0	}5
16		1	
Total		155	

Males 86. Females 69

TABLE II
Initial IQ Distribution

IQ	No.
Untestable	14
0–49	16
50–74	48
75–89	32
90–109	36
110–125	9
Total	155

At follow-up in 1962, it was possible to locate 119 of the 155 children originally studied. Of this group of 119, 4 had died, 5 had moved out of the state, 7 were no longer available within areas close to New York City, 6 were resident in institutions, and 8 refused to participate beyond giving general information about their current status. As a consequence, 89 young adults were immediately available for detailed follow-up investigation. This residual sample comprised 50 males and 39 females, aged 16–28 years, with 80 cases between 18 and 28 years of age.

When the residual sample of 89 was compared with the original sample of 155 children, it was found that, except for some attenuation at the extremes, the distributions of intellectual level and diagnostic category were insignificantly different from those in the original grouping of children. Thus the residual sample adequately reflected the characteristics of the original sample of children studied. As would have been expected, many of the children whose functioning was *worst* had died, been institutionalized or otherwise disappeared from the community. Those who were the *best* functioning had, to some degree, disassociated themselves from being identified as cerebral palsied. Tables III to V summarize the current age levels, diagnostic characteristics and IQ level of the residual sample. No social class bias was reflected in the last cases.

The most frequent diagnostic category in the residual population was still spastic hemiplegia, followed by spastic paraplegia and athetosis. In the younger population, spastic tetraplegia accounted for a significantly large portion of the sample. However, since this group included many of the most handicapped children in both an intellectual and physical sense, many of them have been institutionalized and others have been lost to notice for other reasons. The loss of this subgroup largely

TABLE III
Age of Follow-up Sample

Age in yr.		No.	
15		2	
16	Under 18	0	9
17		7	
18		12	
19	18–20	16	41
20		13	
21		7	
22	21–23	8	21
23		6	
24		6	
25	24–26	9	16
26		1	
27	27–28	1	2
28		1	
Total		89	

Males 50, females 39

TABLE IV
Diagnostic Groups in Follow-up Sample

Diagnosis	No.
Spastic monoplegia	3
Spastic hemiplegia	32
Spastic tetraplegia	8
Spastic triplegia	2
Spastic paraplegia	16
Athetosis	16
Ataxia	7
Mixed cerebral palsy	5
Total	89

TABLE V
Initial IQ of Follow-up Sample

IQ	No.
Untestable	3
0–49	6
50–74	28
75–89	27
90–109	20
110–125	5
Total	89

accounts for the absence from the current sample of children with the lowest IQ. The attenuation of the sample in the IQ range 90–125 stemmed in part from the refusal of some members of this group to participate in the study. When asked, they expressed a strong wish to dissociate themselves from any special population of cerebral palsied children and to be considered as normal individuals.

Five of those studied had been married at the time of follow-up and one of these marriages had terminated in divorce. Of the four intact marriages, two from each sex, two had produced a child and both these children appeared to be normal. In the remaining family groups no issue had occurred.

The social background characteristics of the residual group are summarized in Tables VI, VII and VIII. Data on seven of the families were inadequate for evaluation. The people room ratios (Table VI) and fathers' occupations (Table VII) do not indicate any special degree of familial economic stress.

The group studied was largely a lower middle-class, not specially deprived segment of New York City residents. They were predominantly white, with four Negro and one Puerto Rican. The distribution of native and foreign born, and the distribution of religious preferences, also appeared to parallel those of New York City as a whole. As Table VII indicates, the employment patterns coincided with

those of predominantly working class and lower middle-class segments of the population. Table VIII shows the distribution of educational level among the parents. It adhered more closely to the general population of New York City than did the the parents of the severely retarded adult population studied by Saenger (1957).

TABLE VI
People/Room Ratio of 82 Families

People in family	No. of rooms	No. of families
3	2-2½	1
4	3½	4
5	3-4	3
6-9	3-5½	8
		N = 16
2	2½	1
3	3-3½	9
4	4½	14
5	5	5
6	6	2
7	7	1
		N = 32
2	3-4	4
3	4-6	15
4	5-8	9
5	6-7½	5
6-9	7-10	1
		N = 34

TABLE VII
Current Employment of Fathers

Level of employment	No. of fathers
Unknown	2
Welfare or unemployed	4
Porter, truck helper, freight handler, construction worker	6
Furnace stoker, maintenance worker, factory worker, metal polisher, machine operator, longshoreman	12
Elevator operator, shipping clerk, mail-sorter, arc welder, boiler maker, bakery worker, glass cutter	8
Bus, taxi or truck driver, filling station attendant, transportation system, public service, telephone co., assistant cashier, news-stand, postal employee, counterman, grocery clerk, peddler	23
Bookbinder, typographer, mechanic, machine inspector, carpenter, house superintendent, painter, plumber, beautician	11
Store manager, engineering analyst, retail store owner, post-office superintendent	5
Executive, lawyer, bank clerk, accountant, fireman, policeman, shoe buyer, salesman	11
	N = 82

TABLE VIII

Education Level of Parents of Cerebral Palsied or Retarded Children, Compared with General Adult Population of New York City

Education	Cerebral palsied		Retardates (Saenger 1957)		Population N.Y.C., 1950	
	Father	Mother	Father	Mother	Men	Women
	%	%	%	%	%	%
No school	4	6	13	15	4	3
Some grammar school ..	46	30	38	40	36	35
Completed grammar school	7	12	22	22	17	18
Some high school	23	31	13	11	18	19
Completed high school ..	12	16	7	9	17	18
College	8	5	6	3	8	7

The follow-up examination of the residual sample proceeded in two steps. The first step involved a detailed, lengthy interview conducted in the home. The second involved a psychological and perceptual examination conducted in our laboratories. The present report includes the data derived from both the home interviews and the intellectual evaluations.

The Interview

Each interview took 2–3 hours, and though standardized in content the wording and sequence of the questions were not scheduled. The interviewer elicited information on marital status, social involvement, family organization, schooling, residential stability, extent of physical handicap and degree of self-care, employment and employment opportunities, special skills, stated goals, training and training plans, contacts with hospitals and with treatment and rehabilitation centers, agencies and private physicians, current treatment programs and needs, major intercurrent illnesses, accidents or injuries, and various other factors including sources from which further information could be obtained. Replies were recorded in writing during the interviews.

At the time of the interview, the patient's willingness to be scheduled for detailed psychological testing was explored and appointments were made for such examina-tions. Every interview was conducted in the presence of another member of the family. This practice provided an opportunity for checking the accuracy of information given by the patients and also for observing and recording significant features of the home setting, the patient's role in the home, the relationship of the patient with another member of his family, and the general impression of the level of functioning of this patient as seen through his own eyes as well as those of a member of his family.

The interviews have been analyzed for: (1) Level of employment. (2) Economic status. (3) Self-care status. (4) Educational achievement. (5) Social functioning.

The variables have been related to the initial diagnosis and IQ score. In addition, the relation of each of the current characteristics of functioning to one another has been examined.

Results

Level of Employment

Table IX provides a general picture of the employment status of those in the group over 18 years, whom we shall call adults. The table shows that more than half these young adults are unemployed. Of those who are employed, the primary level of employment is unskilled. A significant number of those in unskilled employment work in sheltered situations or with concessions. Less than one-fifth of the

TABLE IX
Employment Level Distribution: Young Adult Population 18 Years and Over

Employment level	No.
Employed on competitive level ..	15
Employed on non-competitive level	19
In training for competitive employment	6
In training for non-competitive employment	1
Unemployed	39
TOTAL	80

TABLE X
Self-care Status

Self-care status	No.
Completely dependent	6
Needs help frequently; cannot get around independently	10
Self-care except for zippers and laces; gets around fairly well by self	14
Completely independent, but still have abnormal gait and/or physical stigmata	56
Normal	3
TOTAL	89

group are employed in skilled and competitive positions.

A small additional percentage of the sample studied are in training programs for both skilled and competitive and unskilled and sheltered employment.

Economic Status

The employment figures suggest that the cerebral palsied adults in this sample are largely economically dependent. In fact only 3 of the 80 cases in this age group who were interviewed can be described as financially independent. Over 60 per cent of the group (50 cases) are completely dependent on their families for financial support, while an additional 27 contribute partially to their support.

Self-care Status

There is a marked contrast between the level of physical independence that the patients achieved and their economic status. Fifty-six of them are entirely independent in a physical sense (Table X) but still remain stigmatized by either abnormal gait or other visible signs of neuromuscular disturbance. Thirty still need some degree of care, though only 6 of these are completely dependent.

Educational Achievement

Educational achievement, too, stands in marked contrast with economic achievement. Table XI shows that 34 of those interviewed have completed high school, while an additional 15 have either received business school training beyond high school or gone to college. Four have graduated from college and 5 of the 8 who are still in school are attending college. Educational achievement in the group appears adequately to reflect the distribution of intellectual level as well as the social backgrounds of the children.

Social Functioning

The pattern of social functioning in the group resembles that of its economic functioning. When group memberships and involvement in group of community activity were explored, it was found that the patients were characteristically uninvolved. Twenty-two of the 89 were social isolates. In contrast, 17 were actively involved with friends and social organizations. Fourteen of the group had active social involvement, restricted to individuals who were similarly handicapped, and 13 were inactively in this type of group. In the main, the patients tended to function constrictedly in a social sense, and to represent a group of social isolates within the community.

A comparison of their current employment level and their original IQ showed that no cerebral palsied child with an initial IQ under 50 was able to secure employment of any sort as a young adult.

TABLE XI
Educational Achievement

	Entire population	Still attending school	Young adult population (18 yr. and over)
Elementary school incomplete ..	13	--	11
6th grade	1		1
8th grade	10	1	9
J.H.S.	3	..	3
High school incomplete	10	2	9
High school graduate	34	..	31
Business Trade school ..	5		4
College incomplete	1	5	1
College graduate	4		4
TOTALS	81	8	73

In the 50–74 range, 3 were in competitive and 7 in non-competitive employment, and 14 were unemployed. Sixteen of the 42 children with an IQ in the 75–110 range were unemployed; 10 were in competitive employment, 11 in non-competitive employment and 5 in competitive training. In the 110+ range, 2 were in competitive employment, one was in non-competitive employment, and one was unemployed. Although skilled employment was most frequently obtained by those members of the group who were in the intellectually normal or superior range, such employment was by no means confined to this group, and a small proportion of the subjects in the lower IQ ranges were also employed at the skilled level.

When current employment level was related to initial diagnostic category, it appeared that the only diagnostic group in which skilled employment was held was spastic paraplegia (6 in competitive employment, 5 unemployed). Of the patients with athetosis, spastic tetraplegia and spastic hemiplegia, half were employed, but most of them in unskilled or sheltered employment; in the remaining diagnostic groups not one individual was employed, either at a skilled or unskilled level. And none of those with ataxia or mixed cerebral

palsy were even involved in training programs.

When the relationship of employment level to other characteristics of current functioning was studied, the most direct relationship appeared to be between employability and self-care status. Current employment status was related to five levels of self-care; completely dependent; needs help; self-care except for zippers, laces, etc.; completely independent but abnormal gait stigmata; normal. The ratio of employed to unemployed increased as a function of improvement in degree of physical independence. In those cases in which there were no marked physical stigmata and where there was complete independence in self-care, unemployment was at a minimum. In contrast, as degrees of dependency in self-care increased, unemployment rose, until in the group that needed help in getting around and contained persons who could not travel independently, 8 out of 9 individuals were unemployed: the one employed being involved in an unskilled occupation. None of the people who were completely dependent for self-care were employed.

The relationship between employment level and schooling was by no means a simple one. Of the high-school graduates,

13 were unemployed and 17 employed (11 competitive, 6 non-competitive). However, there was no instance of skilled employment in any individual whose schooling had not gone as far as high-school graduation. It appeared, therefore, that with higher education the cerebral palsied young adult would be more likely to find some kind of employment, but even with such educational advantages the likelihood of obtaining skilled employment was remote.

No direct relationship was found between degrees of economic independence at follow-up and earlier IQ. However, no individual with an early IQ under 50 was economically independent or contributing to his economic maintenance, and most of those who had early IQs of 90 or above were making at least some contribution to their economic maintenance. Of the 18 in the IQ range 90–109, 11 were earning a small income, as were 2 of the 4 with an IQ of 110 –. It is worth noting, however, that of the 3 individuals who were entirely independent none were in the upper IQ range. One fell in the 50–74 range and the others had IQs below 90.

When the relation of economic status to initial diagnosis was explored, it appeared that the only 3 individuals in the group who achieved complete economic independence were all spastic hemiplegics. As would be expected from other reports, the cases of ataxia or mixed cerebral palsy had the worst economic outcome. In both these diagnostic groups, no-one made any contribution to his economic maintenance.

The most direct relationship was found between degree of economic independence and current self-care status. The 3 individuals who had become economically independent were also completely independent in self-care, despite some residual manifestations of abnormal gait or other stigmata. Of the 9 who could not get around independently, 8 were completely and 1 almost completely dependent economically. These relationships are consistent with the data on employment and self-care status.

When economic status was related to schooling it was found that of the 3 young adults who were entirely independent in an economic sense, one was a high-school graduate and the remaining 2 had had business and trade school training beyond high school. When a relation was sought between those who contributed to their own economic status and those who were completely dependent, it was found that, among those who had not completed high school, the ratio of contributing to non-contributing individuals was 8 : 27, whereas among those who had completed high school this ratio was 22 : 23.

No simple relationship was found between current self-care status and early IQ level, except for the children who had initially been most defective. Of the 9 with IQs below 50, 5 were completely dependent at follow-up, 2 required a considerable amount of help and could not move around in their environment independently, one took adequate care of himself, and one was able to function comparatively well but with an abnormal gait and other stigmata. Only 2 of the 25 children with IQs above 90 functioned at the two lowest levels of self-care, while 19 functioned at the two highest levels. In general, the current level of self-care status correlated highly with the child's initial intellectual standing.

A comparison of self-care status with initial diagnostic category showed that the 3 children functioning normally at follow-up had initial diagnoses of spastic monoplegia and hemiplegia. In general, children with initial diagnoses of spasticity had the best self-care outcomes. In contrast, the worst outcomes were associated with an initial diagnosis of mixed cerebral palsy; none of the 5 children in this group were independent and 2 were completely

41

dependent. Intermediate between these extremes were the 16 children with athetosis, none of whom were completely independent, but 9 were independent with an abnormal gait or other stigmata.

The interrelation between group membership, sociability and self-care status was strongly marked. Of the 17 children actively involved with friends and social groups, 15 were either completely independent in their self-care, though with some physical stigmata, or totally normal. Only 2 of the 17 required minimal assistance in personal hygiene and dressing. Of the 16 children who had any significant need for help in self-care only 2 had any significant social involvement. One prerequisite for functional social integration appears to be adequacy in self-care. Without such adequacy the cerebral palsied young adult becomes socially isolated or engages in passive non-functional relationships with other people and organizations. Even those who are physically independent show a marked degree of social isolation. Thus, about half the young adults who were capable of independent transportation. in the community did not have any significant social involvement. Of the 56 who were completely independent except for some abnormality in gait and minor physical stigmata, 10 in fact functioned as social isolates. Of the whole group, 22 were socially-isolated, while only 17 were actively involved with friends and social groups. It appeared, therefore, that although the group as a whole had done very well physically, and had acquired a considerable degree of skill in self-care. these achievements were not directly related to the development of personal social functioning or adequate social integration. There were as many social isolates as social participants among the patients with good physical independence.

The relationship of educational achievement to other background and current characteristics is complex. The predictive value of the initial IQ for schooling was highest for the most severely defective groups. No patient with an IQ score below 50 went beyond the 6th grade. Every patient with an IQ score above 110 went at least as far as high school. The most variable school achievements were found in the IQ range between 75 and 110. In the 75 89 range, 4 of the 27 patients went only as far as the 8th grade, 7 had an incomplete high school education, 13 were high school graduates, 2 had a business or trade training, and 1 was a college graduate. In the 90 109 range, 2 went no further than the 8th grade, 1 had an incomplete high school education and 11 graduated, 1 had a business training and 5 an incomplete college education. In the 110 + range, 1 had an incomplete high school and 1 an incomplete college education, and 3 were college graduates.

In contrast to other reports, the relation of school achievement to early diagnosis showed that the spastic group were the only category contributing individuals whose education went beyond high school. Among the 16 athetoids, only 5 completed high school. The worst school progress was found among the 12 ataxic and mixed cases, 6 of whom failed to complete their elementary school education.

The relationship of school achievement to other characteristics may be briefly summarized. There appears to be a direct relationship between school achievement and current self-care status: the higher the self-care level. the greater is the likelihood of schooling being completed at a higher level. This relationship, however, is not of a one-to-one type. More than one-third of the group who were completely independent physically but with some disturbance of gait and stigmata. had not completed high school. several individuals in this group ending in the 8th grade. When economic status is considered, it is found that none of the subjects who had not graduated from high school attained an independent income. However, once again, the relationship is not of a one-to-one type, for none of the subjects who attended college had yet attained financial independence at follow-up.

Conclusions

We can now summarize our findings with respect to the five outcome variables that were separated for analysis. It is clear from the findings that the initial diagnosis of type of cerebral palsy, as well as the initial IQ of the children, have prognostic significance. The spastic groups tended to have the higher IQs, achieved a higher level of schooling, and tended to function on a more independent level in self-care and in a social and economic sense than did the athetoid, ataxic and mixed cerebral palsied groups. Among the spastics, the monoplegics and hemiplegics fared far the best.

When the predictive value of initial IQ findings was examined, it was found that no child with an IQ under 50 had a useful job in later years and that the educational achievement of these children was characteristically poor. Among the children with higher IQs, all those with an IQ of 110 or over went through high school and many entered college. The value of the IQ as a social predictive measure was lowest in children with IQs between 50 and 89. In these children, neither school attendance nor the specific levels of education or work achieved bore any direct relationship to the early IQ.

When the outcome variables related to each other, the strongest relationships were found between self-care and the other aspects of function. High levels of self-care correlated highly with employability, school achievement, general economic status, social integration and interpersonal adequacy in functioning.

The group we studied had done very well in developing their physical abilities. They achieved a high level of self-care and ambulatory independence. However, the stigmatic remnants of childhood cerebral palsy appeared at each point to interfere with maximal social and economic achievement. Only the completely normal group of children who, as adults, were free from physical stigmata and awkwardness in gait or speech obtained full social profit from their physical progress. These had become the normal group in terms of sociability, and had the best economic prospects. The remainder, despite substantial progress in self-care and physical functioning, and substantial educational achievements, were still stigmatized and socially isolated. Consequently, the progress made in the mechanics of functioning have not been reflected in any significant degree of independence in living, social integration or interpersonal functioning. The typical individual at follow-up, therefore, was a young adult with a high-school education, a menial job, financially dependent, unmarried, living at home with his family and minimally involved in community activities and interpersonal relationships.

Acknowledgements: This investigation is supported in part by the National Institutes of Health, National Institute of Child Health and Human Development, Grant 00719; by the Association for the Aid of Crippled Children; and by the National Association for Retarded Children.

The authors wish to thank Dr. William Cooper and the Hospital for Special Surgery (under whose care the patients in this study had originally been) for their co-operation in making the study possible, by making both data and other information available to us.

SUMMARY

A follow-up study of 89 cerebral palsied patients aged 16-28 years relates the original diagnosis and IQ to current employment level, economic status, self-care status, schooling and social functioning. The spastic cases tend to have higher IQs, achieve a higher level of schooling, and be more independent socially, economically and in self-care than the other cerebral palsy groups. Patients with an initial IQ under 50 have only an elementary education and are unemployed; the IQ has less predictive value in the higher ranges. Levels of self-care correlate highly with degree of employability, school achievement, economic status, and degree of social integration.

In agreement with other studies, it is shown that cerebral palsied adults who are potentially employable and capable of social activity are typically unemployed and socially isolated.

REFERENCES

Barsch, R. H. (1962) 'Child-rearing practices of parents of children with cerebral palsy. Part I. Toilet training.' *Cerebr. Palsy Rev.*, **23**, no. 5, 12.
—— (1963) 'Idem. Part II. Sleep and bedtime behaviour.' *Cerebr. Palsy Rev.*, **24**, no. 3, 10.
Bell, A. H. (1962) 'Attitudes of selected rehabilitation workers and other hospital employees toward the physically disabled.' *Psychol. Rep.*, **10**, 103.
Burke, R. D., Zimmerman, J. P. (1960) 'Serving the cerebral palsied adult.' *J. Rehab.*, **26**,
Conference on Rehabilitation Concepts, University of Pennsylvania (1962). Chicago: Amer. Mutual Insurance Alliance.
Crothers, B. (1951) 'Cerebral palsy in relation to development.' *Amer. J. Dis. Child.*, **82**, 1.
—— Paine, R. S. (1959) The Natural History of Cerebral Palsy. London: Oxford Univ. Press.
Curtis, L. W. (1954) Vocational Placement of the Cerebral Palsied. United Cerebral Palsy of NYC Inc.
Davis, F. (1961) 'Deviance disavowal: the management of strained interaction by the visibly handicapped. *Social Problems*, **9**, 120.
Deaver, G. (1958) 'Meeting social, psychological, and vocational problems vital in making the cerebral palsied an economic asset. *Crippled Child*, **36**, no. 1, 8.
Dunsdon, M. J. (1952) The Educability of Cerebral Palsy Children. London: Newnes.
Garrett, J. F., Levine, E. S., eds. (1962) Psychological Practices with the Physically Disabled. New York: Columbia Univ. Press.
Glick, S., Donnell, C. (1955) 'Vocational guidance for the teenager with cerebral palsy.' *Cerebr. Palsy Rev.*, **16**, no. 1, p. 8.
Goffman, E. (1963) Stigma: Notes on the Management of Spoiled Identity. New York: Prentice Hall.
Gurevitz, S., Klapper, Z. S. (1951) 'Techniques for an evaluation of the responses of schizophrenic and cerebral palsied children to the children's apperception test.' *Quart. J. Child Behav.*, **3**, 38.
Hastorf, A. H., Richardson, S. A., Dornbusch, S. M. (1958) In Person Perception and Interpersonal Behavior, ed. by R. Taguiri and L. Petrullo. Stanford, California: Stanford Univ. Press.
Hansen, E. (1960) Cerebral Palsy in Denmark. Copenhagen: Munksgaard.
Heinrich, E., Kriegel, I. (1961) Experiments in Survival. New York: Ass. for Aid of Crippled Children.
Jones, M. H., Wenner, W. H., Toczek, A. M., Barrett, M. I. (1962) 'Prenursery school program for children with cerebral palsy.' *J. Amer. med. Wom. Ass.*, **17**, 713.
Katz, I. (1964) 'Review of evidence relating to effect of desegregation on the intellectual performance of Negroes.' *Amer. Psychol.*, **19**, 381.
Kideon, D. P. (1962) 'Natural history of cerebral palsy.' *Cerebr. Palsy Rev.*, **23**, no. 4, 13.
Koch, F. P. (1958) 'A nursery school for children with cerebral palsy: five-year follow-up study of thirteen children.' *Pediatrics*, **22**, 329.
Krech, K., Crutchfield, R. S. (1948) Theory and Problems of Social Psychology. New York: McGraw-Hill.
Lenard, H. M. (1962) 'Vocational implication for the cerebral palsied.' *Cerebr. Palsy Rev.*, **23**, no. 2, 13.
Machek, O., Collins, H. A. (1961) 'Second year review of evaluating and classifying the vocational potentials of the cerebral palsied.' *Arch. phys. Med. Rehab.*, **42**, 106.
Moir, A. (1960) 'Cerebral palsy and employment experience in Eastern Scotland.' *Rehabilitation*, 37.
Morgan, M. R. (1961) 'Vocational guidance for the handicapped. International seminar in Jerusalem.' *Cerebr. Palsy Bull.*, **3**, 174.
Remboldt, R. R. (1959) 'A changing philosophy regarding cerebral palsy.' William Washington Graves Lectures on Human Constitution.
Richardson, S. A. (1963) 'Some psychological consequences of handicapping.' *Pediatrics*, **32**, 291.
—— Goodman, H., Hastorf, A. H., Dornbusch, S. M. (1961) 'Cultural uniformity in reactions to physical disabilities.' *Amer. Soc. Rev.*, **26**, 241.
Saenger, G. (1962) Follow-up Study of Former Blythedale Patients. New York: Wolff Book Mfg. Co.
—— (1957) 'The adjustment of severely retarded adults in the community.' New York: Report to the New York State Interdepartmental Health Resources Board, Albany, N.Y.
Stephen, E. (1961) 'Assessment, training and employment of adolescents and young adults with cerebral palsy.' *Cerebr. Palsy Bull.*, **3**, 127.
Taylor, E. M. (1955) 'The child with cerebral palsy and his family.' *J. Amer. med. Wom. Ass.*, **10**, 123.
United Nations (1960.) Seminar on Rehabilitation of the Physically Handicapped for Participants from Latin American Countries 1959, Copenhagen, Denmark.
Waldman, A. (1963) 'Employment of the cerebral palsied.' *Cerebr. Palsy Rev.*, **14**, August.
Wortis, H., Cooper, W. (1957) 'The life experience of persons with cerebral palsy.' *Amer. J. phys. Med.*, **36**, 328.
Wright, B. A. (1960) Physical Disability A Psychological Approach. New York: Harper.

MOTOR ACTIVITY IN BRAIN-INJURED CHILDREN

Lillie Pope, Ph.D.

Psychiatry Services, Coney Island Hospital, Brooklyn, New York

Questions have been raised recently [2] as to whether the hyperkinetic behavior so frequently reported as a symptom among children designated as brain-injured refers not to the amount of activity but rather to the lack of focus and direction that characterizes the activity of these children. This study attempts to resolve this question by measuring the amount and quality of motor activity among children between the ages of 7 and 11 who have a medical diagnosis of brain injury or minimal cerebral dysfunction * (but not mental retardation or cerebral palsy). This was done by studying specific acts which constitute motor "activity." Measurements were made with instruments that gave objective multidimensional indices of motor activity.[12]

Studies of kinetic behavior in humans have been handicapped by the technical difficulties of observing, recording, and analyzing the occurrence of multiple si-

---

* The definitions of the terms "brain injury," "brain damage," and "minimal cerebral dysfunction" have been and still are the subject of much discussion. For a brief analysis of this problem of definition and a list of references, see Hertzig et al.[10] and Clements.[4]

Submitted to the JOURNAL *in May 1969.*

This study was supported in part by a grant from United Cerebral Palsy of Queens, Inc. The author wishes to acknowledge her debt to Deborah, Edel and William Siler for technical assistance, to Dr. H. G. Birch, Dr. S. Korn, Dr. M. Pope, and Dr. M. T. Hollinshead for valuable discussions of the work, and to Dr. M. Wachspress for his generous assistance.

AMERICAN JOURNAL OF ORTHOPSYCHIATRY, 1970, Vol. 40. No. 5., pp. 783-794.

multaneous specific elements of behavior. We have until now had very little quantification of levels of activity of children during their early school years; this is unfortunate since it is in these years that restlessness presents a serious educational and medical problem. There have been no objective designations of what constitutes mild, moderate, or excessive degrees of restlessness. In fact, it may be assumed that clinically reported levels vary with tolerance and with the setting in which the restlessness occurs. On the whole, the symptom of restlessness has been treated as a global entity—and has remained undifferentiated quantitatively and qualitatively.

Coordinate to a study of motor activity is an interest in the extent to which the individual demonstrates voluntary inhibitory control of motor behavior.

Clinical observation of children with neurological impairment would seem to indicate that such children are deficient in the degree of control they can exert voluntarily, even where language comprehension is intact and could apparently serve as an effective control mechanism. Preliminary research in the field confirms such clinical observation.[5]

In this present study, the subjects were observed one at a time in four experimental situations. They were first observed in undirected play. They were then assigned a simple task and a difficult task, and measurements were made of the activity profile of the subjects as they performed their tasks. Finally, the subjects were ordered to refrain from moving for a given period of time, and the activity was measured during that period.

SUBJECTS

The experiment used two groups, each consisting of 19 boys between their seventh and eleventh birthdays. Subjects in the experimental group had a medical diagnosis of brain injury or minimal cerebral dysfunction. These Ss were not cerebral palsied or epileptic, and had no accompanying diagnosis of mental retardation or psychosis; their IQ's were between 85 and 115. Within each group, there were as many 7- and 8-year-olds as 9- and 10-year-olds.

Experimental Ss were outpatients in the child psychiatry clinic of a city hospital. Most of the children in the experimental group were receiving drug therapy, but the psychiatrist in charge of each case suspended drug treatment for four or five days prior to the experimental observation in order to eliminate the effect of drugs on the child's behavior

during the period of observation.

The control group consisted of 19 boys with no diagnosis of brain injury or other condition requiring special education, and no known psychiatric history or involvement. It was decided to avoid the usual hospital inpatient or outpatient clinic population because the symptoms or illness responsible for bringing the child to the hospital or clinic could affect his activity level unpredictably. Therefore, control Ss were obtained from the community at large.

Boys were chosen for this study because more boys than girls are diagnosed as having brain injury.[15] The age of the children was restricted to the period before the onset of puberty (i.e. after the seventh but before the eleventh birthday) because hyperactivity has been observed to decrease at puberty.[13]

46

MEASURING INSTRUMENTS

Activity measurements were made by the simultaneous use of two instruments: the accelerometer and the behavior recorder (a keyboard device for recording direct visual observations in a form suitable for computer processing). The accelerometer has been used to measure the overall activity of children older than the age group studied here [13]; the behavior recorder has never been used to record the activity of human subjects.

The accelerometers were worn on the wrist of the writing hand and the ankle of the same side and were used to measure total motor activity, which was operationally defined as the total arm and leg movement as measured by the accelerometers. They were used in this way by Schulman, Kasper, and Throne [13] in their studies of motor activity. The ankle accelerometer was responsive to locomotion, and the wrist accelerometer recorded activity of the hand and arm. Individual readings for each limb were obtained, which were then combined to give a measure of total motor activity.

EXPERIMENTAL AREA

The study was carried out in a hospital ward from which the beds had been removed. The experimental area was 29 feet long and 18 feet wide. The floor of this area was divided into four equal quadrants (zones) by means of crossed tapes pasted to the floor.

Each quadrant of the experimental area contained a table with a surface area of 30 x 60 inches. Each table contained an equal number and assortment of experimental toys, and the tables were arranged in each quadrant so that no area, no table, and no set of toys offered any different attraction. The room was arranged so that the child could move freely, and could play in any area, with any of the toys on the table. One chair was placed in each quadrant so that the child could sit if he wished; it was, however, near a wall and far from the toys.

TOYS

On each table in the experimental area was a group of five different toys. Each table had the same five toys: a friction-operated Greyhound bus, a pinball machine, an "Etch-a-Sketch" toy, a "Tinker Toy" set, and drawing materials.

FORM BOARD FOR SIMPLE AND DIFFICULT TASKS

Simple and difficult tasks in the experiments involved the use of the 10-form Seguin Form Board [1] held at varying angles to the horizontal. A rack with grooves was used to hold the board; by slipping the board into the grooves, the board was supported at a precise angle to the horizontal. In addition to the position in which the board was flat on the table, grooves in the rack supported it at angles of 30°, 60° and 87°.

PROCEDURE

Each child was observed individually through a one-way mirror and his behavior noted on the behavior recorder for a total of 35 minutes in a consecutive sequence of four experimental situations:

I. Undirected Activity in a Playroom

II. Performance of a Simple Task
III. Performance of a Difficult Task
IV. Voluntary Inhibition of Activity

Prior to the experimental observation, each child was given a preliminary warm-up session in which he wore the accelerometers and became accustomed to them, and also met and relaxed with the research assistant (RA) who was to guide him through the experimental situations. Accelerometer readings were noted at the beginning and end of each of the first three experimental situations.

EXPERIMENTAL SITUATIONS

I. Undirected Play: In Experiment I, the child was free to play for 15 minutes in any way he wished with toys available in the playroom. During this period, he was alone in the playroom.

II. Performance of a Simple Task: Following the undirected play, the child was requested to perform a simple task, that of placing the 10 forms of the Seguin Form Board in their proper slots. The forms were on a table 8 feet from the board. For the simple task, the board was presented in three positions: flat on the table, at a 30° angle to the table, and at a 60° angle. The RA remained in the room during this experiment, maintaining a neutral attitude. She never added to her original instructions, nor did she deter the child when he violated her instructions.

III. Performance of a Difficult Task: After finishing the simple task, the subject was requested to perform a difficult task. The form board was presented at an angle of 87°, and the subject was requested once more to insert the forms. In this position, it was possible, but very difficult, to insert the forms so that they did not fall out. Since the experimental area was unchanged, the room contained the toys as they had been left at the termination of Experiments I and II. If a child wearied of attempting to place the forms in the almost vertical form board, and returned to playing with toys, he was not dissuaded from doing so. The ob-

server made note of the time at which the child left the form board task and returned to play with the toys in the play area, and recordings were made of the toys with which he played.

The difficult task experiment was terminated when the stopwatch read 15 minutes; this 15-minute period included performance of the simple as well as the difficult task. Thus, if a child took three minutes to finish the simple task, he had twelve minutes in which to do the difficult task.

IV. Voluntary Inhibition of Activity: The child was requested to sit quietly, without leaving his seat, for five minutes. He sat near the wall, in full view of the toys in the room. The RA was not in the room for this period. The observer recorded the time at which the child rose from his seat.

EXPERIMENTAL BEHAVIOR TO BE OBSERVED

The child's activity in the room was observed and recorded as follows:

Accelerometer Activity

The accelerometer readings were noted for the writing hand and the ankle on the side of the writing hand at the beginning and termination of each of the first three experimental situations.

Activity Noted on the Behavior Recorder

1. *Translational Movement:* Translational movement of the subject across zones was recorded by the observer; the subject's geographical location was thus noted at all times.

2. *Type of Movement within Zones:* The specific behaviors observed were: locomotion, standing, and sitting. These were observed and recorded on the behavior recorder as mutually exclusive activities, and they were timed. The percent

of time in each activity was relative to that experiment's duration.

3. *Tactile Contacts:* The involvement of the child with a toy was judged by a physical contact with the toy.

STATISTICAL TREATMENT OF DATA

A t test of means [8] was applied to every set of measurements. The confidence limit was set at .05. Although in some cases the standard deviations of the samples were markedly different, and normal distribution could not be assumed, the t test has been demonstrated to be sufficiently robust, when sample sizes are equal, to tolerate a waiver of these assumptions.[3, 6]

In the research protocol prepared prior to the study, it was hypothesized that the brain-injured group would differ from the control group in several of the measures to be employed. In these few measures in which directional hypotheses were made, one-tailed tests were used, according to the criteria set by Hayes.[9]

RESULTS

I. UNDIRECTED ACTIVITY IN A PLAYROOM

It appears that, in undirected activity in a playroom the total motor activity of brain-injured children did not differ significantly from that of their normal controls (TABLE 1). However, they spent a greater time uninvolved with any of the stimuli available to them (TABLE 2); but they made contact with more of the toys in the room than did their controls. The average time they spent with each toy was less, and the longest duration of their contacts with toys was briefer than the corresponding time spent by their controls. For the purposes of this study, a child who spends more time in contacts with toys may be said

to have a longer attention span than one who spends a great deal of time uninvolved with the toys or task objects or has contacts of shorter duration. The activity of the brain-injured group was therefore characterized by a shorter attention span, as compared with their controls; the brain-injured group may be said to lack "focus and direction."

Although the stimuli in the four quadrants of the room were identical, and therefore no zone was objectively more attractive than any other, the brain-injured children traversed more zones than did their normal controls. On the average, the experimental group occupied 19.79 zones during this period (S.D. 10.38), while the control group occu-

Table I
ACCELEROMETER READINGS IN EXPERIMENT I [a]

	EXPERIMENTAL GROUP		CONTROL GROUP		t [b]	p
	Mean	S.D.	Mean	S.D.		
Locomotor Activity	83.4	81.5	39.9	39.6	2.04	.05
Activity of Writing Hand	106.9	86.9	77.3	43.6	1.30	n.s.
Total Motor Activity	190.3	161.4	117.2	77.7	1.73	n.s. (.09)

[a] Readings are expressed in Activity Units Per Minute (AUPM).
[b] Two-tailed test; confidence limit set at .05.

Table 2

CONTACTS WITH TOYS IN EXPERIMENT I

| | EXPERIMENTAL GROUP | | CONTROL GROUP | | | |
	Mean	S.D.	Mean	S.D.	t [a]	p
Number of Contacts with Toys	20.16	10.25	14.05	7.52	1.74	.05
Mean Duration of Contacts [b]	.82	.45	1.26	.99	1.73	.05
Longest Contact Made by Each Child [b]	3.34	1.74	4.78	3.05	1.74	.05
Shortest Contact Made by Each Child [b]	.07	.08	.10	.11	1.09	n.s.
Percent Time with No Toys	21.79	11.81	14.47	8.82	2.11	.025

[a] One-tailed test; confidence limit set at .05.
[b] Time in minutes was used to compute these values.

pied 13.53 zones (S.D. 10.84, t=1.76, p.=.04, one-tailed test). The experimental subjects also expended more energy in locomotion as measured by the ankle accelerometer alone than did their controls (TABLE 1). In addition, the experimental subjects spent a *greater proportion of their time* in locomotor activity (TABLE 3).

It is important to note that despite the fact that hyperactivity was reported as a clinical symptom in 18 of the 19 experimental cases, eight of the experimental subjects were less active than the median

for the combined groups in total motor activity.

II. PERFORMANCE OF
A SIMPLE TASK

When subjects were requested to perform a simple task which captured their interest and which required locomotion and manipulation, there were no differences between groups in total motor activity and attention span (TABLE 4). All subjects plunged into the task, and it seemed to absorb all their activity. The presence in the room of the RA during

BEHAVIORAL ACTS IN EXPERIMENT I

| | EXPERIMENTAL GROUP | | CONTROL GROUP | | | |
	Mean	S.D.	Mean	S.D.	t [c]	p
Locomotion [a]	27.35	16.90	12.67	7.44	3.37	.01
Standing [a]	69.94	18.90	86.66	8.34	3.43	.01
Sitting [a]	2.71	6.50	.67	2.84	1.22	n.s.
Dropping or Throwing [b]	1.95	3.78	1.05	1.36	.95	n.s.

[a] Percent of time performing this act.
[b] Number of incidents.
[c] Two-tailed t test; confidence limit set at .05.

Table 4

ACCELEROMETER READINGS IN EXPERIMENT II [a]

	EXPERIMENTAL GROUP		CONTROL GROUP		t [b]	P
	Mean	S.D.	Mean	S.D.		
Locomotor Activity	329.2	167.1	337.7	212.5	.13	n.s.
Activity of Writing Hand	231.8	129.8	217.8	93.0	.37	n.s.
Total Motor Activity	561.0	278.3	555.5	289.0	.06	n.s.

[a] Readings are recorded in Accelerometer Units Per Minute (AUPM).
[b] Two-tailed t test; confidence limit set at .05.

the performance of the task also seemed to have no effect. Apparently the children were absorbed in their work and needed no further guidance from the RA other than the presentation of the task.

Interestingly, the brain injured group spent more time in standing during this experiment (TABLE 5); this may be explained by the greater difficulty they seemed to have in placing the forms in their correct places. Problems in form perception or in dexterity may have caused subjects in this group to stop at the form board a little longer while finding the proper place for each form. In contrast, the control subjects were able to move smoothly and frequently not even to stop while placing the forms in the board, having anticipated the correct position as they approached the board.

III. PERFORMANCE OF A DIFFICULT TASK

The experimental group showed significantly greater total motor activity than the control group when asked to perform a difficult task (TABLE 6). During this period, the experimental group recorded greater locomotor activity on the accelerometers as well as greater total motor activity. The experimental group demonstrated a briefer attention span than the control group, making contact with more objects in the room than did the control group (TABLE 7). No significant differences emerged between groups in the number of translational movements across zones during this experimental situation; this resulted chiefly from the fact that the form board and the table holding the forms were in the same zone. Two corollary measures of loco-

Table 5

BEHAVIORAL ACTS IN EXPERIMENT II

	EXPERIMENTAL GROUP		CONTROL GROUP		t [b]	P
	Mean	S.D.	Mean	S.D.		
Locomotion [a]	77.29	20.33	90.48	10.42	2.45	.02
Standing [a]	22.68	20.30	9.52	10.42	2.45	.02

[a] Percent of time performing the behavioral act.
[b] Two-tailed test; confidence limit set at .05.

Table 6

ACCELEROMETER READINGS IN EXPERIMENT III [a]

	EXPERIMENTAL GROUP		CONTROL GROUP			
	Mean	S.D.	Mean	S.D.	t [b]	p
Locomotor Activity	94.1	87.7	49.7	29.3	2.04	.05
Activity of Writing Hand	103.2	74.9	70.9	39.8	1.62	n.s.
Total Motor Activity	197.3	154.7	120.7	66.1	1.95	.04

[a] Readings are recorded in AUPM (Activity Units Per Minute).
[b] One-tailed t test; confidence limit set at .05.

motor activity were provided by the ankle accelerometer readings and by the percent of time spent in locomotion. These measures indicated that the experimental group displayed greater locomotor activity in this difficult task situation than the control group.

Unexpectedly, the experimental group did not differ from the control group in the length of time it persisted with the difficult task. It had been expected that the experimental subjects would tire of the task more quickly, and leave it to return to play with the toys in the room.

This did not happen. Nine children in the control group and eight in the experimental group remained with the form board for the whole experimental period; others drifted away at varying times, with no differences between groups. This may have been due to the presence in the room of the research assistant; the RA seemed to have had an inhibiting or stabilizing influence on some of the subjects during this portion of the experiment. Some subjects asked for permission to leave the difficult task, but were reluctant to do so because the

Table 7

SPECIFIC ASPECTS OF ACTIVITY IN EXPERIMENT III

	EXPERIMENTAL GROUP		CONTROL GROUP			
	Mean	S.D.	Mean	S.D.	t	p
Locomotion [a, c]	30.81	23.21	17.79	10.42	2.17	.05
Standing [a, c]	68.85	23.85	82.21	10.42	2.18	.05
Dropping or Throwing [b,c]	1.37	1.95	1.00	1.17	.69	n.s.
Number of Contacts with Objects in the Room	17.21	10.89	11.37	6.58	1.95	.05
Time Spent with Forms and Form Board (minutes)	9.15	3.53	9.62	2.16	.48	n.s.

[a] Percent of time devoted to this behavioral act.
[b] Number of incidents.
[c] Two-tailed test; confidence limit set at .05.
[d] One-tailed test; confidence limit set at .05.

RA remained passive, giving them no encouragement. Perhaps personality factors that were independent of the diagnosis of brain injury, such as compulsivity, persistence, and submissiveness to the implicit authority of the adult in the room were greater determinants of the subjects' persistence with the task than the behavioral symptoms for which children had been referred for treatment.

IV. VOLUNTARY INHIBITION OF ACTIVITY

In the final task, when each child was requested to sit for five minutes without leaving his chair, the experimental group demonstrated significantly less voluntary inhibition of activity than did the control group (Experimental Group Mean 1.64 minutes, S.D. 1.84; Control Group Mean 2.04, S.D. 2.02; t=2.17, p=.025, one-tailed test). Whereas nine of the control subjects remained in their seats for the full five minutes, only four of the brain-injured children did so. The brain-injured children were less able to follow instructions, to "heed" in the presence of distractors, or, in the words of parents who bring their children to clinics, "to listen." School and home management problems related to so-called hyperactivity frequently result from precisely the feature observed in this experiment: that the child does not sit still when directed to do so, that he is unable to inhibit activity, and not necessarily that he is indeed more active.

RANK ORDER OF ACCELEROMETER READINGS IN ALL TASKS

An examination of the rank order of all accelerometer readings showed some interesting tendencies. One was that there were between five and ten brain-injured children whose score in each measure of activity was below that of the median for the combined groups. Another observation was that even when there was no significant difference between groups, the experimental group tended to show greater activity. This obtained in all cases except in the performance of a simple task, when a consistently high level of activity was required for performance of the task, in which case no such difference could be noted. Furthermore, in those Ss whose activity was higher than the median for the combined groups, the more active of the experimental group stood out in terms of their activity level; they demonstrated more activity than the controls. Among the controls, several Ss were consistently very active, demonstrating greater activity than most of the experimental Ss.

There was some indication that the more active subjects of the experimental group covered the whole range of ages included in this study, while the more active of the controls seemed to be younger. Since the number of subjects where this occurred was small, a developmental analysis was not made. Further inquiry along these lines is certainly indicated.

DISCUSSION AND SUMMARY

COMPARISON WITH OTHER STUDIES

In order to make meaningful comparisons among the studies of motor activity that have been published, it is important that the groups compared have similar ages and IQ, and that the diagnostic criteria and operational definitions of activity be similar. This is a rather severe restriction. There has been no other study of children of normal intelligence, of early school age, with a diagnosis of brain injury, who are not in a residential setting. The study most closely pertinent to this one was that of Schulman et al.[13]

Schulman studied the total motor activity level of retarded boys of the ages of 11 to 14, using the accelerometer, in various settings. His structured setting was a school which he felt probably tends to reject those students with brain injury who demonstrate poor self-control and who are overactive. His experimental subjects therefore would tend to be the less active of the brain-injured group.

In the present study, the experimental subjects presented the most pressing behavioral problems at school and at home and appeared at the clinic precisely because they were severe management problems. Furthermore, they were younger than those studied by Schulman, and were of normal intelligence: thus, this group was quite different from Schulman's group.

Schulman found no significant differences between the total motor activity level of the brain-injured and their controls. He did find that the activity of different subjects varied in different situations, such as structured activity vs. free activity, day vs. sleep. He found that the activity of the majority of brain-injured children, as measured by the accelerometers, was within normal limits. The present study also found that there was no significant difference between the brain-injured subjects and their controls in total motor activity during the periods of undirected activity and performance of a simple task. Differences did appear during the performance

of a difficult task and in voluntary inhibition of activity. An examination of the rank orders of subjects in all activity measures shows the tremendous overlap in activity level between subjects in the two groups, tending to support Schulman's finding that the activity levels of the majority of the brain-injured children were within the normal range.

Schulman found no evidence that hyperactivity was related to the diagnosis of brain injury in his populations. However, in the present study, a closer view of the activity of the two groups showed distinct differences. When locomotor activity (measured by the ankle accelerometer) is considered, in contrast to total motor activity, there were differences between the two groups; there were also differences in *the proportion of time spent in motion* and in standing still There were differences in how the activity was expended. In this study, the evidence indicates therefore that there are differences in the fine structure of the activity of the two groups, but not in total motor activity, as measured by accelerometers.

SUMMARY

The terms "restlessness" and "hyperactivity" have to some extent been used interchangeably in the literature.[14] If hyperactivity is construed as excessive total motor activity, prior studies indicate no difference in activity level between brain-injured populations and their controls.[13] Even in those studies in which locomotor activity alone is studied (rather than total motor activity), several researchers have found no differences between groups in *some* situations.[11, 15]

In this study, however, it has emerged

that there are significant differences between groups in the percentage of time spent in locomotion as contrasted with standing still.

Thus, while total motor activity level of children of normal intelligence diagnosed as having minimal cerebral dysfunction did not differ from that of their controls during undirected activity in a playroom, their locomotor activity was significantly greater. Furthermore, the total proportion of their time spent in locomotion was greater as well; the greatest difference observed between the two groups was in this area. The results of this study suggest that more precise definitions of restlessness and hyperactivity may be projected. Hyperactivity might be appropriately used to describe an excessive degree of activity, as measured by accelerometers, oxygen consumption, or a similar measuring instrument. Restlessness, in contrast, refers to an excessive *proportion of time spent in motion* as measured for example by the behavior recorder. It is thus possible for a child to be both restless and hyperactive; or to be restless, but not hyperactive; it may even be possible to be hyperactive, but not restless. Thus, the experimental group displayed restlessness rather than hyperactivity.

Furthermore, the behavior of the brain-injured group was less focused than that of the normal controls.

When asked to perform a simple task which involved locomotion and manipulation, the two groups did not differ in total motor activity or in attention to the task. In this situation, the experimental group spent a significantly larger proportion of its time in standing still.

When asked to perform a difficult task, the total motor activity of the experimental group exceeded that of the control group. Locomotor activity, as well as proportion of time spent in locomotion, were both greater for the experimental group in this situation. Thus, the experimental group demonstrated greater restlessness as well as hyperactivity when asked to perform a difficult task.

The brain-injured group demonstrated a lower capacity to obey instructions to sit quietly and inhibit activity.

The behavior recorder used in this study provides a method for making quantitative measurements of the motor activity of human subjects.

The techniques discussed in this study can provide meaningful group norms for the general population, as well as for special groups, such as those with varying levels of mental retardation. Developmental changes in activity level can be studied, and norms developed for each age level.

REFERENCES

1. ANASTASI, A. 1961. Psychological Testing. Macmillan, New York.
2. BIRCH, H., ed. 1964. Brain Damage in Children: the Biological and Social Aspects. Williams & Wilkins, Baltimore.
3. BONEAU, C. 1960. The effects of violations of assumptions underlying the t test. Psychol. Bull. 57:49–64.
4. CLEMENTS, S. 1966. Minimal Brain Dysfunction in Children. U. S. Dept. of Health, Education, Welfare, Washington.
5. COHEN, H., L. TAFT, M. MAHADEVICH, AND H. BIRCH. 1967. Developmental changes in overflow in normal and aberrantly functioning children. J. Pedia. 71:39–47.
6. COHN, J. 1965. Some statistical issues in psychological research. In Handbook of Clinical Psychology, B. Wolman, ed. McGraw-Hill, New York.
7. GARFIELD, J. 1964. Motor impersistence in normal and brain damaged children. Neurol. 14 (7):623–630.
8. GUILFORD, J. 1965. Fundamental Statistics

in Psychology and Education. McGraw-Hill, New York.

9. HAYES, W. 1965. Statistics for Psychologists. Holt, Rinehart, Winston, New York.

10. HERTZIG, M., M. BORTNER, AND H. BIRCH. 1969. Neurologic findings in children educationally designated as "brain-damaged." Amer. J. Orthopsychiat. 39:437–446.

11. HUTT, S., AND C. HUTT. 1964. Hyperactivity in a group of epileptic (and some nonepileptic) brain damaged children. Epilepsia 4:334–351.

12. POPE, L., AND M. POPE. 1969. Measure ment of motor activity. Perceptual and Motor Skills 29:315–319.

13. SCHULMAN, J., J. KASPAR, AND F. THORNE. 1965. Brain Damage and Behavior. Charles C Thomas, Springfield, Ill.

14. STRAUSS, A., AND L. LEHTINEN. 1947. Psychopathology and Education of the Brain Injured Child. Grune & Stratton, New York.

15. TIZARD, B. 1968. Observations of overactive imbecile children in controlled and uncontrolled environments: I. Classroom studies. Amer. J. Ment. Def. 72:541–547.

SECTION III

DISORDERS OF SPEECH AND LANGUAGE DEVELOPMENT

Conditioning of Vocal Response Differentiation in Infants[1]

DONALD K. ROUTH[2]

University of Pittsburgh

The present investigation was aimed at demonstrating the development of differential vocal responding in human, infants by the selective reinforcement of "vowels" or "consonants." Students of learning, including Miller and Dollard (1941), Mowrer (1950), and Skinner (1957), seem to agree

[1] This report is based upon a dissertation submitted in partial fulfillment of the requirements for the PhD degree, Department of Psychology, University of Pittsburgh. The author wishes to express his appreciation to George J. Wischner, who directed the dissertation, and to other members of the dissertation committee; to Anne C. Smith and the staff of the Zoar Home for Mothers and Babies, and the numerous parents who made available experimental space and infant subjects; to W. S. Ray and Harold Bechtoldt for their advice in the statistical analysis of the data; to H. Rubin for advice on the problems of response definition; and to T. Dyehouse and J. Schneider for assistance in determining interobserver reliabilities. Much of the research was carried out while the author was a National Science Foundation Cooperative Graduate Fellow at the University of Pittsburgh. The computer facilities of the Universities of Pittsburgh and Iowa granted machine time for statistical analysis.

[2] Requests for reprints should be sent to the author who is now at the University of Iowa, Departments of Psychology and Pediatrics, Iowa City, Iowa 52240.

that (*a*) conditioning procedures can increase the infant's total production of vocalizations, and (*b*) conditioning can also increase the frequency of a given subclass of vocalizations relative to other vocalizations made by the infant.

Direct evidence favoring the hypothesis that infant vocal responses may be generally increased through conditioning appears in two studies, those of Rheingold, Gewirtz, and Ross (1959) and Weisberg (1963). Rheingold et al. (1959) found that the vocalizations of 3-month-old infants increased under a regime of "social" reinforcement and decreased when this reinforcement was withdrawn. However, these authors could not exclude the possibility that the increase in vocal responding was a function of "elicitation" rather than reinforcement; that is, the infants might have vocalized more simply because of the social stimulation per se and not because the stimulation was contingent on their vocal responses. Weisberg (1963) replicated the Rheingold et al. (1959) study, including a group of infants who received the "social" stimulation with equal frequency but never directly after a vocalization. He concluded that the response-reinforcement contingency was indeed necessary and that conditioning of vocalizations had been demonstrated.

Direct evidence for the conditioning of differential vocal responding in infants has been absent from the literature, though the process is hypothesized by most learning theorists who have considered the issue. Indirect evidence is available in a few infrahuman studies. In one recent study, for example, Burnstein and Wolff (1967) first reinforced guinea pigs for vocal calls in the frequency range of 1,000–2,000 cycles per second, then for calls in the range of 2,000–4,000 cycles per second and finally only for calls in the range of 1,000–2,000 cycles per second once more. In each case these authors found an increased proportion of calls in the reinforced range. The numerous studies of verbal conditioning in adult human subjects are also indirectly relevant, as is the study by Salzinger, Salzinger, Portnoy, Eckman, Bacon, Deutsch, and Zubin (1962) on the conditioning of continuous speech in young children. In these studies, subjects do typically produce a relative rise in the reinforced response category, for example, plural nouns or sentences beginning with a certain pronoun. To the author's knowledge, however, no study of vocal response differentiation in human infants has appeared.

Method

Subjects. Thirty infants ranging in age from 2 to 7 months ($M = 137$ days, $SD = 50$) served as subjects. Of those who were living at home with their parents, 11 were white males, 6 white females, 2 Negro males, and 4 Negro females. All 7 institutional subjects were Negro males. The socioeconomic and educational status of the infants' parents varied quite widely, from university professor to unwed mother. The modal subject was a 4½-month-old white male infant residing in his own home.

Apparatus. The apparatus consisted of a Sears Silvertone tape recorder, a stopwatch, an ordinary plastic reclining infant seat, a pair of mechanical tally counters, and two chairs.

Procedure. Ten subjects were randomly assigned to each of three experimental groups. All subjects were initially given 2 days of base-line recording, referred to as Base-line Day 1 (B_1) and Base-line Day 2 (B_2), in which the experimenter was expressionless and nonresponsive to the infant. On the subsequent 3 days, Conditioning Day 1 (C_1), Conditioning Day 2 (C_2), and Conditioning Day 3 (C_3), all "consonant" re-

sponses were reinforced for the consonant group, all "vowel" responses for the vowel group, and all vocalizations (both consonants and vowels) for the vocalization group. The reinforcement consisted of a smile, three "tsk" sounds, and concurrent light pressure on the infant's abdomen by the experimenter.

After the first 9 subjects had been run it was decided to add extinction procedures. Accordingly, the last 21 subjects were randomly assigned to either the extinction (EX) or nonextinction (NX) conditions, which were carried out after the other procedures on Day C_3. For subjects in the EX condition, the experimenter was expressionless and nonresponsive during the extra recording session, while for subjects in the NX condition the experimenter continued to reinforce the previously reinforced response. For purposes of analysis, subjects were randomly dropped from the EX and NX conditions until each consisted of nine infants, three of whom had been in each of the previous differential treatment groups.

On each of the 5 experimental days there were three recording sessions of 13 minutes each, separated by at least 10 minutes and usually by an hour or more. Recording was begun only if the subject was awake (eyes open) and not crying or fussing. A schedule of recording times was devised for each subject and maintained as closely as possible on all experimental days. A recording session consisted of three 3-minute experimental blocks with the experimenter present and the two intervening 2-minute rest blocks with the experimenter absent. During recording sessions the tape recorder operated continuously at 3¾ inches per second. The subject was strapped into the infant seat and positioned to face the experimenter. All sessions were timed. Subsequently, the number of vowels and consonants were tallied from the magnetic tapes and summed to give a vocalization score.

Response definitions. The following definitions were used: (a) vocalization—a speech sound which is discrete (i.e., preceded and followed by a silence), but excluding all crying (very loud, continuous voiced sounds), fussing (characteristic "aha" or "uhuh" sounds which often precede crying), protesting (discrete, relatively loud whining sounds), coughing, sneezing, vomiting, noisy or congested breathing, hiccoughing, sighing, straining sounds (as during defecation), and whistles; (b) consonant—a vocalization containing in the initial, medial, or final position at least one sound in which the vocal passage is constricted in some way, that is, containing a "closed sound";[3]

---

[3] It may be noted that some English consonants are not closed sounds at all, for example, the phones l, m, n, r, and y. True closed sounds include the phones b, d, f, g, h, k, p, s, t, v, z, etc. All plosives, fricatives, and affricates are closed sounds and would cause any vocalization in which they appeared to be classified as a consonant for purposes of the present study.

(c) vowel—a vocalization containing only "open," voiced sounds, for example, the common English vowel sounds and the semivowels l, m, n, r, y, etc.

One other observer independently tallied the responses for one randomly selected recording session for each of the first eight subjects. Pearson product-moment correlation coefficients between the experimenter and this observer for the experimental blocks within the session were .97 for vocalizations, .81 for consonants, and .95 for vowels. Interobserver correlations for the rest blocks were .97 for vocalizations, .75 for consonants and .96 for vowels. Another observer independently made judgments of consonant versus vowel for all vocalizations in a different, randomly chosen base-line recording session for each of the first eight subjects. Percentage of agreement between the experimenter and the second observer ranged from 73 to 91, with a mean percentage of agreement of 82. No consistent differences were found between observers, all having the most difficulty distinguishing single isolated instances of closed sounds like k or ch.

Results[4]

Figure 1 shows the mean number of consonants produced during experimental blocks on each day by the three groups. It is evident that all groups decreased in consonant production on Day B_2 and then increased on each conditioning day. The overall trials effect, considering the average of the two base-line days, and the three conditioning days, was significant ($F = 11.787$, $df = 3/81$, $p < .01$). The Groups × Trials interaction was also significant ($F = 2.264$, $df = 6/81$, $p < .05$). For the consonant group and the vowel group, the trials effect was significant ($F = 6.968$, $df = 3/27$, $p < .01$, and $F = 3.302$, $df = 3/27$, $p < .05$, respectively), while the trials effect was not significant for the vocalization group ($F = 2.731$, $df = 3/27$, $p > .05$). Essentially the same trends over days, and differences between groups during conditioning, were apparent also in the consonant data for the 2-minute rest blocks (not shown).

Figure 2 shows the mean number of

[4] Additional statistical analysis of the data, including further repeated measures analysis of variance, was performed on all dependent variables. The conclusions to be drawn were essentially similar to those reported. In general, there were numerous violations of the assumptions of constancy of the variance–covariance matrix and homogeneity of the dispersion matrix over days, as revealed by tests suggested by Box (1950).

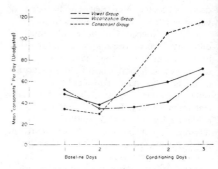

FIG. 1. Mean consonants per day in 3-minute experimental blocks for the vowel, consonant, and vocalization groups as a function of base-line and conditioning procedures

vowels produced during experimental blocks on each day by the three groups. As was the case for consonants, all groups decreased in vowel production on Day B_2, then increased on each conditioning day, the only exception being the vowel group's slight decrease on Day C_2. The rate of vowel production on conditioning days showed a pattern which was the reverse of that for consonant production, being highest in the vowel group, lowest in the consonant group, and intermediate in the vocalization group. The overall trials effect, again considering the average of the two base-line days, and the three conditioning days, was significant

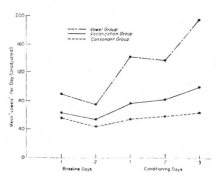

FIG. 2. Mean vowels per day in 3-minute experimental blocks for the vowel, consonant, and vocalization groups as a function of the base-line and conditioning procedures.

$(F = 12.577, df = 3/81, p < .01)$, as was the Groups $\times$ Trials interaction $(F = 2.949, df = 6/81, p < .05)$. Only for the vowel group was the trials effect significant $(F = 8.407, df = 3/37, p < .01)$, while the vocalization group and the consonant group had nonsignificant trials effects $(F = 2.532, df = 3/27, p > .05,$ and $F = 1.851, df = 3/27, p > .05,$ respectively). Again, the same trends over days, and differences between groups on conditioning days, were apparent in the vowel data for 2-minute rest blocks (not shown).

The trend over days with respect to vocalizations was of course the same as for the two subclasses, that is, a decrease on Day B_2 and an increase on each conditioning day. While the vowel group produced the most vocalizations on all 5 days, the other groups tended to overlap, the vocalization group having a higher mean on Days B_1, B_2, and C_1, and the consonant group having a higher mean on Days C_2 and C_3. Again the overall trials effect was significant for the average base-line and the 3 conditioning-day scores $(F = 16.366, df = 3/81, p < .01)$. The Groups $\times$ Trials interaction was nonsignificant $(F = .911, df = 6/81, p > .05)$, and the trials effects for vocalization, consonant, and vowel groups were all significant $(F = 3.100, df = 3/27, p < .05, F = 6.649, df = 3/27, p < .01,$ and $F = 7.605, df = 3/27, p < .01,$ respectively). During 2-minute rest blocks the ordering of groups in vocalization rate was more inconsistent, showing overlapping of all three group curves. The same trend over trials was, however, apparent.

The vowel minus consonant difference score (VCD) was calculated for each subject's performance on each day as an operational measure of response differentiation. The VCD was of course positive if the subject produced more vowels, negative if he produced more consonants. Figure 3 shows the mean VCD score produced during experimental blocks on each day by the three groups. Two of the groups decreased and one increased in VCD on Day B_2. On conditioning days the vowel group tended to move in a positive direction (more vowels than consonants), the consonant group in a negative direction (more consonants than

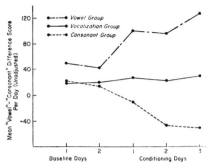

Fig. 3. Mean vowel minus consonant difference scores (VCD) per day in 3-minute experimental blocks for the vowel, consonant, and vocalization groups as a function of the base-line and conditioning procedures.

vowels), while the vocalization group remained at about the same level throughout. Except for Day B_1 there was no overlap in the three group curves. Considering the average base-line score and the scores on the 3 conditioning days, the overall trials effect on VCD was not significant $(F = 1.290, df = 3/81, p > .05)$, while the Groups $\times$ Trials effect was significant $(F = 7.238, df = 6/81, p < .01)$. The vocalization group did not change significantly over trials in VCD score $(F = .240, df = 3/27, p > .05)$. The consonant group's decrease in VCD was significant $(F = 5.181, df = 3/27, p < .01)$, and the vowel group's increase in VCD was significant $(F = 7.131, df = 3/27, p < .01)$. Essentially the same trends over days and group differences were apparent in the VCD scores for 2-minute rest blocks (not shown).

Analysis of covariance was considered to be the most appropriate statistical technique for comparison of the groups' performance on conditioning days, using the combined base-line scores as the adjusting variable in each case. For 3-minute experimental blocks, the 12 Pearson product-moment correlation coefficients between combined base-line scores for consonants, vowels, vocalizations, and VCD scores and the scores on the same variables on each conditioning day ranged from .35 to .75, all positive and all but 2 significant at the

61

.05 level. For 2-minute rest blocks the equivalent correlations were somewhat lower, ranging from .02 to .58. The assumption of homogeneity of regression among groups was found to be violated in only 1 out of 32 tests on the different dependent variables on the 3 conditioning days, combined or separately. The assumption of homogeneity of variance, on the other hand, was found to be violated in 20 out of 32 cases. In the case of vowels, for example, variances were significantly heterogeneous among groups on all 3 conditioning days, combined or separately, for both experimental and rest blocks. Edwards (1962) advises that the F test is sufficiently robust to permit violation of the assumption of homogeneity of variance when the Ns are equal, as is the case for the present study.

The results of analyses of covariance of group differences in production of consonants, vowels, vocalizations, and VCD scores are shown in Table 1. With respect to consonants, Table 1 indicates that the three groups differed significantly during experimental blocks for all conditioning days combined and on Days C_1 and C_2, but not on Day C_3; the groups did not differ significantly in consonant production during rest blocks on any conditioning day. Subsequent F tests of differences between pairs of group means in consonant production gave similar results for Days C_1 and C_2 and for all conditioning days combined, namely, that the consonant group produced significantly more consonant responses than the vowel group, while other differences between pairs of groups were nonsignificant. The F ratios between consonant and vowel groups were 8.519 for combined conditioning days, 14.981 for Day C_1, and 6.312 for Day C_2 ($df = 1/17$, $p < .05$). The F ratios between consonant and vocalization groups were 3.765 for combined conditioning days, 3.035 for Day C_1, and 2.914 for Day C_2 ($df = 1/17$, $p > .05$). The F ratios between vowel and vocalization groups were 1.412 for combined conditioning days, 2.163

TABLE 1

RESULTS OF COVARIANCE ANALYSES OF DIFFERENCES AMONG GROUPS

Source	df	Consonants	Vowels	Vocalizations	VCD scores
		F	F	F	F
3-minute experimental blocks					
Combined days	2/26	5.259*	6.379**	1.021	14.414****
Day C_1	2/26	5.652**	2.298	.526	7.504***
Day C_2	2/26	4.456*	2.473	.344	9.005***
Day C_3	2/26	3.049	11.213***	2.800	13.767****
2-minute rest blocks					
Combined days	2/26	1.085	7.466**	1.796	10.201****
Day C_1	2/26	.426	2.503	1.073	7.778***
Day C_2	2/26	1.568	2.295	.170	6.303**
Day C_3	2/26	.921	8.266**	1.885	6.256**

* $p < .025$.
** $p < .01$.
*** $p < .005$.
**** $p < .001$.

for Day C_1, and 2.546 for Day C_2 ($df = 1/17, p > .05$).

With respect to vowels, Table 1 indicates that the groups differed significantly during experimental and rest blocks on Day C_3 and on combined conditioning days. The groups did not differ significantly in vowel production on Days C_1 or C_2 during either experimental or rest blocks. Subsequent F tests of the differences between pairs of groups showed that for Day C_3 and for combined conditioning days the vowel group produced significantly more vowels than either the consonant or vocalization groups, which did not differ significantly from each other. The F ratios between vowel and consonant groups were 12.521 and 12.463 for experimental and rest-block vowels on combined conditioning days ($df = 1/17, p < .05$), and 25.495 and 8.791 for these variables on Day C_3 ($df = 1/17, p < .05$). The F ratios between vowel and vocalization groups were 5.421 and 7.032 for experimental and rest blocks on combined conditioning days ($df = 1/17, p < .05$), and 1.598 and .098 for Day C_3 ($df = 1/17, p > .05$).

As Table 1 also indicates, there were no significant differences among groups on any conditioning day in total amount of vocalization. To express this another way, one might say that differences in overall rate of vocal responding did not account for variations in the groups' rate of consonant or vowel production.

Finally, Table 1 indicates that the groups differed significantly on VCD scores, the response differentiation measure, on each conditioning day and on combined conditioning days during experimental and rest blocks. Subsequent F tests of differences between pairs of groups showed that the consonant and vowel groups differed significantly for experimental and rest blocks on Day C_1 ($Fs = 7.164$ and 8.770, $df = 1/17, p < .05$), Day C_2 ($Fs = 7.209$ and 7.651, $df = 1/17, p < .05$), Day C_3 ($Fs = 14.684$ and 6.668, $df = 1/17, p < .05$), and on combined conditioning days ($Fs = 13.588$ and 12.167, $df = 1/17, p < .05$). The vocalization and consonant groups differed from each other during experimental but not during rest blocks on Day C_1 ($F = 7.564, df = 1/17, p < .05$, and $F = .058, df = 1/17, p > .05$), Day C_2 ($F = 8.372, df = 1/17, p < .05$, and $F = 2.925, df = 1/17, p > .05$), Day C_3 ($F = 7.377, df = 1/17, p < .05$, and $F = 1.105, df = 1/17, p > .05$), and on combined conditioning days ($F = 9.820, df = 1/17, p < .05$, and $F = 1.945, df = 1/17, p > .05$). The vocalization and vowel groups differed in VCD during experimental blocks only on Day C_3 ($F = 9.066, df = 1/17, p < .05$) and combined conditioning days ($F = 9.066, df = 1/17, p < .05$), but not on Days C_1 or C_2 ($Fs = 3.027$ and 3.170, $df = 1/17, p > .05$); during rest blocks these groups differed on Days C_1, C_2, C_3 and on combined conditioning days ($Fs = 9.267, 5.224, 14.586,$ and 13.848, respectively. $df = 1/17, p < .05$).

Extinction conditions. During the additional recording session on Day C_3, the subjects in the EX condition produced a mean of 15 consonants and 23 vowels, while subjects in the NX condition produced a mean of 17 consonants and 37 vowels. These differences, though in the predicted direction, were not significant (for consonants, $t = .419, df = 16, p > .05$; for vowels, $t = .701, df = 16, p > .05$).

Age and other individual differences. Age was not, in general, found to relate to the dependent variables of the present study. The Pearson product-moment correlation coefficient between age and total number of base-line vocalizations, for example, was .003 ($p > .05$). The number of subjects in individual experimental conditions was felt to be too small to provide meaningful information about the relationship between age and the degree of response differentiation developed.

In the present subject population, sex and race differences were confounded with institutional status to the extent that comparisons of males and females and Negroes and whites were not felt to be justified. No obvious differences emerged from inspection of the data.

Discussion

The infant subjects in the present study tended during conditioning to increase their production of vocal responses, including both "consonants" and "vowels," relative to base-line levels, whether they were reinforced for either subclass alone or for all vocalizations. This observation is in line with the findings of Rheingold et al. (1959).

The three experimental treatments of the present study produced significantly different effects on the groups' consonant production, vowel production, and on response differentiation as measured by the VCD score. The subjects tended to increase their production of the "reinforced" class of vocal responses more than their production of the "non-reinforced" class. Also, the increase from base-line to conditioning days and the response differentiation which developed generalized significantly from the experimental blocks to the rest blocks.

It seems reasonable to interpret the results in conditioning terms, to speak of the processes of acquisition, stimulus generalization and discrimination, response generalization and differentiation, and extinction, as a function of the reinforcement or nonreinforcement of the different response classes. In the present study, as in the Rheingold et al. (1959) and Weisberg (1963) studies, the subjects increased their production of the reinforced response class (acquisition). The subjects also tended to increase the frequency of a nonreinforced response class which was similar to the reinforced response (response generalization), but to some extent to produce a selectively greater increase in the reinforced response class (response differentiation). The increase in vocal responses during rest blocks relative to the rest-block base lines may be viewed as stimulus generalization; that is, the stimulus situation in the rest blocks was the same as that in the experimental blocks with the exception of the experimenter's presence or absence. It was not possible, in the present study, to observe whether stimulus discrimination occurred. The relatively greater increase in the reinforced response class during rest blocks, as indicated by VCD scores, may be seen as the generalization of response differentiation. And, finally, the direction of the nonsignificant difference between EX and NX subjects might be interpreted as the beginning of an extinction process.

There were differences between the present study and the Rheingold et al. (1959) and Weisberg (1963) studies in the age of the subjects and also in the response definitions used. As an extension of the two studies, the present work has demonstrated conclusively the phenomenon of response differentiation in vocal responding of young infants. Suggestive evidence for the phenomena of stimulus and response generalization was also provided. The failure of the present study to demonstrate the extinction phenomenon is possibly due to the brevity of the extinction session.

The hypothesis that the so-called reinforcing stimulus (smile, stroking the abdomen, "tsk" sounds) might actually have elicited vocalizations is not tenable because it could not account for the production of more consonants by one group and more vowels by another. Interpretations of the present results in terms of growth, adaptation, or sensitization might similarly account for the increase of responses over days but not for the differential effects of the treatments on consonant and vowel production. In addition, a "growth" hypothesis would have to deal with the lack of observed relationship between age and base-line vocalizations.

In conclusion, it appears that not only the total rate of vocal production but also the qualitatively specific components of infant vocalizations may be modified by conditioning procedures. These results are consistent with a conditioning theory of language acquisition.

REFERENCES

Box, G. E. P. Problems in the analysis of growth and wear curves. *Biometrics*, 1950, **6**, 362–389.
Burnstein, D. D., & Wolff, P. C. Vocal conditioning in the guinea pig. *Psychonomic Science*, 1967, **8**, 39–40.
Edwards, A. L. *Experimental design in psychological research.* (Rev. ed.) New York: Holt, Rinehart & Winston, 1962.
Miller, N. E., & Dollard, J. *Social learning and imitation.* New Haven: Yale University Press, 1941.
Mowrer, O. H. *Learning theory and personality dynamics.* New York: Ronald Press, 1950.
Rheingold, H. L., Gewirtz, J. L., & Ross, H. W. Social conditioning of vocalizations in the in-

fant. *Journal of Comparative and Physiological Psychology*, 1959, **52**, 68–73.

SALZINGER, S., SALZINGER, K., PORTNOY, S., ECKMAN, J., BACON, P., DEUTSCH, M., & ZUBIN, J. Operant conditioning of continuous speech in young children. *Child Development*, 1962, **33**, 683–695.

SKINNER, B. F. *Verbal behavior*. New York: Appleton-Century-Crofts, 1957.

WEISBERG, P. Social and nonsocial conditioning of infant vocalizations. *Child Development*, 1963, **34**, 377–388.

UNDERSTANDING LANGUAGE WITHOUT ABILITY TO SPEAK:

A CASE REPORT [1]

ERIC H. LENNEBERG

Harvard University

Infants' random babbling is generally considered to play a major—by some, an essential—role in the acquisition and development of language. In fact, many psychologists believe that the main reason for the failure of mammals other than man to learn to speak or even to bring their vocalizations under new and varied stimulus control is due to their scanty random vocalizations. Recently it was discovered that dolphins make a great variety of vocal tract produced noises and, to be sure, the hope was soon expressed that these animals may with proper training learn to converse with their trainers in English. Incidentally, this hope was shared by Dr. Doolittle, Hugh Lofting's charming literary creation.

Our understanding of human behavior is often greatly enlightened by careful investigations of clinical aberrations and in many instances disease or congenital abnormalities provide conditions that may replace the crucial experiments on children that our superego forbids us to plan and perform. No psychological theory on verbal behavior can be successful unless it takes into consideration and accounts for the pathological variations that may be observed clinically. In the present paper I will present the case of a child who is typical of a large group of children with deficits in their motor execution of language skills but who can learn to understand language even in the total absence of articulation. This and similar clinical material forces us to review our theoretical formulations concerning the role of babbling and echoic responses in the acquisition of language and to review once more the relationship between understanding and speaking a language.

CASE REPORT

This is an 8-year-old boy who has a congenital disability for the acquisition of motor speech skills (anarthria) which, however, has not

impaired his ability to learn to understand language.

Medical History

The mother, at the time of subject's birth, was a para I, gravida II white housewife who had enjoyed good health. Throughout her second pregnancy she suffered from a mild chronic bronchitis but gestation was otherwise unremarkable. The baby was born 2 weeks prematurely by dates. Delivery was spontaneous, preceded by 6 hours of labor though the birth was precipitous. No other complications were recorded. The birth weight was 4 pounds 10 ounces. Good respiration was established within half a minute at which time the baby cried vigorously. He had good color and was at no time cyanotic or jaundiced. The following abnormalities were noted at birth: he had bilateral club feet (talipes equino varus on left and metatarsus varus on right) and a fine white line in a sagittal direction on the upper lip. Otherwise the physical examination was reported to be within normal limits. The mother was told that the placenta had been too small to nourish the fetus adequately but no pathological report is available. The baby was placed in an incubator for 2 weeks and remained in the newborn nursery at the hospital for 2 months. He sat at 9 months and walked only at 2 years of age, earlier development having been handicapped by casts and corrective shoes. He has never been heard to use any words. He has had the usual complement of inoculations and there have been no severe diseases. At age 2 he fell on his head and required two stitches; the incident had no sequelae. The first pediatric examination recorded in the hospital chart (age 2 years) revealed anomalies of the eyes in addition to the anomalies of feet and lip. There was a right ptosis and a convergent strabismus.

Family History

The family history is noncontributory. The subject is the second of three children; both siblings are intelligent and well. The mother is

[1] This paper was written while the author was a National Institute of Mental Health Career Investigator (Grant M-2921).

JOURNAL OF ABNORMAL AND SOCIAL PSYCHOLOGY, 1962, Vol. 65. pp. 419-425.

now divorced and lives with the subject's grandmother. A home visit revealed a warm and socially adequate climate.

Physical and Laboratory Examinations

When first seen by the author the child had been brought to a neurological service with a chief complaint of failure to develop speech. He was then 3 years and 9 months, of markedly small stature but with a head circumference normal for his chronological age (49.6 centimeters). Anomalies of the eyes had been corrected surgically. He had single palmar creases in both hands but no other mongoloid stigmata. The only other abnormal finding on examination was an enlarged heart; no murmurs were heard. His oral cavity was of normal configuration and he had no difficulties in chewing, swallowing, sucking, blowing, or licking. Laryngoscopy was negative. On radiological evidence his bone age was 2:8 according to Todd's standards. A skull series was normal. All laboratory tests were negative, and there were no signs of hypothyroidism or inborn errors of metabolism. An electroencephalogram was read as nondiagnostic though it was noted that activity in the right temporal area was less rhythmic than in the left.

Psychological Tests

Tests were performed at 4, 5, and 8 years. Merrill-Palmer, WISC, Bender Visual Motor Gestalt, and Leiter International Performance tests were used, the examinations being administered by three different psychologists and at two different clinics. The subject always related easily to the examiner and gave no signs of emotional disturbance or psychiatric disease. IQs were consistently in the 72–83 range but might have been consistently biased by the subject's inability to express himself verbally. He always gives an alert impression, reacts quickly to verbal instructions, and has always shown an adequate concentration span with little signs of distractibility or hyperactivity. At his most recent test no evidence of "organic" deficits was obtained although some "immaturity in his drawings" was noted. He is slightly retarded in his mental development but the deficit is definitely in the educable range and cannot explain his inability to speak.

Voice and Speech

The child's crying and laughter have always sounded normal. He is also able to make other noises, for instance short cough-like grunts accompanying his pantomimed communications.

While playing alone he will readily make noises that sound somewhat like Swiss yodeling (though he has never had any experience with these sounds!) and which do not resemble any kind of vocalization heard among normal American children. (Samples of these sounds are reproduced in a documentary film.) When the author first saw him he appeared to have some difficulty in bringing his voicing mechanism under voluntary control. For instance, he was unable to make the pointer of the VU meter in an Ampex tape recorder jump by emitting grunts into a microphone even though he was fully aware of the logical connection between sound and deflection of the pointer and was fascinated by it. He would hold on to the microphone and move his head and lips toward it as if to prompt himself for the action; after a few futile attempts and with signs of rising frustration he would in desperation end up gesturing to the examiner's mouth inviting him to make the needle jump, or else simply resort to clapping his hands and accomplish his end this way. In recent years he seems to have learned to control his vocal apparatus to a greater extent. He has had speech training for a considerable length of time and can now repeat a few words after the speech therapist or his mother but the words are still barely intelligible and are never produced without the support from the speech correctionist or the mother (samples are reproduced in the film).

Some of the spontaneous sounds emitted by the patient at 4 years were analyzed spectrographically.[2] The spectrograms are grossly abnormal for a child of this age and resemble those of a neonate in a number of respects, such as the unsteadiness in the formant pattern, the intermittent bursts of nonharmonic overtones, and the almost random change in resonance distribution over the spectrum (Lenneberg, 1961). The spectrograms may be interpreted either as grossly immature or as evidence of a fixed central nervous system abnormality implicating the basic mechanisms for speech synergism.

From the patient's first visit to the clinic it

[2] A 5-page table giving a transcript of commands, questions, and statements with classification of subject's response and a figure showing frequency cycles per second have been deposited with the American Documentation Institute. Order Document No. 7317 from ADI Auxiliary Publications Project, Photoduplication Service, Library of Congress, Washington 25, D. C., remitting in advance $2.50 for microfilm or $6.25 for photocopies. Make checks payable to: Chief, Photoduplication Service, Library of Congress.

has been obvious that he had a normal and adequate understanding of spoken language. He has been seen more than 20 times since then and the finding of full comprehension has been confirmed by neurologists, psychologists, speech therapists, medical residents, and other hospital personnel. A number of tape recordings have been made of interviews including a visit to the patient's home. Most of the examinations were done without the presence of his mother. At one time a short series of instructions were tape recorded and transmitted to the patient through earphones. He followed the instructions without being able to see the examiner.

Demonstration Film

At age 8 years his capacity to comprehend was fully documented in a 16-millimeter sound film which is publicly available.[3] The film was not rehearsed and the examiner had been known to the patient by sight only. The demonstration includes the following items: ability to chew, swallow, and suck; sounds emitted while playing at age 4; tape recordings of mother's "conversation" with subject, recorded during a home visit; following commands and answering questions by nodding; a short story is told followed by questions on it which are couched in complex grammatical constructions such as the passive voice.

Interpretation

It is tempting to explain the patient's responses to verbal instructions by extralinguistic means. Perhaps he is merely responding to visual cues given by the examiner and has, in fact, not learned to understand English! Could children with his type of abnormality develop perceptual skills such as were observed in von Osten's

[3] *The Acquisition of Language in a Speechless Child,* 16-millimeter sound film. Running time 18 minutes, distributed by Psychological Cinema Register, Pennsylvania State University.

famous horse, der kluge Hans, who supposedly could stamp his hoof in response to questions posed to him in German, but who, upon close examination by the psychologist Pfungst, had merely learned to observe the questioner, picking up minute motor cues related to posture and respiratory patterns which signaled to him whether to stop or to continue to stamp his hoof? There is direct evidence against this hypothesis. The child described can react to tape recorded instructions in the absence of any observer. Further, his responses do not merely consist of nodding but also of doing things which could under no circumstance be conveyed by inadvertent motor cues. In the film which documents the case, it is clear that the child frequently follows commands without looking at the examiner. Out of the 45 responses only 3 times was there vacillation between correct and incorrect answers and the last answer in each case is correct. On the other hand, there was no hesitation in the 3 instances when incorrect answers were given. There is no reason to assume that this child has superhuman ability to respond to visual cues instead of assuming that he has learned what every other child of his age has learned, namely, to understand English. Table 1 summarizes the child's performance. It is the result of a panel of three judges who scrutinized the film, viewing each command and its execution individually and with as many repetitions as was necessary in order to determine by unanimous agreement whether there was any likelihood of extralinguistic cuing.

Finally, we must consider the possibility that this patient had no understanding of syntactic connections but merely responded to key words in the commands and questions. This possibility is extremely unlikely in the face of his understanding of such sentences as "Take the block and put it on the bottle." "Is it time to eat breakfast now?" Was the black cat fed by the nice lady?"

TABLE 1

Number of Subject's Correct, Indecisive, and Incorrect Responses

Type of response required	Classification of subject's response						
	Correct		Indecisive		Incorrect		
	No cue possible	Cue possible or certain	No cue possible	Cue possible or certain	No cue possible	Cue possible or certain	Total
Action	19	5	0	0	2	2	28
Yes-No nodding	2	11	0	3	0	1	17
Total	21	16	0	3	2	3	45

Diagnosis

The hospital's clinical diagnosis is multiple congenital anomalies, which, however, is a waste-basket classification and of no heuristic value. Certainly it does not explain the absence of motor speech. The two most common causes for this deficit, peripheral deafness and severe emotional disturbance, may be readily ruled out on clinical evidence. Nor may we assume that the patient's mental retardation is a sufficient cause since the degree of deficiency revealed in his psychological tests is not ordinarily accompanied by any marked speech deficit. Patients with an IQ as low as 25 to 35 have a wide repertoire of sounds and frequently use a vocabulary of 50 or more words. Some authorities would classify this patient as having congenital or developmental motor aphasia. I am not in favor of such a classification on terminological grounds. Aphasia has come to designate loss of speech in persons who had been fluent before the onset of disease or trauma. The condition occurs in children (Guttmann, 1942) as well as in adults and presents a symptomatology that is distinct from any developmental condition. However, the most important reason for rejecting the term aphasia for cases such as described here is that aphasia has traditionally been applied to cortical and subcortical lesions. The present case, on the other hand, gives every indication of an abnormality on a lower level, probably mesencephalic, because of the association with the ocular abnormalities and the discoordination as seen in the spectrograms. The term congenital anarthria better characterizes the condition. Psychological tests make cortical or subcortical damage also unlikely and his excellent understanding of language supports this view.

DISCUSSION

Failure to Learn to Understand Despite Babbling and Imitative Facility

The case reported makes it clear that hearing oneself babble is not a necessary factor in the acquisition of understanding; apparently, hearing oneself babble is also not a sufficient factor. In a language acquisition study on home-raised mongoloid children (research in progress) I have gathered empirical evidence that these children are excellent imitators who babble abundantly and freely. In all cases they have a speaking command of at least single word utterances; yet their understanding of complex commands and questions (such as used in the demonstration film) is frequently defective (usually if

their IQ is about 50 or below). Here the vocal play is present and motivation is provided through interaction with parents, but it does not enable these children to overcome their inborn cerebral deficit.

Relationship between Speaking and Understanding

We must now pose the problem: if the secondary reinforcement provided by hearing oneself babble is neither necessary nor sufficient for an acquisition of understanding of language, could learning to speak be an entirely independent task, justifying a theory that applies to it alone, but not to the learning of understanding? We will see that the answer to this question is a qualified *no*.

The case presented here—by no means unique —is particularly dramatic because of the vast discrepancy between understanding and speaking; a similar phenomenon in more attenuated form is extremely common. Understanding normally precedes speaking by several weeks or even months. The discrepancy is regularly increased in literally all types of developmental speech disorders and is best illustrated in a condition known in the profession as Delayed Speech. Pertinent are also those children who have structural deformities in the oral cavity or pharynx and who produce unintelligible speech for years—sometimes throughout life—without the slightest impairment of understanding. Congenitally deaf children also learn to comprehend language in the absence of vocal skills. Understanding in all of these circumstances is definitely prior to and in that sense independent from speaking.

However, there is no clear evidence that speaking is ever present in the absence of understanding. Speaking is to be understood here as the production of utterances that are bona fide examples of a natural language (such as English) with presumptive evidence of autonomous composition of grammatically acceptable sentences. An empirical test of speaking without understanding might be as follows: a child acquires nothing but words that have no meaning to him (by blind imitation) and learns the formal principles governing the generation of sentences. He will now utter sentences out of context and irrelevant to situations by established common sense standards; he would also have to be demonstrably incapable ever to respond appropriately to commands formulated in natural language. My assertion is that such a condition has never been described as a congenital, developmental problem (Mark, 1962). (Adventitious conditions such as sensory aphasia in the adult, are problems in *partial loss, not partial acquisition* of language and are therefore not relevant to this discussion. Nor could case reports of psychotic children be adduced reliably because even if their utterances are primarily echolalic, there are usually indications that the child does understand, at least at times, what is said to him. In fact, this is usually the basis of the therapy given them.) It is thus likely that the vocal production of language is dependent upon the understanding of language but not vice versa. Though there is no conclusive proof of this hypothesis, there are theoretical considerations that make this likely. In order to make this latter point clear, a few general remarks on the nature of grammar are indispensable. My discussion will lean heavily on Chomsky's (1957) and Chomsky and Miller's (1962) work.

Wherever the word *imitation* is used in connection with language learning it is assumed that subjects learn more than passive mirroring of sentences heard. The novel creation of sentences is a universally accepted fact. At first it was thought that this phenomenon could be accounted for by postulating that grammar simply reflected transitional probabilities between words. In this model the learning of grammar was thought to be like the learning of probabilities. Such learning has been demonstrated to occur for a great many mammals. If this model were acceptable, a child's exposure to certain contingencies should enable him to learn grammar in the absence of "understanding" the relationship between words. Chomsky has offered formal proof against left-to-right probabilistic models, and has shown how a different model can overcome some of the basic difficulties encountered by Markovian grammars. We shall not concern ourselves here with the mathematical detail but shall merely demonstrate by a few examples (most of them suggested by Chomsky) that grammar simply cannot be explained in terms of learned sequential contingencies, and that therefore the understanding and producing of sentences cannot be equated with probability learning.

Consider the following two strings of words, (a) colorless green ideas sleep furiously, (b) furiously sleep ideas green colorless. In terms of transitional probabilities they are indistinguishable. Both sentences can only occur in a zero order of approximation to English. However, we can discriminate between them from the point of view of grammaticality. Sentence a strikes us as a possible sentence, whereas b does not.

The difference between a and b could not possibly be due to association by contiguity for obvious reasons (Miller, Galanter, & Pribram, 1960). Nor is the sequence of form class markers -*less, -s, -ly* the hallmark of grammaticalness as shown by the sentence, (c) friendly young dogs seem harmless, which is grammatical though it reverses the order of the markers.

In order to account for the difference in our perception of a and b we might try to see whether sequential contingencies do exist, but instead of on the level of words, on the level of parts of speech (actually proposed by Jenkins & Palermo, 1961). If this were so the essence of the transitional probability model would be saved and the principal underlying the formation of sentences would still be simple enough to allow of the possibility of speaking without understanding. Unfortunately this model is no more successful in accounting for "sentencehood" than any other Markovian device. If we compare the strings, (d) occasionally call warfare useless, (e) useless warfare call occasionally, we find that now d is perceived as more grammatical than e though the order of parts of speech in d is that of b above which we rejected as less grammatical. This example shows that the traditional categorization in terms of parts of speech is certainly not successful in reinstating a Markovian model.[4]

Mowrer (1960) has proposed that simple contiguity of words is sufficient explanation for the complex meaning that is conveyed by a sentence. Osgood (1957) on the other hand believes that grammatical order can be set aside by motivational factors and that with an increase of motivation word order would correlate with order of importance of words. Doubt is cast on both views, however, by comparison of sentences such as, (f) the fox chases the dog, (g) the dog chases the fox, which clearly make either position untenable. A child whose task it is to learn to produce sentences such as f and g in the appropriate physical environment must necessarily learn some principal of concatenation which goes *beyond* recognition of contiguity. It would be tempting to maintain that the principle to be learned is something like "First noun phrase is the actor or subject in a sentence." Yet, the patterning involved must be more complex and in a sense more abstract still, for

[4] Nor is there any hope that eventually more efficient categories might be discovered since Chomsky's (1957) criticism is leveled against all finite state sentence generating devices. Compare his argument concerning mirror-image languages, and Miller's (1960) argument.

even a preschool child would understand the sentence, (*h*) the fox is chased by the dog, as belonging to *g* and not to *f*. To explain this phenomenon we would now have to postulate that in addition to the principle above, the child would also have to learn that the presence of the morphemes *is, -ed, by* signals a reversal of the original principle. But sentence (*i*) the fox is interested by virtue of his nature in chasing the dog, eliminates this possibility because this sentence is understood as similar in meaning to *f* instead of *g* despite the presence of morphemes *is, -ed, by* occurring in essentially the same sequential order as in *h*. In other words, if we must learn to compose sentences that conform to English grammar, we can only learn to apply the structural principles of sentence formation by first learning to understand and to group sentences in accordance with similarity or differences in meaning. It is not possible to explain the grammatical phenomena demonstrated in the test sentences above by assuming that the entire sentence is in one way or another associated with the complex natural situation to which it refers. Sentences without any referential meaning such as, (*j*) A v's C, (*k*) C v's A, (*l*) C is v'ed by A, (*m*) A is v'ed by C, can easily be grouped in terms of similarity and dissimilarity of meaning. Therefore, the word *meaning* in this context refers to grammatical understanding and not to an association between a symbol and a physical stimulus.

Obviously, we do not yet have a satisfactory model that might explain how grammar is learned. All we can say is that a child learns to produce novel sentences after hearing a number of utterances which were produced by formal laws of generation in addition to a number of other determining factors: he must be able to abstract the formal laws through observation (or be equipped to accept sentences as an input and recognize invariant patterns of complex relationship) before he can apply them to the production of new sentences. It is particularly important to realize that what the child learns during acquisition of grammar is the peculiar formal relationship that obtains between a number of different grammatical patterns, i.e., the relationship between active-passive, declarative-interrogative-negative, and many other similar relationships called *rules of transformation* (Chomsky, 1957; Harris, 1957). It is this latter ability—and only this—that enables any speaker of English to group the Sentences *f* through *i* according to similarity in meaning. The psychological process involved here is more similar to the operations by which we know that:

$$w \; (\sqrt{w} \times \sqrt{w})$$

and

$$\frac{w^6}{w^4}$$

can both be represented by w^2 than to an operation by which we know that the symbol S_4 is next in line to be generated after a train of symbols S_1, S_2, S_3, has been produced. This point is illustrated by Chomsky's examples of structural ambiguity. There are rules of transformations which convert sentences of the form (*n*) one visits relatives, (*o*) relatives are visiting, into a phrase, (*p*) visiting relatives. Because of the two different transformational origins this phrase is ambiguous and, when used in a sentence, may render that entire sentence ambiguous: (*q*) visiting relatives can be a nuisance.

The conclusion of this discussion is that *knowing a language* may be, and ordinarily is, manifested by two distinct behavioral manifestations: understanding and speaking. Upon careful analysis, however, both of these manifestations depend upon the application and use of a single set of grammatical rules; in the case of understanding, the rules are applied to the analysis, i.e., processing and organizing of input data; in the case of speaking, the same rules are applied to the organization of output data or responses. In the process of language learning, the acquisition of grammatical rules must occur first in connection with analysing incoming sentences; then with producing outgoing sentences. The most important point here is, however, that *knowing* a natural language is dependent upon the *acquisition of a single set of organizing principles* and that this set of principles is merely reflected in understanding and speaking but is not identical with these skills.

Summary

A case was presented, typical of a larger category of patients, where an organic defect prevented the acquisition of the motor skill necessary for *speaking a language*, but evidence was presented for the acquisition of grammatical skills as required for a complete *understanding of language*. Theories on the acquisition of speech and language must account for both motor and grammatical skills. Present theories assert that babbling, hearing oneself vocalize, and imitation are the cornerstones of speech development. These phenomena primarily relate to the development of the motor skills involved which, however, never develop in isolation, i.e., without simultaneous acquisition of grammatical skills. The case presented together with the language deficit in certain Mongoloids clearly shows that babbling, hearing oneself talk, and imitation are neither sufficient nor necessary factors in the acquisition of grammar and since the motor skills alone are never shaped into "speaking without grammar," i.e., parroting without understanding, it is concluded that the present theories are inadequate.

REFERENCES

CHOMSKY, N. *Syntactic structures.* Hague: Mouton, 1957.

CHOMSKY, N., & MILLER, G. A. Introduction to the formal analysis of natural languages. In D. Luce, E. Galanter, & R. Bush (Eds.), *Mathematical psychology.* 1962, in press.

GUTTMANN, E. Aphasia in children. *Brain,* 1942, **65**, 205–219.

HARRIS, Z. S. Co-occurrence and transformation in linguistic structure. *Language,* 1957, **33**, 283–340.

JENKINS, J. J., & PALERMO, D. S. Mediation processes and the acquisition of linguistic structure. Paper read at SSRC conference in Cambridge, Massachusetts, October 1961.

LENNEBERG, E. H. Speech as a motor skill with special reference to nonaphasic disorders. Paper read at SSRC conference in Cambridge, Massachusetts, October 1961.

MARK, H. J. Elementary thinking and the classification of behavior. *Science,* 1962, **135**, 75–87.

MILLER, G. A. Plans for speaking. In G. A. Miller, E. Galanter, & K. H. Pribram (Eds.), *Plans and the structure of behavior.* New York: Holt, 1960. Pp. 139–158.

MILLER, G. A., GALANTER, E., & PRIBRAM, K. H. *Plans and the structure of behavior.* New York: Holt, 1960.

MOWRER, O. H. *Learning theory and the symbolic processes.* New York: Wiley, 1960.

OSGOOD, C. E. Motivational dynamics of language behavior. In M. R. Jones (Ed.), *Nebraska symposium on motivation: 1957.* Lincoln: Univer. Nebraska Press, 1957. Pp. 348–424.

SECTION IV

MENTAL RETARDATION

MENTAL DEFICIENCY—DEVELOPMENT OF A CONCEPT

Johs. Clausen [1]

Department of Research, The Training School at Vineland [2]

DURING the last century there have been profound changes in the concept of mental deficiency. An attempt to discern the trend of these changes may bring some of the current problems of this field into sharper focus. The purpose of the present article is to outline the historical changes of concepts regarding mental deficiency, to present for discussion a point of view on definition, and to consider some of the implications of such definition on diagnostic practices. Although many of the propositions offered here have been presented previously, the persistent lack of uniformity in the field justifies their restatement.

Doll (1941) has said: "The *concept* of mental deficiency today is clear enough; the diffi-

culty lies rather in the inadequate employment of means by which the accepted definitions are satisfied." It may, however, be necessary to modify the definition in order to achieve agreement on how the definition is satisfied.

The present article contains a brief historical outline to show how the concept of mental deficiency has changed with time and to indicate the origin from which the present day concept has evolved. It does not claim to be an exhaustive historical treatise, in that several such detailed accounts are already available (Ireland, 1900; Barr, 1904; Nowrey, 1945; Penrose, 1949; E. E. Doll, 1962). Whitney (e.g., 1953) has contributed to this journal several biographical sketches of individuals associated with the early period of the deficiency problem in the USA, and Milligan (1961) has reviewed the history of the American Association on Mental Deficiency.

Early History:

The history of mental deficiency is, of course, almost as long as the history of man-

[1] My thanks are due to Dr. Kathleen Young and Dr. Henry E. King of Western Psychiatric Institute and Clinic, Pittsburgh, Pennsylvania and to Dr. Mortimer Garrison, Jr. of The Woods Schools, Langhorn, Pennsylvania, who read the manuscripts and made many valuable suggestions. I also acknowledge the helpful assistance of my wife, Mrs. Martha M. Clausen, in improving the language of the article.

[2] Now at the New York State Institute for Basic Research in Mental Retardation, Staten Island, New York.

AMERICAN JOURNAL OF MENTAL DEFICIENCY, 1967, Vol. 71., pp. 727-745.

kind. Prior to the period of the Renaissance, only the most severe forms of deficiency were recognized. Deficient individuals were variously treated as being "les enfants du bon Dieu," or were killed off as a burden on society. The first attempt at a definition seems to have been presented by Sir Anthony Fitz-Herbert in New Natura Brevium in 1534, and focused on the ability of a person to understand what is for his profit and what is for his loss. According to Nowrey (1945), a distinction between idiocy and insanity was first made by John Locke in 1690: "Herein seems to lie the difference between idiots and madmen, that madmen put wrong ideas together and reason from them, but idiots make very few or no propositions and reason scarce at all."

The first systematic study of a mentally deficient person was Itard's (1932) account of the *Wild Boy of Aveyron* found in 1798. A youth was found wandering in the woods and was turned over to Itard for training. Against the background of Rousseauian philosophy with its slogan of "return to nature," it was quite challenging to find a boy who had never left nature. Thus it was a concern with prevailing philosophical trends rather than a professed interest in idiots which sparked this historical event. Itard, who was a physician at the national institute for the deaf and dumb in Paris, approached the problem through the teaching methods which were being used for the deaf and dumb, the so-called physiological method. The objective of this method was to activate the nervous system by a carefully planned program of sensory stimulation, and of developing sensory discrimination through the education of each sensory modality separately. Great emphasis was put on the role of sensory experience in intellectual development.

The outcome of Itard's efforts with the "Wild Boy" was not spectacular, but the attempt resulted in an awakening of interest in idiots. In 1837 Seguin, a pupil of Itard's, opened a school for idiots in Paris using the physiological educational approach. The first asylum for idiots in England was established in 1840, due to the efforts of the philanthropist Andrew Reed. At about the same time Guggenbühl organized a training school for idiots in Switzerland. In Berlin, Saegert (1845) became interested in the education of idiots, and the first German state institution for the training of idiots was established in 1844, pioneered by Ettmüller.

By 1850, when Seguin left France for the USA where he became a moving force in the education of the mentally deficient, Samuel G. Howe—Director of the Perkins Institute for the Blind—had already used the physiological education approach in the training of blind idiots. A training school for idiots had been established in Massachusetts in 1848 by Hervey B. Wilbur. By 1876 twelve institutions, private or state, were in operation within this country. These institutions were not organized as permanent custodial institutions, but as training schools from which the trainees were to return to the community.

In the first phase of the mental deficiency movement idiocy was of primary concern. The term derives from a Greek word meaning persons who do not take part in public life, those who do not hold office. It did not, therefore, have the narrow connotation of present day usage. Through time, however, the meaning became severely restricted so that a need arose for a term applying to less handicapped individuals. A distinction between imbecility and idiocy in terms of severity of impairment was made in 1838 by Esquirol. The origin of the term imbecile is the Latin *imbecillis,* meaning weak, feeble, without strength.

In 1860 Duncan introduced the classification of simpletons. The simpletons were described as having ". . . nearly all the faculties to a certain degree, but indicate their alliance to the true idiot by their physiological deficiencies and general inertia of mind" (From Penrose, 1949, p. 6). Thus, since the beginning of the Nineteenth Century the field of mental deficiency has been characterized by a continuous expansion of the concepts.

Definitions:

The many definitions of mental deficiency which have been offered, reflect different concerns of their authors with respect to causes and/or manifestations: organic impairment, arrested development, social inadequacy, level of intelligence, and even cultural factors. Seguin (1866, p. 39) defined idiocy as ". . . a specific infirmity of the cranio-spinal axis, produced by deficiency of nutrition in utero and in neo-nati." He noted that nutritional deficiency in the first period of life had not been fully investigated, and he added the following comment to his definition: "It (idiocy) incapacitates mostly the functions which give rise to the reflex, instinctive, and conscious phenomena of life; consequently, the idiot moves, feels, understands, wills, but imperfectly; does nothing, thinks of nothing, cares for nothing (extreme cases), he is a minor, legally irresponsible; isolated, without associations; a soul shut up in imperfect organs, an innocent."

In the first comprehensive text-book on mental deficiency, *The Mental Affections of Children. Idiocy, Imbecility, and Insanity,* published in 1900 by Ireland, the following definitions were offered (p. 1) "Idiocy is mental deficiency, or extreme stupidity, depending upon malnutrition or disease of the nervous centers, occurring either before birth or before the evolution of the mental faculties in childhood. The word imbecility is generally used to denote a less decided degree of mental incapacity."

In the first edition of Tredgold's book *Mental Deficiency,* (1908, p. 2) mental deficiency or amentia, was defined as ". . . a state of mental defect from birth, or from an early age, due to incomplete cerebral development, in consequence of which the person affected is unable to perform his duties as a member of society in the position of life to which he is born." It is interesting to note that Tredgold, whose primary concern was with pathological and biological aspects of mental deficiency, used the consequences of organic impairment on social adaptability as the criterion of deficiency. Thus Tredgold, as well as Ireland, regarded mental deficiency as a behavioral manifestation of organic causes. Tredgold's text-book which has appeared in seven editions between the years of 1908 and 1947, has had most profound influence in the field.

Penrose (1949) obviously preferred a biological criterion. He stated (p. 35): "Instead of basing diagnosis of defect upon social incompetence, it is possible in some cases to use the criterion of physical diagnosis. Thus it is fairly safe to assume, without making any test of intelligence or of social adaptation, that a mongolian child, a microcephalic, a phenylketonuric, or an untreated cretin will be a potentially certifiable defective." While this is true in general, recent reports of phenylketonuric individuals with normal intelligence (Tischler et al., 1961) suggests the danger of pressing this argument too far. Penrose realized the difficulties of a biological criterion, and accepted as supplementary criteria social adaptation and level of intelligence. Jervis (1952) suggested that "mental deficiency may be defined, from a medical point of view, as a condition of arrested or incomplete mental development induced by disease or injury before adolescence or arising from genetic causes."

While there has been a continuous tradition of biological definitions of mental deficiency, other definitions have existed as well. Legal definitions have been prominent in England. In the USA, however, such definitions have seldom been referred to in the professional literature, although many states have legal definitions of mental deficiency, often established in relation to sterilization acts. In most British books which pertain to the subject, reference is regularly made to legal definitions, specifically to the work of the British Royal Commission of 1904 and 1957, and to the British Mental Deficiency Act of 1913 and 1927. The British Education Act of 1921 and 1944, and the Woods report of 1929 are reviewed. In the British Mental Deficiency Act of 1927 mental deficiency was defined as ". . . a condition of arrested or incomplete development of mind existing before the age of eighteen years, whether arising from inherent causes or induced by disease or injury" (From Clarke & Clarke, 1958, p. 45). Basically, this is a biological definition.

Tredgold, as mentioned above, was concerned primarily with biological aspects of mental deficiency, but felt compelled to define the concept in terms of social inadequacy. Many subsequent authors followed Tredgold's lead in using social adequacy as the criterion: e.g., Goddard (1914), Porteus (1921), Penrose (1949), and Wallin (1949). Doll (1941) was an advocate of multiple criteria for mental deficiency, and warned against a single criterion definition. According to Doll (1941), the complete concept of mental deficiency should include: 1. social incompetence, 2. mental incompetence, 3. deficiency of development, 4. constitutional origin, 5. duration to adulthood, and 6. essential incurability. One of Doll's prime achievements was the development of a social maturity scale which provides a quantitative measurement for the social adequacy dimension (1953).

Kuhlman (1941) defined mental deficiency as ". . . a mental condition resulting from a subnormal rate of development of some or all mental functions." He seemed to have preferred a definition in terms of social inadequacy, but observed that degree of inadequacy could be but roughly estimated for any given case. He suggested (1924) a compromise by drawing a line for degree of mental deficiency below which every case was regarded as deficient, irrespective of any other consideration. He suggested an IQ of 75 to be used as the critical value. The recent

official AAMD definition (Heber, 1961) also made reference to adaptive behavior: "Mental retardation refers to subaverage general intellectual functioning which originates during the developmental period and is associated with impairment in adaptative behavior." Subaverage intellectual functioning is further defined as less than one standard deviation below the population mean. This can be a very broad definition, depending upon whether one stresses intellectual functioning or adaptive behavior. The problem is further discussed below.

It was characteristic of the early period that mental deficiency was regarded as a result of organic factors—genetic factors or injury—manifesting themselves in an individual's inability to take care of, and provide for, himself. Different views were introduced by the development of other events. In 1907 Binet and Simon published their famous intelligence test. Soon afterwards it was translated into English and introduced into the USA by Goddard to be used in appraising mental development of the mentally deficient. Thus a tool was provided to quantify mental ability and to define mental deficiency in terms of MA or IQ.

Goddard's work on psychometric measures for deficients led to his introduction of the term moron for designating the high grade deficients. This contributed to a firm inclusion of such individuals in the overall concept, in accordance with Duncan's earlier suggestions. Goddard regarded the term moron to be identical with the term feebleminded as it was used in England. Whereas Tredgold was conspicuously silent regarding Goddard's work, he expressed the opinion that the term moron included the lowest stratum of what he called "dullards," whom he did not regard as being deficient.

Because of shortcomings of the testing technique, most of the authorities on mental deficiency have rejected a psychometric definition: Tredgold, Goddard, Porteus, Penrose, Doll, and Clarke & Clarke. Porteus (e.g.,

1933), a durable critic of traditional intelligence tests, criticized severely the use of IQ as criterion of mental deficiency, calling it *"reductio ad absurdum."* Among proponents for a psychometric definition of mental deficiency were Hollingworth and Wechsler. Hollingworth (1926, p. 40) stated: ". . . it will be apparent that the only entirely satisfactory practice would be to speak of [subnormal] individuals simply in terms of the IQ (intelligence quotient), without introducing words which convey the idea of a distinct entity." According to Wechsler (1958, p. 49), "The definition of mental deficiency in terms of attained mental age or IQ represented a marked step forward. . . ." Some of the definitions adopted by state legislatures are in terms of IQ. In clinical practice, the designation of mental deficiency seems to be made most often on a psychometric basis, in spite of the objections of the many authorities.

For the period between 1921 and 1944, the British Educational Act regarded as mentally defective children who could not benefit from education in ordinary public elementary schools. This was a strictly behavioral definition, as it did not relate the condition of mental deficiency to central nervous system impairment. Thus, for a while, two sets of criteria for mental deficiency were accepted: social inadequacy and educational failure.

The recognition of the importance of cultural and social factors for mental development, also has served to modify the original concept. While the primary consequence of these factors are for etiology, they also have significance for definition. One of the most consistent advocates for the importance of cultural and social factors is Sarason (1959). He stated (p. 21) that: "The relation between test scores and cultural background is often overlooked," and his distinction between mental retardation and mental deficiency is related to these factors. Boring (1965) recently argued emphatically for recognition of the social factors in mental deficiency. It seems

reasonable to believe that psychoanalysis, with its emphasis on consequences of early experience, on traumatic events, and on the potential of emotional conflicts for impairment of intellectual functions, has fostered certain attitudes toward mental deficiency. Adherents to the psychoanalytical school have traditionally emphasized experiential factors rather than biological ones. In assessing deficient subjects, they would be likely to look for external rather than organic causes. While this development is difficult to document, it seems likely that the psychoanalytical school has played a role in shaping opinions which were in opposition to those represented by Tredgold.

As the concept of mental deficiency became broader, the social problems connected with the condition became recognized, and the general attitude toward the condition changed. In the early part of the Nineteenth Century deficient individuals inspired pity; they appealed to people's sympathy. There was great optimism as to what idiots could do if only they were properly trained. It seems that the Wild Boy from Aveyron was received with considerable enthusiasm. Eventually the relationship between mental deficiency on the one side and poverty, insanity, criminality, and prostitution on the other was emphasized. The period between 1900 and 1946 has been referred to as the "alarmist period." The British Mental Deficiency Act of 1927 included a definition of moral defectives, as ". . . persons in whose case there exists mental defectiveness coupled with strongly vicious or criminal propensities and who require care, supervision, and control for the protection of others." (From Clarke & Clarke, 1958, p. 46). Goddard (1926) estimated that 25 to 50% of the prison population was mentally defective. In his book "The Kallikak Family" (1912), he stressed the relationship between mental deficiency and anti-social tendencies as well as their genetic mode of propagation. He saw dire consequences for society in that the deficients had a tendency to have more offspring than the responsible and the more intelligent part of the population. Goddard was a protagonist for sterilization as a measure to halt this development. Today, the problems involved here seem to be attacked more vigorously from the social side. In mental deficiency, as a field of investigation, no particular concern is now shown with regard to criminality. It may be that criminologists are more concerned with mental deficiency.

In a recent article Reed (1965) argued that the higher birthrate of people with low IQ is a statistical fallacy, resulting from the exclusion of childless married couples in the surveys. If these individuals be included, the high IQ section of the population has a slightly higher number of offsprings than has the low IQ section.

The Russian tradition in mental deficiency has differed from the West European and American. Luria may well be quoted as the most eloquent spokesman for the Russian school. He contended (1961) that academic failure is not an acceptable criterion for mental deficiency; that children may fail for various reasons: 1. *Educationally backward children* who may be intellectually normal, but may have adopted a negative attitude toward learning because of emotional conflicts or interruption of education due to illness. 2. *Astenic children* who have suffered from general infection or from malnutrition. These children are not defective, but because they become quickly exhausted, they need medical treatment and special curriculum in sanatorium schools. 3. *Children with partial defects,* e.g., slight loss of hearing, who may have developed a defect in language acquisition and as a consequence a defect in abstract thinking and intellectual processes. In contrast to these three categories are "the truly feebleminded children" who have suffered brain injury in the intrauterine period, period of delivery, or in the earliest years. The following subgroups are listed: 1. Those with residual or general brain disease resulting in

generally arrested development; 2. Those with neurodynamic disturbances—imbalanced individuals, some excitable and restless and some torpid and inhibited, and 3. Those with additional focal syndrome resulting in symptoms of acoustic, visual, or kinesthetic disability. The "truly feebleminded children" distinguish themselves from the others by certain psychophysiological characteristics which indicate impairment of the orienting reflex. Luria rejected a psychometric criterion since several children with the same IQ may belong to different categories and therefore require different treatment. In other words, he demanded that the diagnostic classification indicate the etiology and the treatment to be administered.

The psychophysiological investigations of Luria and the Russian school are extremely interesting, but the data available in translation do not completely document an objective system for differentiation of the various categories. It is most desirable that investigators in this country pursue the leads provided by the Russian scientists.

The orientations surveyed here are not always mutually exclusive, nor are they equal in their impact on the field. Through time there has been a shift in emphasis from the original position of exclusive consideration of organic factors (disease, injury, genetics) to recognition of cultural and social factors. All these orientations have become gradually more inclusive, resulting in an enlargement of the concept.

Rate of Incidence:

Parallel with the broadening of the definition, an increase in incidence rate is to be expected. According to Ireland (1900), surveys around 1890 with respect to the number of idiots in the population varied from 0.30% in the Canton of Bern to 0.04% in Sweden. A special inquiry in Denmark in 1888–89, supposed to have been more accurate than most such censuses, indicated 0.2% of idiots and imbeciles combined in the population. The first systematic attempt to obtain reliable data on incidence rate was that of the English Royal Commission of 1904. An aggregate population of 3,873,151 was surveyed and was found to embrace 0.023% idiots, 0.081% imbeciles, and 0.357% feeble-minded (morons); a total of 0.46% defectives. A ministerial commission in France in 1907 found ca. 1% of the population to be defective. In 1929 Lewis reported a survey of 622,880 people in England (The Wood Report) and found 0.86% defectives (0.04% idiots, 0.17% imbeciles, and 0.65% feebleminded [morons]). A Scotch survey of 1933 estimated the incidence rate to be between 1.5 and 3%, and a Swedish survey (Dahlberg, 1937) found that 3% of the boys and 1.7% of the girls required education in special classes. Estimates in various counties of England and Wales in 1951 varied from 0.040 to 0.579%.

Around the turn of the century the incidence rate of the feebleminded individuals in the USA was reported to be 0.15% although Fernald suggested 0.20% as a more correct estimate. In the various counties in the USA, surveys from 1915 to 1917 ranged from 0.340 to 0.735%. Goddard (1911) shocked the world by finding 3% of a school population to be feebleminded on the basis of Binet-Simon test scores. Apparently a psychometric criterion was used on this occasion. Terman (1919), also using psychometric criteria, estimated from 2 to 3% of school children to be deficient. Doll (1956) estimated 1% of the total population and 2% of school population to be deficient. In the recent survey in Onondaga County (New York State Department of Mental Hygiene, 1955), it was found: "One per cent of all children under 18 years of age were reported as retarded, measured by an intelligence quotient less than 75. . . . Including children known to have intelligence quotients greater than 75, a total of 3.5 per cent was referred to as 'possibly retarded.' " These figures pose the question of why only 1% of the population have IQs below 75 and why

individuals with IQs above 75 are referred to as retarded.

The Presidential Panel (1962) estimated 3% of the population to be in the deficient category, a figure as high as that given by Goddard in 1911. There is no statement, however, as to how this estimate was obtained. If one were to accept a psychometric definition using an IQ of 75 as the critical value, one would have 6.7% of the population classified as deficient. According to the official AAMD definition of 1961, the part of the population falling below 1 SD of the mean (15.9%), are potential candidates for a diagnosis of mental deficiency, to be further determined by whether or not they show impairment of adaptive behavior. It appears that nobody has yet made a population survey using this definition.

As pointed out by Tizard (1953), in addition to differences in definition, results of surveys often reflect the different techniques which have been used in the survey: psychometric studies, field studies, or followup investigations of individuals once diagnosed as subnormal.

Several studies (see Clarke & Clarke, 1958, p. 28; and Masland, Sarason, & Gladwin, 1959, p. 140) have found the 10-14 age group to have particularly high incidence rate. According to Penrose (1949, p. 20) this may be due to either the rigid standards of scholastic environment during the school years, the lack of standardized tests for adults, or higher mortality among the defectives. Differences also are found for various locations, particularly between urban and rural areas.

The recent estimates of incidence rate do not seem to be based on very solid data. Most of them are not results of population census or statistical criteria in terms of IQ. Usually it is difficult to determine which criteria have been used.

The present survey shows that there has been an increase in reported number of mentally deficient individuals. It is difficult, however, to ferret out the various contributing factors and to estimate their relative effect on the total number. At least the following factors must be considered: the expanding definition and the criteria used in surveys and estimates; increased alertness to the problem; improved diagnostic facilities; and differential practices of birth control—less used by defectives themselves or by culturally deprived individuals where probability for deficiency is enhanced.

Since social inadequacy has been advocated as the crucial issue in mental deficiency, it is conceivable that the broadening concept and the increase in incidence rate are related to social factors. To a large extent the changes in definition and incidence outlined above, have taken place in a period when industry was becoming more highly mechanized, when human rights were being more vigorously asserted, when society was beginning to show greater concern for those of its members who could not adequately take care of themselves, when education and literacy were becoming widespread, and when the democratic form of government was bestowing on the common man political responsibilities. These changes made living more complicated, and increased the demands made on the individual. Thus the changes in concept may reflect a stricter screening. It is also conceivable that the differences observed between Russia and the Western World, are related to differences in political systems; e.g., a more centrally controlled society may reduce discordance between a limited individual and a normal one by placement in school and occupation. Thus the problem of the higher grade defective may be de-emphasized.

While the relationship between mental deficiency and social-political factors seems obvious, it is a difficult problem to verify by concrete data. In the more than 50 years since Goddard's claim of an incidence rate of 3%, the figure has not increased, though the complexity of living conditions has certainly increased.

Degree of Deficiency:

Traditionally the mentally deficient population is subdivided according to degree, form, or clinical variety (or etiology). Each of these types of classification will be considered here in turn.

It was, of course, early recognized that there are different degrees of deficiency, which gave rise to differential terminology in the field. In keeping with English tradition, the British Mental Deficiency Act of 1927 defined the subcategories in terms of social adequacy. Idiots were defined as mental defectives ". . . of such a degree that they are unable to guard themselves against common physical dangers"; imbeciles as mental defectives ". . . so pronounced that they are incapable of managing themselves or their affairs, or, in the case of children, of being taught to do so"; and the feebleminded as having degree of deficiency ". . . so pronounced that they require care, supervision, and control for their own protection or for the protection of others, or, in the case of children, that they appear to be permanently incapable by reason of such defectiveness of receiving proper benefit from the instruction in ordinary schools" (Quoted from Tredgold, 1947, pp. 60–62).

In the USA the psychometric tradition prevailed. Goddard (1914) regarded social responsibility as the main criterion for mental deficiency, but felt that such responsibility should vary with the level of intelligence. Thus he accepted the classification adopted by the American Association for the Study of the Feebleminded. According to this, idiots were individuals having MAs below 2, imbeciles had MAs between 3 and 7, and morons had MAs between 7 and 12. The critical MAs were very soon translated into IQ terms, varying 5 or perhaps 10 points among the various authors. The following is a typical classification: idiots, IQ 0–25; imbeciles, IQ 25–50; morons, IQ 50–70. It is commonly estimated that about 5% of the mentally deficient are idiots, 20% imbeciles, and 75% morons.

Apparently as a reaction against the stigma felt to be associated with these terms, the Diagnostic and Statistical Manual of the American Psychiatric Association (1952) classified mental deficiency in terms of Mild, Moderate, and Severe; and the AAMD Manual (Heber, 1961) introduced four levels of subnormal intelligence: Profound, Severe, Moderate, and Mild; defined in terms of standard deviation units. Through measurement by standard intelligence tests, these categories were described in the Report of the Presidential Panel (1962) as follows: Profound, IQ below 20; Severe, IQ 20–35; Moderate, IQ 35–50; and Mild, IQ 50–70. These figures do not correspond to the definition of the Manual, since the mild category should extend to 1 SD below the mean, and a standard intelligence test does not have an SD of 30, but approximately half of this. It is interesting to note that there has been less objection to defining the degree of mental deficiency in terms of IQ than there has been in defining the total field.

A rather recently introduced subdivision is a distinction between trainable and educable mental deficients. The AAMD Manual estimated the IQ range for trainables to be between 25 or 30 and 50, and the range for educable to be between 50 and 70, 75, or 80. Again it is a subdivision of the condition in terms of intelligence scores. These terms have been more used among educators than among any other groups concerned with mental deficiency, but there seems to be general acceptance of their usage.

The general problem of subcategories according to level of intelligence is relatively uncomplicated. No assumptions are made other than those related to the normal distribution of IQ scores. One is here concerned with the lower extreme of the normal distribution curve, and a decreasing number of subjects are found as one moves away from the mean. No assumptions are made that the idiots are in all respects only quantitatively different from the morons. It is a matter of placing critical dividing points on a continuum, and it is understood that the subdivision is arbitrary. Thus the subdivision is a matter of convention rather than differentiation according to a specific criterion. As long as the conventions are adhered to, it does not particularly matter where the dividing lines are placed. Consistency in use is the most important consideration.

Sarason (1959) objected to this type of subdivision on the grounds that the use of a label tends to attribute to the subject all the characteristics that have been associated with the label. He said that calling a subject an imbecile does not give more information about the person than stating that his IQ is 30. While improper use of a label should be avoided, grouping of subjects often has practical advantages. Arbitrary subdivision of continua is constantly made by psychologists without serious problems.

Forms of Mental Deficiency:

For almost a century the mentally deficient have been subdivided in a dichotomic fashion. Such grouping would naturally be broad and indistinct. Originally (e.g., Tredgold) the resulting categories were referred to as etiological groups, but it seems more consistent with the modern use of this term to reserve etiology for categorizing according to diseases and dysfunctions which presumably provoked the condition, i.e., the more specific clinical categories.

In 1887 Down divided the defectives according to classes of causes, congenital and accidental. This scheme also was advocated in 1895 by Shuttleworth. Tredgold (1908) suggested the terms intrinsic and extrinsic, which are apparently synonymous with the phrases primary and secondary amentia that he later adopted. Primary amentia referred to any condition of the germ plasm which should result in imperfect development of the brain. Tredgold estimated that 80% of the defectives could be included in this category. Secondary amentia denoted prevention of full development of the brain by adverse factors of the environment, and embraced 20% of the deficient·population. Tredgold emphasized that this terminology was not identical with that of the congenital-acquired dichotomy, since environmental factors may be operating in utero, making a condition congenital, but not germinal in origin. Lewis (1933) introduced a modification of these schemes by a division into pathological and subcultural types. He designated all conditions of organic (or biological) origin as pathological, whether they resulted from injury or disease. Lewis assumed that pathological cases were exogenous in origin and accounted for the slight skewness toward the lower values found in the empirical distribution curves of IQ. The subcultural group included mentally deficient individuals where no organic factors were found. These were from the lower extreme of the normal distribution curve, and included the higher grade deficient subjects. Lewis assumed that genetic factors were responsible for the condition, although he recognized that environmental factors could also be of influence. Lewis' term subcultural is unfortunate since it can be interpreted as being synonymous with cultural deprivation. Penrose suggested that "physiological" would have been more appropriate.

Strauss and Lehtinen (1947) preferred to divide the deficient population into the categories of endogenous and exogenous. By exogenous defectives they understood cases who had received injury of the brain before, during, or after birth, and they assumed specific manifestations of the brain injury in terms of motor, perceptual, cognitive, and emotional behavior. By endogenous defectives, they understood cases where organic signs cannot be found, a category corresponding to Lewis' subcultural group. As synonymous with endogenous-exogenous the terms familial-organic have sometimes been used.

In 1952 Riggs and Rain presented a classification system which was organized along the organic-familial dimension. The merit of this attempt was to standardize the terms. They found that it was difficult to maintain the dichotomy because of the quality and the amount of information available. Six categories emerged: Organic, Familial, Mixed, Unclassified, Unknown, and Mongoloids. By including the last group they showed that their system was a mixture of a traditional dichotomic scheme and consideration of clinical categories.

Dichotomic subdivisions have existed for a long period·of time in mental deficiency. On the surface there is considerable similarity among these division schemes, but in actuality they reflect profound changes in concept. Gradually, the importance of social factors has gained increased recognition. Similarly, the proportion of mental deficients estimated to be genetically determined has been reduced from 80 to 29 per cent (Clarke & Clarke, 1958).

The justification for assuming that there are two different basic forms of mental deficiency may be questioned on two accounts: the differential symptomatology which makes such diagnostic division feasible; and the problem of consequent functional distinction between the groups of individuals assigned to the two categories. In the individual case it is often very difficult to decide whether genetic factors are present or whether social factors have been operating. In examining for injuries of the CNS there is always the possibility that more refined techniques than those employed may have revealed such injuries. Current practices of surveying a child's medical history in an attempt to find specific events, such as prolonged high temperature, with which to associate the deficient condition, is not very satisfactory. Particularly not since the same event may have occurred in the history of a normal child.

Experimental evidence of functional differences between classifications is far from conclusive. Werner and Strauss, (e.g., 1939, 1941, 1942) reported differences in performance level between endogenous and exogenous subjects for a number of tasks. Several investigators have failed to corroborate these findings (see Clausen, 1966a) and results from The Training School laboratory have not confirmed such differences when subjects were grouped according to Riggs and Rain's classification system. Even profiles of WAIS and PMA subscores do not seem to differ among subgroups (Clausen, 1965). Clarke (Clarke & Clarke, 1958, p. 63) has remarked that ". . . some of the psychological tests which Strauss regards as diagnostic of brain injury are not universally considered as of good validity." It should be noted that when Werner and Strauss compared endogenous and exogenous groups, they were comparing groups which initially were not equivalent but differed with respect to degree of deficiency. To compensate for this they selected subject groups with regard to IQ. In other words they selected the lowest section of the endogenous and the highest section of the exogenous groups. In this way they did not have representative samples of the groups they were comparing. It appears that they ignored the major differences in level between endogenous and exogenous in order to focus on minor and questionable differences in matched groups.

Graham et al. (1962) were not successful in differentiating traits resulting from brain injury or maladjustment.

An alternative to the dichotomic approach may be the emphasizing of the interaction between organic and social factors in deficients. In another article (Clausen, 1966c) the point has been argued that whereas mental deficiency may result from many different causes, these causes do not appear to make their specific stamp on the individual so that a characteristic structure of abilities evolves. One may rather assume that the same central mechanism (or mechanisms) which permeates practically all functions may be impaired in the mentally deficient—which impairment may be brought about by genetic factors, injury, disease, nutritional state, or cultural factors. Interaction between genetic and en-

vironmental factors in the etiology of mental deficiency has been suggested by several other authors (Clarke & Clarke, 1958; Sarason, 1959, p. 35; Spitz, 1965). A. D. B. Clarke (p. 85) said ". . . nowadays it is better realized that nature and nurture reciprocally interact and cannot be conceived of apart."

The point of view is promoted that a distinction of two basic forms of deficiency cannot be effected with sufficient precision and with sufficient support in experimental results to lend it purpose. This should not be construed to mean that attempts to differentiate deficient subjects is to be abandoned. Until such differentiation has been demonstrated, however, the use of a classification system which infers the establishment of this differentiation, serves little purpose.

Etiological Classification:

The use of etiology as a term for clinical categories, i.e., specific diseases causing or associated with the condition, has been preferred. New diseases have been continuously identified, again a story of expansion, from cretinism to homocystinuria. One cannot, however, relate all cases of mental deficiency to specific diseases or symptoms of diseases. As has been pointed out by O'Connor (1958, p. 25): "A clear diagnostic medical criterion is generally lacking."

The distinction between forms of mental deficiency and etiological classification was not made originally. Tredgold (1908) listed three clinical varieties under primary amentia: Simple, microcephalic, and mongolian which were supposed to include 80% of the deficient population, indicating frequent use of Simple Variety. The secondary amentia was subdivided into Disease of the brain and Defective nutrition of the brain. Under Disease of the brain he listed the following varieties: Epilepsy; Vascular, Toxic, or Inflammatory Impairment; Syphilis; and Infantile cerebral degeneration. Defective nutrition of the brain was related to Cretinism; to Amentia due to nutritional defect; and to Amentia due to isolation or sense deprivation. Essentially the same organization was maintained in the 7th edition of Tredgold's book (1947). The main difference was that the secondary amentia was subdivided into Traumatic, Infective, Degenerative, and Deprivative categories.

Several listings and groupings of diseases which are associated with mental deficiency have appeared in the literature (e.g., Masland, 1958). The most authoritative is the medical classification in the AAMD Manual (Heber, 1961). According to this system, there are eight groups of causes of mental deficiency: 1. Infection, 2. Intoxication, 3. Trauma or Physical agent, 4. Disorder of metabolism, growth or nutrition, 5. New growth, 6. Unknown prenatal influence, 7. Unknown or uncertain causes with structural reactions alone manifest, and 8. Uncertain (or presumed psychologic) cause with functional reactions alone manifest. With subcategories this classification includes a total of 90 items.

The AAMD classification is not a medical classification in the strict sense, since it includes the category of psychological causes which embraces cultural factors. For this reason we have preferred to refer to it as an etiological classification system.

The main developmental trend with regard to etiological factors is that we have learned to identify more diseases which are associated with mental deficiency. It is, however, not only a question of expanding the list but also a matter of modifying its internal composition. Whitney (1949) pointed out that since 1880 accidental factors have been reduced, birth injury has been reduced from 14–20% to 3–5%, and opium and diphtheria are no longer mentioned as etiological factors. On the other hand, encephalitis which was not mentioned in 1880, is today a common cause. Cretinism was the only endocrine condition recognized at that time, whereas today endocrine conditions account for more than 5% of all defective cases—with cretinism essentially out of the

picture. Although improved medical practices have reduced incidence rate of mental deficiency, this may be counterbalanced by new hazards. Pharmacological agents and radiation are some of the factors whose influence, with respect to mental deficiency, is difficult to assess at the moment.

There is no doubt that whenever possible the designation of mental deficiency should be supplemented with a medical diagnosis. It should be noted that—as was the case in assigning individuals to forms of deficiency—this is not always easy. Often the medical diagnosis has to be made on the basis of a medical history, rather than from signs which are present at the moment. Such histories are not always sufficiently accurate or complete for the purpose. Secondly, a great number of cases must be classified by exclusion rather than on the basis of positive evidence. Thus the AAMD classification system tends to accumulate a large number of subjects within the category of presumed psychological causes. While the significance of medical classification for medical treatment and theoretical orientation is beyond question, there is the further problem of the significance of such classification for the training program. This question does not appear to have been the subject of much discussion but there seems to be a tendency to assume that each category possesses a specific behavioral pattern, as Werner and Strauss claimed for the brain-injured. Actually, there are not much data available to substantiate this assumption. Doll (1946, p. 853) observed that "These clinical types may be thought of as more or less definite syndromes in the sense that they severally represent similarities of etiology, attributes, course, and treatment." He did not, however, discuss the attributes which characterize the various clinical types. In an earlier publication (Doll et al., 1932), Doll described some psychological characteristics of birth-injured children, but he did not attempt to differentiate these in characteristics from other clinical types. Investigations from this laboratory (Clausen, 1965, 1966a, 1966b, in preparation) were not successful in establishing relationships between etiology and ability pattern, either from the approach of comparing—for a variety of measures—etiological subgroups (Riggs & Rain's, as well as the AAMD classification system), or from the approach of subdividing, on the basis of ability patterns, a heterogeneous sample of deficients into homogeneous subgroups.

An observation of Doll (1946, p. 853) is important in this connection: "It should be noted, however, that the feeblemindedness itself may have a variable relationship to different clinical types. For example, while mental deficiency is assumed always to accompany mongolism or microcephaly, it only sometimes results from or is accompanied by birth lesion or hydrocephalus."

In the opinion of the present author, the primary diagnosis is mental deficiency, with medical diagnosis as a subscript when available information makes this feasible. This position should not be construed to indicate an underestimation of the importance of medical examination of the deficients, nor is it a rejection of the interaction between biological factors and behavioral manifestations. It is the author's opinion that the significance of research in mental deficiency centers around this relationship. At present, however, there is very limited information concerning it. A statement about etiology in mental deficiency is very often a speculative proposition. It does not indicate much about behavioral attributes of the individual and does not suggest much with respect to specific treatment or to training program. The point of view presented here is consistent with the position previously taken (Clausen, 1966a, 1966c) with respect to the impairment of a central function (or central functions) in a large section of the mentally deficient population.

The conclusion that etiological categories are not reflected in behavioral manifestation, has to be regarded as a preliminary one. It is one of the most crucial tasks of this field to accomplish differentiation of subgroups. The lack of success with the problem to date may result from insufficient precision of our measuring tools, from failure to include the behavioral characteristics which are significant in this respect, or from other shortcomings of approach. It is of utmost importance to continue to probe for behavioral differences between etiological categories. There is no point, however, in assuming differentiation which has not been demonstrated. There seems to be very limited knowledge as to the tailoring of treatment and training programs for etiological categories, hence it may be argued that the grouping serves no purpose. When it comes to drawing samples for research, however, it is essential to operate with as well defined groups as possible.

Terminology:

Parallel with the changes in concept has come a change in the meaning of some of the terms: Originally the term *familial* referred to cases with genetic factors. Doll (1946), for instance, used familial feeblemindedness as synonymous with primary amentia. In 1939 Strauss discussed the alternative explanations for familial deficients, genetic factors or social deprivation, thereby indicating the two different meanings of the word. Sarason (1959, p. 16) talked about familial-cultural factors. The AAMD Manual (Heber, 1961) defined familial as "Pertaining to a strong tendency to occur among more than one member of an affected family." A person's bias with respect to the nature-nurture controversy provides a rather free hand with this type of definition. It would appear that most psychologists today would associate familial with cultural-economic factors.

The terms mental deficiency and mental retardation have been used synonymously as well as in relationship to dichotomic grouping. The professional organization—the AAMD—both in the title of the organization and of its journal has used the term deficiency, and the official Manual defines deficiency as a synonym for retardation. The organizers of a symposium of the Association for Research in Nervous and Mental Disease (Kolb et al., 1962) and many others, have used the terms interchangeably. Sarason (1959) has argued for separate definitions: Mental deficiency would apply to cases where organic factors were found to be the cause of the condition; Mental retardation would be used for cases where organic signs are not present but where there is reason to believe that social factors are operating. The World Health Organization has adopted this distinction, as have many individuals, e.g., E. E. Doll (1962).

The lack of standard terminology is exemplified by the fact that within a single volume (Masland, Sarason, & Gladwin, 1958) Sarason and Gladwin distinguished between mental retardation and mental deficiency, while Masland used mental retardation as a generic term.

If the attempt to distinguish between major types of deficiency in a primary classification system should be abandoned, there would be no need to differentiate between mental deficiency and mental retardation. The question then arises as to which of the two phrases would best serve as a generic term for the field. Although not specifically stated, there are indications that retardation is preferred over deficiency because of less harsh implications. Retardation, however, may be rejected because it suggests a delay in development rather than in deficiency of attainment, implying that individuals so described will ultimately reach the level of the normals. Our own research (Clausen, 1966a) has shown that mentally deficient subjects in the IQ range of 50 to 75 at the age of 20–24 years, for a great variety of functions, do not reach the performance level of normal 8–10 year olds. Already in 1926, Hollingworth argued (p. 39) that " 'Backward' and 'retarded' vaguely and erroneously imply that the condition is one which will disappear with time . . ." True retardates—defined in terms of delayed development—are probably to be found among the so-called borderline cases or dull normals. They would only be distinguished from the deficients in retrospect. For these reasons a uniform description of the field by the term mental deficiency is advocated.

Discussion:

The lack of standard diagnostic practice in the field of mental deficiency was very evident in the handbook which the American Medical Association recently published for the primary physician (Gardner, Tarjan, & Richmond, 1965). The definition used in the handbook was Kidd's (1964) modification of the AAMD definition. This modification was offered by Kidd to make the formulation of the AAMD definition more specific while maintaining the underlying concepts. In the handbook (p. 1) it was stated that ". . . in most cases the physician can make no specific etiologic diagnosis," and that only between 10 and 25% of the retarded are likely to be identified first in the physician's office. The remaining 75–80%, however, are still claimed to be the concern of the primary physician. This, in spite of extremely vague diagnostic guidelines, leaves considerable latitude for personal preferences on the part of the practicing physician as to when the diagnosis should be applied.

Diagnostic entanglement is not a monopoly held by mental deficiency. It seems to exist more generally in the area of behavioral disorder. King (1965) made the following observation: "Under the pressure of practical need, and in the absence of either a systematic taxonomy of human behavior or adequate test methods that might serve as a basis for defining disordered states, what has grown up to fill the needs of most modern societies has been a system for identifying deviant behavior, and forming it into classes, that is based on mixed criteria of normality drawn in unequaled proportions from legal, medical, moral, social, and biologic sources."

The term diagnosis in relation to mental deficiency seems to have been used in two different meanings. The term has been used to denote the classification or recognition of a deficient state. This is a problem of defining a human condition which represents the extreme of a normal distribution. No natural distinctions exist, and the dividing line between the deficient and normal behavior has to be arbitrary, according to practical rather than scientific criteria. In this connection diagnosis is used in its original sense: apart + knowledge, to distinguish, to differentiate. It is this use of the term which is most relevant to a discussion of the concept of mental deficiency and which corresponds to a view of mental deficiency as a condition rather than a disease. Pertinent here is Clarke's (1957) remark that: "The concept of mental deficiency is thus not a scientific one, but rather social, legal and administrative." Subordinate to this broad use of the term, diagnosis is used in the more traditional medical sense: related to a disease where the concern is with the nature of the disease, its symptoms, and prognosis. Since only a fraction of the mentally deficient can be diagnosed in this way, the term should preferably be used with a prefix such as medical diagnosis, clinical diagnosis, differential diagnosis, etc., as the case may be. It seems that a considerable amount of confusion may be avoided by distinguishing between the two levels of diagnosis, and it may even be that such distinction is applicable for other areas of behavioral disorder.

It has frequently been stated that mental deficiency should be considered a condition rather than a disease. This being the case, the condition is one of mental deficit. Even when formulating a definition from a medical point of view, Jervis (1952) used the phrase "arrested or incomplete mental development."

If mental deficiency is to be considered as a uniform field, it is necessary to find a common denominator for all individuals classified as deficient. At the present stage of knowledge, it seems that in intellectual functioning alone has this common element been in any way approached. The mental deficit must be of sufficient degree to interfere with a person's educational progress, adaptation to social norms, establishment of interpersonal relationships, and to employability (ability to support himself). The diagnosis, therefore, is made on the basis of behavioral rather than pathologic observation. Traditionally these deficiencies have been subsumed under the term social incompetence. We are not, however, concerned with social incompetence as such. Social incompetence may result from a variety of reasons: neurotic behavior, psychotic involvement, crippling diseases, etc. The essential concern is a social incompetence caused by intellectual deficit. It would be a well defined field if only the amount of intellectual deficit and degree of social competency could be objectively assessed. Unfortunately, as has been pointed out by many authors, (e.g., Clarke & Clarke, 1958; Penrose, 1949; Sarason, 1959) social competency is an elusive concept which varies with time, location, and social strata. Doll's Social Maturity Scale notwithstanding, social adequacy is a very difficult dimension to handle for diagnostic purposes. Standard intelligence scales may be the best predictors of whether social inadequacy is likely to occur on the basis of intellectual deficit. The measurement of mental ability, the unique contribution of psychology, may well be the most adequate instrument in defining mental deficiency. The objections against a psychometric definition of mental deficiency have been that such scales lack in validity, that they may be heavily influenced by social factors, and that they are not infallible predictors of future development. With respect to validity, the intelligence scales are probably the best tool available—as compared to subjective estimate of development potential, or judgment of social inadequacy, which by necessity must vary with examiner and circumstances. Sarason

(1959) has very forcefully argued the importance of social factors in test performance, a point which can hardly be rejected. The primary concern in the diagnosis of mental deficiency, however, may be regarded to be the functional level of the individual at the moment, rather than etiology. It is the existing condition which determines whether or not an individual should receive special treatment or special training. Whether this results from genetic factors, from CNS damage, or home condition is of secondary importance. These factors would probably be more closely related to prognosis.

If a psychometric definition of mental deficiency should be adopted, this would perhaps require some modification of the present assumptions about the IQ concept. One might have to relax the traditional rigidity as to the constancy of the IQ. Doll (1946) has already argued that IQ does not have the same constancy in deficients as in normals, because of a different rate of development. One might have to be somewhat more guarded with respect to prediction, but should be able to avoid gross errors by annual re-examinations, at least during the critical years. One of Sarason's (1959, p. 1) arguments against a psychometric definition of mental deficiency is: "The child with an I.Q. of 68 or 69 is automatically labeled mentally defective and then takes on *in the thinking of the clinician* all the characteristics that have been associated with the label. In other words, the child takes on the characteristics of the class or category of mentally defective individuals not because these characteristics were observed but because he has been labeled." If there are logical reasons for a psychometric definition, then rigidity of the examiners cannot be a valid argument. Rather one should go to work on the training of the clinicians. Opposition to a psychometric definition by psychologists may lessen when more facts about behavioral characteristics of the deficients become available. Studies from this laboratory (Clausen, 1966a)

showed that the mean score of 50 variables (sensory, motor, perceptual, and complex mental tasks) has a high correlation with IQ in mental deficients, higher than in normals. We have found, in other words, that IQ is a reasonable predictor of a general ability level and it seems justifiable to assume that scholastic achievement and employability are related to this general ability level.

The latest official American definition—presented in the AAMD manual—includes the two phrases "general intellectual functioning" and "impairment in adaptive behavior." Instruments for obtaining measures of general intellectual functioning are readily available. Adaptive behavior, however, is ill defined; guidelines are poor; and for all practical purposes one is still limited to a subjective evaluation of "social adequacy." It seems that only the name, rather than the content, has changed in comparison to previous definitions. Under such circumstances it seems likely that the clinicians ignore the adaptive behavior and make their diagnoses on the basis of the general intellectual functioning alone. Thus the acceptance of a psychometric definition of mental deficiency may simply mean the legalizing of widespread current practices.

The term "general intellectual functioning" has been used in the same sense as it was used in the AAMD definition. There may be some question as to how the level of such general intellectual functioning is best determined, either by IQ alone or supplemented by other measures of abilities. The former has the advantage of the single measure's certitude but relatively narrow base, while the latter is broader based, but presents the problem of combining scores. This, however, may be regarded as a practical problem of secondary importance relative to the question as to the type of criterion which should be adopted.

The adoption of a psychometric criterion will not solve all diagnostic problems. It will still be necessary to exercise clinical judgment, even if the objective is to reduce judgment to a minimum.

If a psychometric definition of mental deficiency is accepted, it becomes a question as to the critical point for distinguishing mental deficients from normals. This is a crucial question, because it is the borderline case which poses the most serious problem for diagnosis. A low-IQ individual will be diagnosed mentally deficient regardless of what definition is used—because there is a relationship between intellectual capacity and social adequacy, and because of a relationship between low intellectual capacity and known pathology. With regard to intellectual functioning the AAMD Manual recommends 1 SD below the mean. This seems to be a very liberal definition, as it potentially includes ⅙ of the total population within the category of mental deficiency. It would appear that when a person with an IQ of 85 (about 1 SD below the mean, corresponding to the AAMD Manual definition) shows impairment of adaptive behavior, the maladaption is caused by factors other than intellectual, and the person should therefore not be classified as mentally deficient. Garfield and Wittson (1960) have also made some critical comments to the AAMD definition on the grounds that it is too inclusive. It is the opinion of the present writer that the traditional cut-off point of 70 or 75—corresponding to about 2 SD below the mean—is more adequate on the grounds that it is primarily below this level that individuals show impairment of adaptive behavior, caused by low level of general intellectual functioning.

The placement of the dividing line between mental deficiency and normalcy has important practical consequences as it determines which per cent of the population would fall in the deficient category. Also, the broader the definition, the more emphasis has to be put on treatment factors such as environmental manipulations in the form of special schooling, training, and occupational selection. It is the borderline cases which have the greater chance to learn to be more self sufficient in terms of social standards, if maximum utilization of their potentials is achieved.

The population selected on the basis of a psychometric criterion would presumably differ from that selected on the basis of criteria such as Doll's, since he used a more specific and a more restrictive definition. It may well be that the difference is not as great as one might have expected. It would be interesting to determine the amount of overlap when two such criteria were employed—separately for various IQ levels.

A psychometric definition as recommended here comes close to what Luria (1961), accuses an American definition of being. While Luria's work demands respect and admiration, it must be observed that the Russian definition of oligophrenia is much narrower than any current American definition of mental deficiency. In demanding demonstrable impairment of CNS, it includes only a portion of what would in this country be considered as organics. Luria has primarily scorned the psychometric criterion for mental deficiency since it might include subnormal functioning caused by sensory impairment. One may counter that in the USA sensory impairment should be recognized as such by routine screening, at least at kindergarten age. If, however, this has not been the case, and if this neglect has resulted in interference with intellectual development, such children may be regarded as deficient on the basis of their functioning level at the moment. The effect of the sensory deprivation is essentially the same as the effect of genetic, metabolic, traumatic, cultural, etc. factors. That the treatment would consist of corrective devices for the sensory functioning is another question.

In summary: A psychometric definition of mental deficiency is proposed in that other criteria seem insufficient, lack precision, and evade definition. This definition stresses the functional level of the individual at the moment, and therefore loses something with regard to prediction. The psychological aspects of mental deficiency—emphasizing a condition rather than a disease—become the paramount content of the concept. To this diagnosis should be added an indication of severity of deficiency and—whenever possible —a subscript of etiology, particularly indicating the medical or biological factors which seem to have led to the condition.

The proposed definition does not entail an abrupt change in orientation, but purports to be more in conformity with reality. It discards some refinements which do not seem to be supported by present knowledge. There is no particular satisfaction in getting rid of these refinements, and the increased heterogeniety that it may introduce in the deficient population is decidedly not an advantage. It seems, however, to better reflect our position at the moment. The present situation demands intensive work on causative factors in mental deficiency, on the establishment of solid facts regarding behavioral characteristics of the mentally deficient, and regarding the relationship between biological factors and their behavioral manifestations.

N.Y.S. Institute for Basic Research
in Mental Retardation
Forest Hill Road
Staten Island, New York 10314

REFERENCES

Barr, M. W. *Mental defectives, their history, treatment and training.* Philadelphia: Blakiston, 1904.

Binet, A., & Simon, T. *The development of intelligence in children.* English translation by Elizabeth S. Kite. Baltimore: Williams & Wilkins, 1916.

Boring, E. G. The classes of stupidity. Review of Stevens and Heber: Mental retardation. A review of research. *Scient. Amer.,* 1965, 213, 113–119.

Clarke, A. D. B. The social adjustment of the mentally deficient. I. Recent English research. *Amer. J. ment. Defic.,* 1957, 62, 295–299.

Clarke, A. M., & Clarke, A. D. B. *Mental deficiency. The changing outlook.* Glencoe, Ill.: The Free Press, 1958.

Clausen, J. PMA subscores in retardates and normals: pattern, scatter, correlations, and relation to etiology. *Amer. J. ment. Defic.,* 1965, 70, 232–247.

Clausen, J. *Ability structure and subgroups in mental retardation.* Washington, D. C.: Spartan, 1966. (a)

Clausen, J. Threshold for pure tone and speech in retardates. *Amer. J. ment. Defic.,* 1966, 70, 556–562. (b)

Clausen, J. Assessment of behavioral characteristics in mental retardates. Paper presented at Amer. Assoc. Psychopath. Convention, New York, Feb. 18–20, 1966. (c)

Clausen, J. Performance level in relation to EEG, neurological, and etiological subcategories. Manuscript, in preparation.

Committee on nomenclature and statistics of the American Psychiatric Association. *Diagnostic and statistical manual.* Mental Disorders. Washington, D. C.: Amer. Psychiat. Assoc., 1952.

Dahlberg, G. On the frequency of mental deficiency. *Uppsala Läkareförenings Förhandlingar,* 1937, 5, 439–443.

Doll, E. A. The essentials of an inclusive concept of mental deficiency. *Amer. J. ment. Defic.,* 1941, 46, 214–219.

Doll, E. A. The feeble-minded child. In L. Carmichael (ed.), *Manual of child psychology.* New York: John Wiley, 1946. Pp. 845–885.

Doll, E. A. *The measurement of social competence.* Philadelphia: Educational Test Bureau, 1953.

Doll, E. A. Mental Deficiency. *Encyclopaedia Britannica,* 1956, 15, 257–260.

Doll, E. A., Phelps, W. M., & Melcher, R. T. *Mental deficiency due to birth injuries.* New York: Macmillan, 1932.

Doll, E. E. A historical survey of research and management of mental retardation in the United States. In E. P. Trapp & P. Himelstein (eds.), *Readings on the exceptional child.* New York: Appleton-Century-Crofts, 1962. Pp. 21–68.

Down, J. L. *Mental afflictions of childhood and youth.* London: Churchill, 1887.

Duncan, P. M. *First report of the Eastern Counties' Asylum for Idiots and Imbeciles.* Colchester: Essex and West Suffolk Gazette, 1860.

Gardner, G. E., Tarjan, G., & Richmond, J. B. *Mental retardation. A handbook for the primary physician.* Chicago: Amer. Med. Assoc., 1965.

Garfield, S. L., & Wittson, C. Some reactions to the revised "Manual on terminology and classification in mental retardation." *Amer. J. ment. Defic.,* 1960, 64, 951–953.

Goddard, H. H. Two thousand normal children measured by the Binet measuring scale of intelligence. *Ped. Sem.,* 1911, 18, 231–258.

Goddard, H. H. *The Kallikak family.* New York: Macmillan, 1912.

Goddard, H. H. *Feeble-mindedness, its causes and consequences.* New York: Macmillan, 1914.

Graham, F. K., Ernhart, C. B., Thurston, D., & Craft, M. Development three years after perinatal anoxia and other potentially damaging new born experiences. *Psychol. Monogr.,* 1962, 76, (3, Whole No. 522).

Heber, R. A manual on terminology and classification in mental retardation. *Amer. J. ment. Defic.* Monogr. Suppl. (Second ed.) 1961.

Hollingworth, L. S. *The psychology of subnormal children.* New York: Macmillan, 1926.

Ireland, W. W. *The mental affections of children. Idiocy, imbecility, and insanity.* Philadelphia: Blakiston, 1900.

Itard, J. M. G. *The wild boy of Aveyron* (Trans. by G. and M. Humphrey). New York: Appleton-Century, 1932.

Jervis, G. A. Medical aspects of mental deficiency. *Amer. J. ment. Defic.,* 1952, 57, 175–188.

Kidd, J. W. Toward a more precise definition of mental retardation. *Ment. Retard.,* 1964, 2, 209–212.

King, H. E. Psychomotor changes with age, psychopathology and brain damage. In A. T. Welford & J. E. Birren (eds.) *Behavior, aging and the nervous system.* Springfield, Ill.: Charles C Thomas, 1965. Pp. 476–525.

Kolb, L. C., Masland, R. L., & Cooke, R. E. *Mental retardation.* Res. Publ. Assoc. nerv. ment. Dis., Volume 39. Baltimore: Williams & Wilkins, 1962.

Kuhlman, F. Mental deficiency, feeble-mindedness, and defective delinquency. *Amer. Assoc. Study Feebleminded,* 1924, 29, 58–70.

Kuhlman, F. Definition of mental deficiency. *Amer. J. ment. Defic.,* 1941, 46, 206–213.

Lewis, E. O. *Report on an investigation into the incidence of mental defect in six areas, 1925–1927.* Report of the Mental Deficiency Committee, Part IV. London: H. M. Stationary Office, 1929.

Lewis, E. O. Types of mental deficiency and their social significance. *J. ment. Sci.,* 1933, 79, 298–304.

Luria, A. R. An objective approach to the study of the abnormal child. *Amer. J. Orthopsychiat.,* 1961, 31, 1–16.

Masland, R. L., Sarason, S. B., & Gladwin, T. *Mental subnormality.* New York: Basic Books, 1958.

Milligan, G. E. History of the American Association on Mental Deficiency. *Amer. J. ment. Defic.,* 1961, 66, 357–369.

New York State Department of Mental Hygiene, Mental Health Research Unit. Technical Report: *A special census of suspected-referred mental retardation,* Onondaga County, N. Y. Syracuse, N. Y., 1955.

Nowrey, J. E. A brief synopsis of mental deficiency. *Amer. J. ment. Defic.,* 1945, 49, 319–357.

O'Connor, N. O. The prevalence of mental defect. In A. M. Clarke & A. D. B. Clarke (eds.) *Mental deficiency. The changing outlook.* Glencoe, Ill.: The Free Press, 1958. Pp. 21–39.

Penrose, L. S. *The biology of mental defect.* New York: Grune & Stratton, 1949.

Porteus, S. D. A new definition of feeble-mindedness. In *Recent studies from the Vineland Laboratory.* Vineland, N. J.: The Training School, 1921. Pp. 1–4.

Porteus, S. D. *The Maze Test and mental differences.* Vineland, N. J.: Smith Publishing House, 1933.

President's Panel on Mental Retardation. *A proposed program for national action to combat mental retardation.* Washington, D. C.: U. S. Government Printing Office, 1962.

Reed, S. C. The evolution of human intelligence. *Amer. Scientist,* 1965, 53, 317–326.

Riggs, M. M. & Cassel, M. E. A classification system for the mentally retarded, Part II: Reliability, *Trng. Sch. Bull.,* 1952, 49, 151–168.

Riggs, M. M. & Rain, M. E. A classification system for the mentally retarded, Part I: Description. *Trng. Sch. Bull.,* 1952, 49, 75–84.

Saegert, K. W. *Über die Heilung der Blödsinningen auf intellektuellem Wege.* Berlin: Schröder, 1845/46.

Sarason, S. B. Psychological problems in mental deficiency (3rd ed.). New York: Harper, 1959.

Seguin, E. *Idiocy and its treatment by the physiological method.* New York: William Wood, 1866.

Shuttleworth, G. E. *Mentally deficient children: Their treatment and training.* London: H. K. Lewis, 1895.

Spitz, H. H. The age of alchemy. *Ment. Retard.,* 1965, 3, 26–27.

Strauss, A. A. Typology in mental deficiency. *Proc. Amer. Assoc. ment. Defic.,* 1939, 44, 85–90.

Strauss, A. A. & Lehtinen, L. E. *Psychopathology and education of the brain-injured child.* New York: Grune & Stratton, 1947.

Strauss, A. A. & Werner, H. The mental organization of the brain-injured mentally defective child. *Amer. J. Psychiat.,* 1941, 97, 1194–1203.

Strauss, A. A., & Werner, H. Disorders of conceptual thinking in the brain-injured child. *J. nerv. ment. Dis.,* 1942, 96, 153–172.

Terman, L. M. *The intelligence of school children.* Boston: Houghton Mifflin, 1919.

Tischer, B., Gibson, W. C., McGeer, E. G., & Nuttall, J. Degrees of mental retardation in phenylketonuria. *Amer. J. ment. Defic.,* 1961, 65, 726–738.

Tizard, J. The prevalence of mental subnormality. *Bull. World Hlth. Org.,* 1953, 9, 423–440.

Tredgold, A. F. *Mental deficiency.* London: Bailliera. Tindall, & Fox, 1908, First ed. New York: William Wood, 1914, Second ed. Baltimore: Williams & Wilkins, 1947, Seventh ed.

Wallin, J. E. W. *Children with mental and physical handicaps.* New York: Prentice-Hall, 1949.

Wechsler, D. *The measurement and appraisal of adult intelligence.* Baltimore: Williams & Wilkins, 1958.

Werner, H. & Strauss, A. A. Types of visuo-motor activity in their relation to low and high performance ages. *Proc. Amer. Assoc. ment. Defic.,* 1939, 44, 163–168.

Werner, H., & Strauss, A. A. Pathology of figure-background relation in the child. *J. abnorm. soc. Psychol.,* 1941, 36, 236–248.

Whitney, E. A. Mental deficiency in the 1880's and 1940's. *Amer. J. ment. Defic.,* 1949, 54, 151–154.

Whitney, E. A. Some stalwarts of the past. *Amer. J. ment. Defic.,* 1953, 57, 345–360.

DNA (Cell Number) and Protein in Neonatal Brain: Alteration by Maternal Dietary Protein Restriction

Stephen Zamenhof

Edith van Marthens

Frank L. Margolis

The effects of malnutrition on development have been extensively studied. For brain, such studies were concerned mainly with the effects on weight or size (*1, 2*), which, however, depend on factors (such as lipids, water content) that do not reflect the number of brain cells. Winick and Noble (*3*) and Dickerson *et al.* (*4*) investigated the effect of malnutrition after birth on the DNA content of the brain. If the malnutrition occurred from birth to weaning, the animals (rats, pigs) exhibited a permanent brain DNA deficiency. The influence of malnutrition on learning behavior of rats has also been studied (*5, 6*). Many investigators have implied that protein deprivation before and after birth results in mental impairment in children (for reviews see *7*).

For the understanding of this influence of malnutrition on behavior, the study of changes in the number of brain cells is of interest. Whereas, in the rat the number of glial cells and the total number of brain cells increases for some time after birth (*8, 9*), the number of neurons does not increase (*8, 10, 11*), with the possible exception of short-axoned neurons (*11*). Thus, we studied the effect of maternal malnutrition before and during gestation, on the amount of brain DNA (brain cell number) in newborn animals.

Our report is a continuation of previous studies (*12, 13*) of factors influencing the amount of DNA in the brain, which reflects the number of brain cells because the DNA content of a diploid cell of a given species is constant; our

SCIENCE, 1968, Vol. 160., pp. 322-323

eventual purpose is the elucidation of the relation between alterations in brain cell number and behavior.

We used albino rats derived from the Sprague-Dawley strain; these rats have been bred in our laboratory for at least ten generations; the females were virgin, 3 months old, and weighed 200 to 260 g. The animals were maintained (i) on powdered diets containing either 8 percent or 27 percent protein (14) by a pair-feeding schedule (intake 16 g/day); or (ii) another group was maintained on pelleted diet (15) as desired (16 g/day). The protein was casein. Both protein diets contained the same amounts of fats (10 percent) and salts (4 percent). In addition, the 8 percent protein diet contained 78 percent starch, and the 27 percent protein diet contained 59 percent starch. To both diets, 2.2 percent of Vitamin Diet Fortification Mixture in Dextrose (14) was added to a week's supply. The females were kept on these diets for 1 month before mating and throughout gestation. The restriction was such as to still permit full-term gestation (16) and normal number in litter.

The newborns were weighed, and then killed by decapitation, within 6 hours of delivery. The brains (cerebral hemispheres) were immediately removed without cerebellum and olfactory lobes (13) and weighed; they were then frozen and subsequently used for the analysis. DNA was determined by a modification of diphenylamine colorimetric method (12, 17), and protein was determined by a modification of Folin colorimetric method (18).

The results (Table 1) show first that the rats on two different full diets exhibited differences in body and brain weights, but the total amount of DNA [and therefore total brain cell number (19)] was the same. Thus, cell number is a more constant indicator; the brain weight cannot be used as a measure of brain cell number.

As expected (2, 6), dietary protein restriction of the mother resulted in considerably (30 percent) lower body weights of the newborn offspring; however, in contrast to previous experiments (2), in which the dietary restriction was during gestation only, in our experiments in which the restriction was also imposed 1 month before mating, the brain weights were also considerably

Table 1. The effect of restriction of maternal dietary protein on weight and content of brain of newborns. Diet A, full pellet; B, full diet, containing 27 percent protein; C, restricted containing 8 percent protein.

| Diet | Number of animals | | Offspring weights (g) | | Brain content of offspring | |
	Mothers	Off-spring	Body	Brain*	DNA (μg)	Protein (mg)
A	5	41	5.7 ± 0.4	0.159 ± 0.071	544 ± 20	
B	4	32	6.38 ± .4	.181 ± .014	546 ± 22	9.29 ± 0.43
C	4	31	4.46 ± .22	.139 ± .081	491 ± 29	7.45 ± .57
		Decrease† (%)				
			30	23	10	19.8
		Probability				
			P<.001	P<.001	P<.001	P<.001

* Cerebral hemispheres, without cerebellum and olfactory lobes.   † Difference between 27 percent and 8 percent protein groups.

* ± standard deviation

(23 percent) lower. This decrease is reflected in comparable percentage decrease in total protein content. All these changes are statistically significant.

The restriction also resulted in a significantly lower (10 percent) DNA content, that is, significantly lower total brain cell number. However, this difference is less pronounced than the difference in brain weight which again indicates that the latter cannot be used as a measure of the former.

Since at birth the brain cells are reported to be predominantly neurons [8], it is likely that the decrease has indeed affected the number of neurons. Since, as discussed above, the neurons essentially do not divide any more after birth, any neuron deficiency at birth may persist throughout the life of the animal. Such deficiency may contribute to the impaired behavior of the offspring of protein-deficient mothers that has been reported in the literature.

The change in protein content, twice as large as that in DNA, indicates that not only the number of cells was altered but also the cells are qualitatively different. Whether these qualitative changes are irreversible or whether they merely represent a delay in maturation is still not known. However, when evaluated at 3 months of age, the experimental animals manifested abnormalities of gait and response to environmental stimuli.

STEPHEN ZAMENHOF
EDITH VAN MARTHENS
FRANK L. MARGOLIS
Department of Medical Microbiology and Immunology and
Department of Biological Chemistry, University of California School of Medicine, Los Angeles 90024

References and Notes

1. P. Gruenwald, *Biol. Neonatorum* **5**, 215 (1963); R. E. Brown, *Develop. Med. Child Neurol.* **8**, 512 (1966).
2. F. J. Zeman, *J. Nutr.* **93**, 167 (1967).
3. M. Winick and A. Noble, *ibid.* **89**, 300 (1966); **91**, 179 (1967).
4. J. W. T. Dickerson, J. Dobbing, R. A. McCance, *Proc. Roy. Soc. London, Ser. B* **166**, 396 (1967).
5. R. M. Barnes, S. R. Cunnold, R. R. Zimmerman, H. Simmons, R. B. McLeod, L. Krook, *J. Nutr.* **89**, 399 (1966).
6. D. F. Caldwell and J. A. Churchill, *J. Neurol.* **17**, 95 (1967).
7. R. Barnes, *Fed. Proc.* **26**, 144 (1967); D. Baird, *ibid.*, p. 134.
8. K. R. Brizee, J. Vogt, X. Kharetchko, *Progr. Brain Res.* **4**, 136 (1963).
9. M. Winick and A. Noble, *Develop. Biol.* **12**, 451 (1965).
10. J. B. Angevine and R. L. Sidman, *Nature* **192**, 766 (1961); M. Berry, A. W. Rogers, J. T. Eayrs, *ibid.* **203**, 591 (1964).
11. J. Altman and G. D. Das, *J. Comp. Neurol.* **126**, 337 (1966).
12. S. Zamenhof, H. Bursztyn, K. Rich, P. J. Zamenhof, *J. Neurochem.* **11**, 505 (1964).
13. S. Zamenhof, J. Mosley, E. Schuller, *Science* **152**, 1396 (1966).
14. Nutritional Biochemicals, Cleveland, Ohio.
15. Wayne Mousebreeder Block, Allied Mills, Chicago, Ill.
16. J. W. Millen, *The Nutritional Basis for Reproduction* (Thomas, Springfield, Ill., 1962).
17. F. L. Margolis, in preparation. The current absolute values of DNA are higher than those reported in reference (*13*) due to an improved extraction procedure.
18. O. H. Lowry, N. J. Rosebrough, A. L. Farr, R. J. Randall, *J. Biol. Chem.* **193**, 265 (1951).
19. From the DNA values per brain, the numbers of total brain cells could be calculated by dividing by a (constant) DNA content per cell (6×10^{-6} μg), on the basis of evidence that the cells in cerebral hemispheres are essentially diploid.
20. Supported by NIH grant HD-01909 and American Cancer Society grant E-474.

CHILDHOOD

LEAD POISONING. .

an eradicable disease

JANE S. LIN-FU

In the history of modern medicine, few child-hood diseases occupy a position as unique as lead poisoning. It is a preventable disease. The etiology, pathogenesis, epidemiology, and symptomatology have all been well defined. Methods for screening, diagnosis, and treatment have long been available. In the past three decades, concerted efforts to conquer infectious diseases have resulted in the development of vaccines for such viral diseases as polio and measles, the discovery of many antibiotics for bacterial and other infections, and the systematic application of these therapeutic agents, but little has been done to eradicate lead poisoning. Yet this man-made disease exists in epidemic proportions in many cities.

While mortality and morbidity associated with such diseases as polio, tuberculosis, meningitis, and pneumonia have declined sharply, lead poisoning has continued to take a high toll among children. Silently, almost unnoticed, it causes the needless death of many children and leaves many more with mental retardation, cerebral palsy, convulsive seizures, blindness, learning defects, behavior disorders, kidney diseases, and other handicaps.

Lead poisoning, or plumbism, is largely an occupational disease in adults. But in children it is almost invariably caused by repeated ingestion of chips and flakes of lead-containing paint and plaster from the walls, windowsills, and woodwork of dilapidated pre-World War II houses. Because of its roots in dilapi-

CHILDREN, 1970, Vol. 17. No. 1., pp. 2-9.

dated housing in old urban neighborhoods, it has a high incidence only among children living in city slums. In these areas, accessibility to flaking and peeling lead paint and broken plaster, lack of knowledge among parents that ingestion of lead paint is dangerous and even lethal, frequent inadequate parental supervision of young children, and a high incidence of pica (a perverted appetite for nonfood items such as dirt, paper, paint, and plaster) all set the stage for lead poisoning.

Children between 1 and 6 years old are the main victims, and those between 1 and 3 years of age comprise 85 to 90 percent of the cases. Boys and girls are affected equally. A high incidence is reported among Negroes and Puerto Ricans, probably because such a large proportion of these ethnic groups live in "lead belts." Lead poisoning occurs the year round, but lead encephalopathy (brain injury caused by lead), a very serious complication, is much more frequent during the summer. Some cases occur in winter when leaded battery casings are burned for fuel and the fumes are inhaled or there is prolonged contact with the ashes.

Nobody knows how many children in the United States are exposed to this health hazard and how many are actually poisoned, for many cases of lead poisoning are never diagnosed. But since the problem is closely related to poor housing conditions, an educated guess may be made on the basis of the number of old deteriorating houses in the United States and the known prevalence rate of lead poisoning among children living in such houses. According to the 1960 Housing Census, 30.6 million of the occupied housing units in the United States were built in or before 1939, when lead paint was still commonly used for interiors. Of these units, 5.6 million were classified as deteriorating and 1.8 million as dilapidated.

Although since the 1940's lead pigment has been replaced by titanium in interior paints, recent surveys in Baltimore, Philadelphia, and Minneapolis revealed that from 40 to over 80 percent of houses in selected slum areas still contain dangerous quantities of flaking lead paint that was applied many years ago. Surveys have indicated that among children living in such dwellings from 10 to 25 percent of those between 1 and 6 years of age have absorbed potentially dangerous quantities of lead, although clinical symptoms of lead poisoning have been present in only 2 to 5 percent of the children.[1] It is thus apparent that childhood lead poisoning is disturbingly

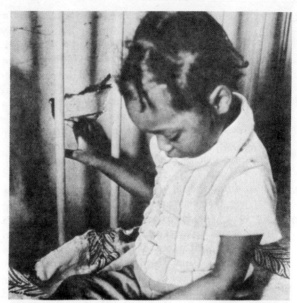

All the ingredients for an incipient case of lead poisoning are present in this picture—old peeling plaster containing lead-based paint within reach of a toddler, who, like most children of her age, is likely to pick up and eat anything.

prevalent in well delineated areas in many old cities.

Equally disturbing are the mortality and morbidity associated with this disease. Until the advent of chelating agents—therapeutic agents that bind the lead ions and remove them from the body—about two-thirds of the children with lead encephalopathy died. Even with the use of chelating agents, first BAL (British anti-lewisite) and later EDTA (ethylene-diaminetetracetate), the fatality rate remained a shocking 30 percent for many years. More recently, with the use of BAL and EDTA in combination and other supportive therapy, the fatality rate has been reduced to less than 5 percent.

But the reduction of the fatality rate in treated cases is neither evidence of adequate control of the disease nor a cause for complacency, because many of the survivors are left severely handicapped. A follow-up study of 425 children in Chicago who were treated for lead poisoning revealed that 39 percent had some kind of neurological sequelae. Among the 59 children in this group who before treatment presented symptoms of lead encephalopathy, 82 percent were left with handicaps: 54 percent had recurrent seizures, 38 percent were mentally retarded, 13 percent had cerebral palsy, and 6 percent had optic atrophy. Some had multiple handicaps.[2]

In Queensland, Australia, extensive epidemiological studies have demonstrated a high incidence of chronic kidney disease among patients who had lead poisoning in childhood 10 to 40 years ago. Half of these patients with kidney damage also suffered from gouty arthritis and many had severe high blood pressure, mental impairment, and various kinds of psychiatric disorders.[3]

Thus far studies on the effect of increased lead exposure have focused largely on the sequelae of overt poisoning. Little is known and little has been done to determine whether or not damage to the body occurs at a low level of exposure. Although clinical symptoms of lead poisoning often do not appear until the blood lead level is .06 mg/100 gm. of blood or higher, it is generally agreed that the normal blood lead level should not exceed .04 mg/100 gm. Recently it has been suggested that chronic debilitation and damage, which may not be recognized for many years, may result from an intake of lead far below what has been assumed to be dangerous, and that lead may be harmful to the body even in the absence of clinical symptoms.

Lack of awareness

The foregoing facts about lead poisoning pose a compelling question: How can a disease so prevalent and with such serious results escape attention of both the public at large and the Nation's health workers? In looking for an answer, one must first realize that lead poisoning in children is an illness rooted in social, economic, educational, psychological, cultural, medical, and even political factors. A direct result of a child's environment, it is prevalent only among children whose families are least able to improve their living conditions and who are not generally informed. The well-informed segments of the population are seldom affected.

Moreover, the answer is that many health workers who work among the poor are not aware that lead poisoning in children is still a problem. They apparently think that the mandatory use of lead-free paint for toys, furniture, and interiors of dwellings during the past quarter century has eliminated the problem. Furthermore, childhood lead poisoning is a disease that health workers may not recognize, even though it exists in epidemic proportions, because it has no distinctive clinical features. The symptoms of childhood lead poisoning are nonspecific. Anemia, listlessness, excessive irritability, loss of appetite, abdominal pain, constipation—signs and symptoms that appear before obvious evidence of encephalopathy, such as vomiting and convulsions—can all be misinterpreted as indications of some other illness. Because children who suffer from lead poisoning come from the slums, their anemia may be considered to be the result of inadequate nutrition; their listlessness and excessive irritability, to be the results of a pathological home environment; their abdominal pain and vomiting, to be symptoms of indigestion or gastroenteritis. Even convulsions may be regarded as signs of epilepsy rather than as evidence of lead encephalopathy.

Routine physical examination, blood count, and urinalysis will not provide an unsuspecting health worker with the correct diagnosis. Unless the worker inquires specifically whether the child has eaten chips of paint or plaster and draws a blood specimen for lead determination, he is likely to miss the diagnosis altogether and treat the child for something else, only to be confronted later with the same patient, who may then exhibit signs of brain injury, which may already be irreversible. In cities with a high incidence of lead poisoning, certain hospitals serving children from known "lead belts" report few or no cases of the disease.

Inadequate housing codes

In addition to poor housing conditions and a general lack of awareness of the problem, other elements contribute to the persistence of lead poisoning. Many cities in which lead poisoning is a public health problem do not have health or housing codes adequate to protect tenants from exposure to lead paint. Even in cities with codes specifically prohibiting lead paint in the interior of dwellings, enforcement of such codes is generally far from satisfactory. The currently available methods of paint removal are expensive and many landlords are not willing to undertake this expense. In cities with large slum areas and insufficient housing for people of low income, city officials sometimes hesitate to enforce the housing codes, reasoning that too rigorous enforcement would compel the landlords to abandon their slum buildings, thereby creating more problems for the city. Even when city officials are interested in enforcing codes, they frequently do not have enough inspectors and sanitarians to carry out the necessary procedures for enforcement—inspection of houses, collection of paint specimens, testing for lead content, and reinspection.

Another reason housing codes are not effective is that enforcement relies primarily on the criminal process, usually in the form of misdemeanor prosecution in the lower criminal courts. Criminal prosecution in such cases is fraught with many procedural and conceptual difficulties. First, summonses are often improperly served, being sent by mail rather than delivered by hand. Even when a landlord has been properly served with a criminal summons, he may fail to appear in court and thus force a postponement. Because a criminal court cannot proceed with a case until the defendant appears in court, housing cases often remain pending for months or even years. When the landlords do appear in court, adjournments and delays are frequent. Furthermore, proving the guilt of the offender beyond a reasonable doubt may be a long and complicated procedure in a lead poisoning case.[4]

When a landlord is found guilty, there is still the so-called "conceptual hurdle"—the reluctance of criminal courts to recognize a housing violation as a true "crime." A distinction is often made between the so-called "true crime" such as murder, assault, and robbery, and the "social welfare offenses" or crimes of omission, which consist of failure to meet health and safety standards. Penalties imposed for the latter offenses are generally minimal and inconsequential. In New York City, for example, while the city's statutes allow the imposition of fines ranging up to $1,000 per violation and provide for jail sentences of up to 1 year for repeated offenders against the housing code, in practice, jail sentences have practically never been imposed. In 1965 the average fine per case was less than $14; the average fine per violation was about 50 cents. Of the cases that did draw fines, many involved violations that had been uncorrected for years. Such inconsequential penalties convince many landlords that it is cheaper to pay the fine than to do the repair.[4]

Failure to get rid of lead paint in a house where a

child is known to have developed lead poisoning usually means that a treated child returns to the same hazardous environment to be exposed to another episode of poisoning. The recurrence rate is high in lead poisoning. Among survivors of acute lead encephalopathy who are reexposed to an environment that contains lead paint, the incidence of severe permanent brain damage is almost 100 percent. *Thus early casefinding and treatment programs are virtually meaningless when treated children are returned to their old environment.* Even when a lead-free home is found for a treated child, this merely solves the problem·for that particular child; it presents no solution to the problem of lead poisoning in general. If the lead paint in the house is not removed, the lethal heritage will soon pass on to other families with children, and lead poisoning among children multiplies.

Steps to eradication

While the obstacles to the eradication of lead poisoning are tremendous, they are not insurmountable. Slum clearance combined with provision of adequate housing for the poor is the most effective means of eliminating lead poisoning. But even before this measure is undertaken on the scale required, lead poisoning may be reduced through education, early detection, treatment, and follow-up programs that include removal of lead from houses wherever it is found. A few cities have demonstrated the value of such methods.

In Chicago, for example, there is a massive screening program for lead poisoning operated through the coordinated effort of local officials, health workers, and the community.

In the summer of 1965 a Citizens Committee to End Lead Poisoning was founded after the discovery of several cases of lead poisoning in the East Garfield Park District. With the help of the American Friends Service Committee, the Chicago Board of Health, and the Medical Committee for Human Rights, an educational and casefinding program was launched. A group of dedicated teenagers carried on a door-to-door campaign in the area, collecting urine specimens from children to be tested for lead poisoning.

In December of the same year the Chicago Board of Health announced plans for a large-scale screening program, and by the next September, 30,000 urine specimens had been tested. In October 1966 the Board of Health began an extensive casefinding program based on blood lead determination by atomic absorption spectroscopy—a screening method far superior to the urine test used earlier. The program has been conducted through the OEO-sponsored Chicago Committee for Urban Opportunity and supported in part by the Children's Bureau and State funds. Community representatives, working out of Urban Progress Centers, go from door to door distributing leaflets and alerting parents to the hazards and symptoms of lead poisoning. They also arrange for all children in the family between 9 months and 5 years of age to have a blood lead test made in the Urban Progress Center by a Board of Health physician. The Lead Poisoning Clinic, headed by Dr. Henrietta K. Sachs, was established for the diagnosis and treatment of children found in the screening program to have elevated blood lead levels.

By October 31, 1969, over 120,000 children had been tested, and over 1,500 children had been treated.

As a result of this intensive program, the incidence of elevated blood lead levels among children from the same areas declined from 8.5 percent in 1967 to 3.8 percent in 1968. Along with a rise in the number of cases of the disease that were detected came a decline in the fatality rate. In 1963, the first year the disease was made reportable, 203 cases of lead poisoning were reported in Chicago and the fatality rate was 2.9 percent. In 1968 the number of reported cases rose to 702 while the fatality rate dropped to 1.3 percent. But because many children were returned to the homes in which they had developed lead poisoning, some recurrence among treated children was reported.

Similar figures have been reported from New York City where physicians from all medical agencies in the city are encouraged to send blood specimens on all suspected cases of lead poisoning to the city health department laboratory for prompt and accurate blood lead analysis. In 1954, New York City reported 80 cases of lead poisoning and a fatality rate of 15 percent; in 1968, the fatality rate was less than 1 percent in the 725 cases reported. The city health department is currently working with the lead poisoning screening programs of the Montefiore Hospital and of the federally supported comprehensive health care projects for children and youth at the Albert Einstein College of Medicine, the Jewish Hospital and Medical Center of Brooklyn, the Brookdale Hospital Center in Brooklyn, and Roosevelt Hospital. Because approximately 75 percent of the children with lead poisoning reported in New York City are from families receiving public assistance, plans are underway to mail with public assistance checks a leaflet on lead poisoning written in both English and Spanish. It has also been proposed that the leaflet be mailed with birth certificates so parents will become aware of the problem before their children reach the age of risk.

In Philadelphia, lead poisoning was made a reportable disease in 1950. But from 1950 to 1960 only 278 cases were reported; these cases involved 53 deaths. In 1961 the Electric Storage Battery Co. began to provide free blood lead determinations for suspected cases. As a result, 109 cases and seven deaths were reported during 1961.

In 1966 the Philadelphia City Council adopted an ordinance amending the Health Code and the Board of Health issued regulations regarding the labeling, application, and removal of lead paint. In reported cases in which lead paint in the interior of dwellings proves to be the source of poisoning, the Board of Health requires all loose paint to be removed wherever found and all intact lead paint accessible to children to be removed down to the bare surface of the wall. Premises may not be repainted until they are approved on reinspection.

Since the ordinance and regulations became effective, approximately 400 properties have been made safe in this way. During the same period—1967 to 1968—there were 176 cases of lead poisoning and two deaths reported.

In 1968, a urine screening program for lead poisoning among children 1 to 3 years of age was initiated in the child health conferences of three district health centers in Philadelphia's high-risk areas.

Baltimore was one of the first cities to recognize lead poisoning in children as a public health problem. For more than 30 years, it has demonstrated an interest in this problem through continuous detection and prevention programs that include enforcement of health and housing codes, epidemiological surveys, and intensive educational campaigns. Aided by the Property Owners' Association, the health department has obtained good cooperation from landlords.

Unlike other cities that have detected increasing numbers of cases, in recent years, as awareness of the disease has increased, Baltimore has reported a steady decline since 1958 when 133 cases and 10 deaths were reported. In 1968 only 13 cases and no deaths were reported. Only one death was reported for each of the years 1964, 1966, and 1967, and none in 1965. These figures probably do not represent the real incidence and fatality rate of lead poisoning in Baltimore, and should be interpreted with caution. It may not be entirely unreasonable, however, to speculate that the continuous existence of the various programs for many years, along with paint removal from many dwellings, has yielded encouraging results.

Voluntary action

Two years ago, the Urban League of Rochester, N.Y., persuaded 22 youths from its Project Uplift Youth Incentives Program to assist the Rochester Committee for Scientific Information (RCSI) in its study of lead poisoning. The young people collected paint samples from slum homes and turned them over to RCSI for analysis. Since then Project Uplift has assigned smaller groups of youths to work with the Rochester Neighborhood Health Center and with doctors from the University of Rochester's Strong Memorial Hospital Department of Pediatrics. Last summer the young people and the Rochester Neighborhood Health Center distributed material explaining the campaign to all families registered with the health center. Teams, of two teenagers each, visited the homes to find out whether the children had eaten paint and to collect paint samples. If a paint sample showed a dangerous content of lead, the teenagers collected urine samples from the young children living in those dwellings for testing for lead poisoning. Subsequently, those children whose urine showed positive results were examined thoroughly. Nearly 7 percent of the children tested thus far have been found to have dangerous levels of lead in their systems.

In New York City the New York Scientists' Committee for Public Information has called the public's attention to lead poisoning by sponsoring meetings both for the population at risk and for health and community workers.

In Minneapolis the University of Minnesota Biomedical Student Committee for Social Responsibility and the Minnesota Committee for Environmental Information have sponsored a program to determine the prevalence of lead poisoning in one area of the city. Two University of Minnesota research assistants conducted a survey in early 1969 and found that 40 percent of the houses they examined had chipping interior paint with dangerous lead content. On the basis of this finding, a screening program was begun for children in the high-risk areas. In the summer of 1969 the Minneapolis City Council passed an ordinance prohibiting the use of lead paint in dwellings.

Many comprehensive health care projects for children sponsored by the Children's Bureau have set up programs to control lead poisoning. Among these are projects at the Hill Health Center in New Haven, the Children's Hospital of the District of Columbia, and the ones in New York City already mentioned.

The Johns Hopkins University School of Medicine has received a grant from the Children's Bureau for an urgently needed study of tests used in screening children for lead poisoning. The goal is to develop a simple, quick method of determining the amount of lead in human blood for use in large-scale screening programs. At present blood lead determination, in which a physician or skilled technician must puncture the vein to draw enough blood for analysis, is the only reliable test available. The successful use of this test with more than 120,000 children in Chicago is evidence of its feasibility as a large-scale method of screening for lead poisoning. However, scientists are seeking a quicker, but equally reliable, method that will require only the small amount of blood obtained from a finger prick.

The two currently used urine tests are far from satisfactory; the coproporphyrin test is often negative in lead poisoning and positive in other diseases, while the ALA (delta aminolevulinic acid) test is found to correlate poorly with blood lead levels. Moreover, it is difficult to collect urine from children from 1 to 3 years of age, the age group with the highest incidence of lead poisoning. Determination of the level of lead in hair has also been suggested as another screening test. Because the usefulness of this test has been questioned, further evaluation of it is needed.

In 1969 the Lead Industry Association published a booklet entitled "Facts About Lead and Pediatrics," presenting seven steps to the prevention of lead poisoning. The booklet is being distributed to physicians, public health authorities, social workers, city officials, and others who can help achieve prevention and control of the disease in children.

The recent upsurge of interest in childhood lead poisioning among Federal and local agencies, citizens' groups and government officials, health and community workers, and private and public institutions encourages the hope for an eventual end of this preventable manmade disease. But much more needs to be done.

Steps ahead

The ideal solution to childhood lead poisoning is slum clearance and urban renewal with the provision of adequate housing for families of low incomes. But this goal cannot be achieved quickly. Meanwhile, control and prevention must depend on other means, such as:

1. Public education through all channels and all media of communication to point out the dangers of paint eating, to acquaint the public with the symptoms of lead poisoning, and to urge parents to seek help whenever lead poisoning is suspected, even in the absence of symptoms. Many parents who are aware that their children eat paint do not know that this is dangerous. Among women who themselves eat clay or starch—a common practice in certain cultural groups—a child's paint eating may not receive attention.

2. Education of physicians, nurses, social workers and all other health workers on the prevalence of lead poisoning among children so that they will always have an index of suspicion. Health workers should routinely inquire about pica and paint ingestion in all children 1 to 6 years old, particularly those from high-risk neighborhoods, and should look for lead poisoning even before overt symptoms appear.

3. Mass screening programs in "lead belts" for all children between 1 and 6 years of age, using blood lead determination, the only reliable screening test.

4. Immediate referral of children found to have elevated blood lead levels to a medical center for diag-

nosis and treatment if necessary; prevention of a treated child's reexposure to lead in the home; and followup and retesting of all treated children who continue to be exposed. The prevention of reexposures means that health workers must work closely with housing authorities to see that lead paint is removed from every dwelling where poisoning has occurred.

5. The establishment of effective health and housing codes pertaining to lead and lead poisoning and the diligent enforcement of these codes. Where codes are not enforced, court action may be necessary. In New York City, for example, where the health department is said rarely to invoke a law allowing it to

A member of Project Uplift, a teenage volunteer organization sponsored by the Urban League of Rochester, N.Y., collects a sample of peeling plaster from an innercity dwelling for analysis to determine whether the paint contains lead.

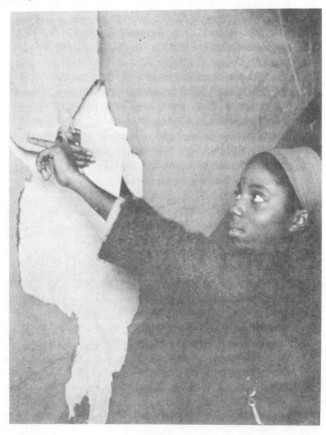

require landlords to correct lead hazards, a neighbor-hood health center is seeking court orders for land-lords to repair as common law nuisances dwellings where children have suffered lead poisoning. Other measures that have been advocated are withholding rents to make the necessary repairs or fining land-lords for each day the violations remain uncorrected.[5]

6. A concerted effort by research institutions to develop a simple, practical, and relatively inexpen-sive method for paint removal. The expense of cur-rently available methods to make paint inaccessible to children—either by paint removal through burn-ing, scraping, and sanding, or by covering the old paint with plasterboard or fiberglass—is an impor-tant deterrent to correction by landlords.

Research is also urgently needed to accomplish the following objectives:

● Development of a simple portable device for lead detection to make it possible systematically to iden-tify houses containing lead paint. At present detec-tion of lead paint in houses involves collection of paint samples and chemical analysis of such samples.

● Evaluation of available screening tests for lead poisoning and development of a reliable, simple, in-expensive method to determine blood lead level.

● Prospective studies of children with elevated blood lead levels who are "asymptomatic," to deter-mine the subtle effects of lead that do not become im-mediately apparent.

● A uniform reporting system for all screening programs to facilitiate the collection of pertinent data, exchange of information, and comparison of results.

● Improved methods of treatment to reduce not only the number of deaths from lead poisoning, but also the residual effects in survivors.

● Increased knowledge about the causes and cures of pica to reduce the incidence of lead ingestion.

THE ESTIMATED COST of treatment and institutional-ization to the age of 60 of a person who incurs severe permanent brain damage from lead poisoning in childhood is about $222,000. Complete removal of old lead paint from an average rowhouse with 10 windows, two doors, and baseboards would cost $250 to $300; replacement of window and door units and baseboards in such a house would cost $600 to $1,200.[6] These figures show only the difference in dollar costs between preventing lead poisoning through paint removal and permitting severe brain damage to occur in children. They do not take into consideration the suffering and heartache of affected families or the loss of useful manpower to the Nation.

Until society recognizes that permitting children to be killed and crippled by lead through paint ingestion is a crime not very different from permitting massacre and maiming of children by the use of lead bullets, this needless manmade disease will continue to victimize children.

Jane S. Lin-Fu, M.D., now with the Maternal and Child Health Service in the Health Services and Mental Health Administration, Public Health Service, was for 6 years pediatric consultant with the Children's Bureau. Her many writings on the medical problems affecting children include "New Hope for Babies of Rh Negative Mothers," which appeared in the January–Februrary 1969 issue of CHILDREN.

[1] Lin-Fu, Jane S.: Lead poisoning in children. U.S. Department of Health, Education, and Welfare, Social and Rehabilitation Service, Children's Bureau, Washington, D.C. C. B. Publication 452. 1967.

[2] Perlstein, M. A.; Attala, R.: Neurologic sequelae of plumbism in children. *Clinical Pediatrics,* May 1966.

[3] Emmerson, Bryan T.: Long-term effects of lead poisoning. Paper given at a conference on lead poisoning in children, Rockefeller University, New York, N.Y., May 25, 1969.

[4] New York University School of Law: Housing rights for the poor: rights and remedies. Project on Social Welfare Law Supplement No. 1. New York, N.Y. 1967.

[5] Urvant, Penny: Health advocates. *Public Health Reports,* September 1969.

[6] Chisolm, J. J., Jr.: Acute lead poisoning. Paper given at a conference on lead poisoning in children, Rockefeller University, New York, N.Y., May 25, 1969.

Rh Factor: Prevention of Isoimmunization and Clinical Trial on Mothers

VINCENT J. FREDA
JOHN G. GORMAN
WILLIAM POLLACK

The observation by Theobald Smith in 1909 (1), that in the presence of passive antibody the corresponding antigen will not immunize, has been confirmed and studied by others (2). From these many reports there emerged the new immunological principle that passive immunity strongly suppresses active immunity. But apparently a specific practical use for it as a means of suppressing the immune response has not been considered before.

Levine (3) has established that if the mother has an existing circulating antibody directed against the baby's red cells—for example, antibody to A that would be present in group O, Rh-negative mothers with a group A, Rh-positive baby—then immunization to Rh by pregnancy is uncommon. It is extremely difficult to immunize Rh-negative volunteers to Rh with injection of ABO-incompatible Rh-positive cells or with ABO-compatible cells which have been coated in vitro with an excess of antibody to Rh_0 (4).

In 1960 we put this principle to use and initiated a program to determine whether initial immunization of Rh-negative mothers could be prevented by the passive administration of Rh antibody immediately after childbirth (5). At the same time, quite independently and by another approach, Finn et al.

(6) began experimental work, guided by this identical concept.

We first procured a sterile preparation of γG-globulin containing very large amounts of antibody to Rh. Starting with pooled serum with high titer from a small number of donors, γG-immunoglobulin to Rh factor was prepared, filtered, and packaged sterile in 5-ml vials as a 16.5 percent solution suitable for intramuscular injection. This material was pure γG, free from γM-globulin (19S). The method of processing has the effect of increasing the original antibody titer (to Rh) about 100-fold even though 75 percent of the original antibody activity present in fractions I, III, and IV is excluded in the process. Intramuscular injection of Rh-negative individuals with 5 ml of this material has produced artificial titers of antibody up to 1:128, 1 ml up to 1:32, and 0.1 ml up to 1:2.

First used in 1961, approximately 200 doses of our material have now been given to more than 120 Rh-negative individuals, with no resulting side effects. Apart from the possible accidental use in an Rh-positive individual, this material should be as safe as the commercial γ-globulin currently used for the prevention of rubella, hepatitis, and other such diseases. The experi-

SCIENCE, 1966, Vol. 151., pp. 828-829., Copyright 1966 by the American Association for the Advancement of Science.

If γ-globulin has been that it does not transfer serum hepatitis.

In our first study, at Sing Sing Prison (5), there were nine Rh-negative male volunteers; four were treated with γG to Rh before each red cell stimulus and five acted as controls. All received an injection of 2 ml of Rh-positive blood each month for 5 months, and their blood was examined for a year. None of the treated group were immunized, but four out of the five controls became highly immunized to the Rh factor after this intensive stimulus. The second trial was then begun with 27 Rh-negative men (14 in the treated group, and 13 in the control group). On day 1 of the study all 27 men received intravenous injections of 10 ml of Rh-positive blood. Then 3 days after this red cell stimulus, the treated group (14 men chosen randomly) received intramuscular injections of 5 ml of γG to Rh. All were observed for 6 months; at 6 months none of the treated men were immunized and 6 of the 13 controls were immunized. After this, 11 of each group were given a second stimulus of 5 ml of Rh-positive blood, and the treated groups were again given 5 ml of the γG, this time 2 days after the red cell stimulus. Six months later (18 months after the start of the experiment) none of the treated men were immunized, and two more of the control group—for a total of 8 of the 13 original controls—were now immunized to the Rh factor.

Ten months after the second injection the lack of immunity in the γG-protected group was tested in nine of these men by a third antigenic stimulus of 1 ml of Rh-positive blood without the γG cover. If any of these men had attained even an extremely low level of immunity from their two earlier antigenic stimuli, they would be expected to make an accelerated or secondary immune response to this third Rh-provoking stimulus. All failed to show antibodies to Rh in their serum 24 weeks later (5). This meant that the

suppression of antibody formation was complete, and that the men had not been left in a primed state or sensitized by their two previous (γG-covered) antigenic stimuli with Rh-positive red blood cells. Subsequently 8 of the original 14 treated volunteers received a fourth and fifth antigenic stimulus of 10 ml of Rh-positive blood without the γG-globulin cover and two of the eight are now actively immunized to Rh. Thus it is not a question that they

Table 1. Summary of results (numbers) of trials of γG-immunoglobulin to Rh in male volunteers.

Subjects	1st trial 1962–63	2nd trial 1963–65
Test groups		
Actively immunized	0	0
Volunteer	4	14
Control groups		
Actively immunized	4	8
Volunteer	5	13

could not be immunized at all to Rh, but rather that they were indeed protected on the previous occasions by the γG cover.

These results showed, first of all, that our γG to Rh was quite safe. There were no side effects whatsoever. It provided complete suppression of immunization to the Rh factor in subjects heavily stimulated with Rh-positive cells (that is, with circulating antigen). It could be given up to 72 hours after the red cells and still provide a complete effect. It also did not support the suggestion of Cohen and Allton that under certain conditions passive antibody might enhance rather than suppress immunity. Such enhancement would be disastrous if it were inadvertently caused in Rh-negative mothers. We have not yet seen any sign of enhancement, and our own studies have since been extended to lower doses (that is, as little as 0.0001 ml of γG-globulin intramuscularly).

Because of the favorable findings of

the male volunteer study, a trial in Rh-negative mothers was begun in April 1964. In this trial, which is still continuing, 4.5 ml of γG to the Rh_0 factor is injected intramuscularly into non-

Patients*	Immune antibodies present	No immune antibodies present
Protected†	0	48
Control	7	52
Total	7	100

* From the Rh Antepartum Clinic of the Columbia-Presbyterian Medical Center, New York City.
† In each of these protected patients the passively administered antibody had completely disappeared by about 6 months after delivery, at which time (and afterwards) no antibody could be detected by the saline, enzyme, or the "antiglobulin" methods; presumably these mothers have been protected. Two of these mothers have now been delivered of a subsequent Rh-positive, ABO-compatible, unaffected infant and have received their second injection of γG-globulin to Rh factor.

immunized Rh-negative mothers within 72 hours of delivery of an ABO-compatible Rh-positive baby. These mothers and noninjected controls are being examined at intervals with antibody screening (Table 2). In this study, the results of Kleihauer testing for fetal cells do not have any influence on whether or not a mother is admitted to the study, all mothers at risk being included.

Of 174 mothers (84 protected and 90 controls) admitted to date to the clinical trial, 107 have been followed for periods of approximately 6 months to 1½ years after delivery. That no protected mother had become actively immunized was proved in every case: no antibody at all (either passive or active) could be demonstrated in each mother's serum when tested 6 months or more after delivery by both the indirect "antiglobulin" and saline methods and also by the enzyme technique. Because the presence of passive antibody might obscure early active antibody formation we did not consider any results of our clinical trial valid until the "protected" mothers had been followed until all passive antibody had disappeared. In another study (8), lack of active immunity was presumed in some mothers with passive antibody still present at 3 months after delivery, if no antibody could be demonstrated by the "saline" method. The absence of "saline" antibody is not a strictly valid criterion for nonimmunity because in our studies on male volunteers, over the past 3½ years, it was not at all uncommon for active immunization to the Rh factor to occur without the appearance of "saline" antibodies.

The positive trend of our results is now being confirmed by the results of others (8, 9). However, the final proof of the complete efficacy of this preparation will come only when the results from a number of subsequent Rh-positive pregnancies are known. In any event, the outlook is fairly promising that γG-immunoglobulin to the Rh factor will soon become a practical public health measure for the prevention of Rh hemolytic disease of the newborn.

SECTION V

SPECIFIC ACADEMIC DIFFICULTIES

Learning to Read

Eleanor J. Gibson

Educators and the public have exhibited a keen interest in the teaching of reading ever since free public education became a fact (*1*). Either because of or despite their interest, this most important subject has been remarkably susceptible to the influence of fads and fashions and curiously unaffected by disciplined experimental and theoretical psychology. The psychologists have traditionally pursued the study of verbal learning by means of experiments with nonsense syllables and the like—that is, materials carefully divested of useful information. And the educators, who found little in this work that seemed relevant to the classroom, have stayed with the classroom; when they performed experiments, the method was apt to be a gross comparison of classes privileged and unprivileged with respect to the latest fad. The result has been two cultures: the pure scientists in the laboratory, and the practical teachers ignorant of the progress that has been made in the theory of human learning and in methods of studying it.

That this split was unfortunate is clear enough. True, most children do learn to read. But some learn to read badly, so that school systems must provide remedial clinics; and a small proportion (but still a large number of future citizens) remain functional illiterates. The fashions which have led to classroom experiments, such as the "whole word" method, emphasis on context and pictures for "meaning," the "flash" method, "speed reading," revised alphabets, the "return" to "phonics," and so on, have done little to change the situation.

Yet a systematic approach to the understanding of reading skill is possible. The psychologist has only to treat reading as a learning problem, to apply ingenuity in theory construction and ex-

The author is senior research associate in psychology at Cornell University. This article is adapted from a paper read at a conference on Perceptual and Linguistic Aspects of Reading, sponsored by the Committee on Learning and the Educational Process of the Social Science Research Council and held at the Center for Advanced Study in the Behavioral Sciences, Palo Alto, California, 31 October 1963.

SCIENCE, 1965, Vol. 148., pp. 1066-1072.

perimental design to this fundamental activity on which the rest of man's education depends. A beginning has recently been made in this direction, and it can be expected that a number of theoretical and experimental studies of reading will be forthcoming (2).

Analysis of the Reading Process

A prerequisite to good research on reading is a psychological analysis of the reading process. What is it that a skilled reader has learned? Knowing this (or having a pretty good idea of it), one may consider how the skill is learned, and next how it could best be taught. Hypotheses designed to answer all three of these questions can then be tested by experiment.

There are several ways of characterizing the behavior we call reading. It is receiving communication; it is making discriminative responses to graphic symbols; it is decoding graphic symbols to speech; and it is getting meaning from the printed page. A child in the early stages of acquiring reading skill may not be doing all these things, however. Some aspects of reading must be mastered before others and have an essential function in a sequence of development of the final skill. The average child, when he begins learning to read, has already mastered to a marvelous extent the art of communication. He can speak and understand his own language in a fairly complex way, employing units of language organized in a hierarchy and with a grammatical structure. Since a writing system must correspond to the spoken one, and since speech is prior to writing, the framework and unit structure of speech will determine more or less the structure of the writing system, though the rules of

correspondence vary for different languages and writing systems. Some alphabetic writing systems have nearly perfect single-letter-to-sound correspondences, but some, like English, have far more complex correspondence between spelling patterns and speech patterns. Whatever the nature of the correspondences, it is vital to a proper analysis of the reading task that they be understood. And it is vital to remember, as well, that the first stage in the child's mastery of reading is learning to communicate by means of spoken language.

Once a child begins his progression from spoken language to written language, there are, I think, three phases of learning to be considered. They present three different kinds of learning tasks, and they are roughly sequential, though there must be considerable overlapping. These three phases are: learning to differentiate graphic symbols; learning to decode letters to sounds ("map" the letters into sounds); and using progressively higher-order units of structure. I shall consider these three stages in order and in some detail and describe experiments exploring each stage.

Differentiation of Written Symbols

Making any discriminative response to printed characters is considered by some a kind of reading. A very young child, or even a monkey, can be taught to point to a patch of yellow color, rather than a patch of blue, when the printed characters YELLOW are presented. Various people, in recent popular publications, have seriously suggested teaching infants to respond discriminatively in this way to letter patterns, implying that this is teaching them to "read." Such responses are not reading, however; reading entails decoding to speech. Letters are, essentially, an instruction to produce a given speech sound.

Nevertheless, differentiation of written characters from one another is a logically preliminary stage to decoding them to speech. The learning problem is one of discriminating and recognizing a set of line figures, all very similar in a number of ways (for example, all are tracings on paper) and each differing from all the others in one or more features (as straight versus curved). The differentiating features must remain invariant under certain transformations (size, brightness, and perspective transformations and less easily described ones produced by different type faces and handwriting). They must therefore be relational, so that these transformations will not destroy them.

It might be questioned whether learning is necessary for these figures to be discriminated from one another. This question has been investigated by Gibson, Gibson, Pick, and Osser (3). In order to trace the development of letter differentiation as it is related to those features of letters which are critical for the task, we designed specified transformations for each of a group of standard, artificial letter-like forms comparable to printed Roman capitals. Variants were constructed from each standard figure to yield the following 12 transformations for each one: three degrees of transformation from line to curve; five transformations of rotation or reversal; two perspective transformations; and two topological transformations (see Fig. 1 for examples). All of these except the perspective transformations we considered critical for discriminating letters. For example, contrast v and u; c and u; o and c.

The discrimination task required the subject to match a standard figure against all of its transformations and some copies of it and to select only identical copies. An error score (the number of times an item that was not an identical copy was selected) was obtained for each child, and the errors were classified according to the type of transformation. The subjects were children aged 4 through 8 years. As would be expected, the visual discrimination of these letter-like forms improved from age 4 to age 8, but the slopes of the error curves were different, depending on the transformation to be discriminated (Fig. 2). In other words, some transformations are harder to discriminate than others, and improvement occurs at different rates for different transformations. Even the youngest subjects made relatively few errors involving changes of break or close, and among the 8-year-olds these errors dropped to zero. Errors for perspective transformations were very numerous among 4-year-olds and still numerous among 8-year-olds. Errors for rotations and reversals started high but dropped to nearly zero by 8 years. Errors for changes from line to curve were relatively numerous (depending on the number of changes) among the youngest children and showed a rapid drop among the older— almost to zero for the 8-year-olds.

The experiment was replicated with the same transformations of real letters on the 5-year-old group. The correlation between confusions of the same transformations for real letters and for the letter-like forms was very high ($r = +.87$), so the effect of a given transformation has generality (is not specific to a given form).

What happens, in the years from 4 to 8, to produce or hamper improvement in discrimination? Our re-

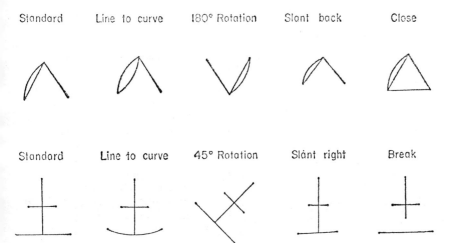

Fig. 1. Examples of letter-like figures illustrating different types of transformation.

sults suggest that the children have learned the features or dimensions of difference which are critical for differentiating letters. Some differences are critical, such as break versus close, line versus curve, and rotations and reversals; but some, such as the perspective transformations, are not, and must in fact be tolerated. The child of 4 does not start "cold" upon this task, because some of his previous experience with distinctive features of objects and pictures will transfer to letter differentiation. But the set of letters has a unique feature pattern for each of its members, so learning of the distinctive features goes on during the period we investigated.

Table 1. Number of errors made in transfer stage by groups with three types of training.

Group	Type of training		Errors
	Standards	Transfor-mations	
E1	Same	Different	69
E2	Different	Same	39
C	Different	Different	101

If this interpretation is correct, it would be useful to know just what the distinctive features of letters are. What dimensions of difference must a child learn to detect in order to perceive each letter as unique? Gibson, Osser, Schiff, and Smith (4) investigated this question. Our method was to draw up a chart of the features of a given set of letters (5), test to see which of these letters were most frequently confused by prereading children. and compare the errors in the resulting "confusion matrix" with those predicted by the feature chart.

A set of distinctive features for letters must be relational in the sense that each feature presents a contrast which is invariant under certain transformations, and it must yield a unique pattern for each letter. The set must also be reasonably economical. Two feature lists which satisfy these requirements for a specified type face were tried out against the results of a confusion matrix obtained with the same type (simplified Roman capitals available on a sign-typewriter).

119

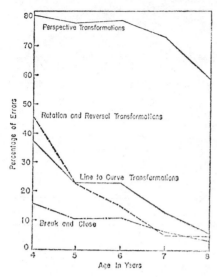

Fig. 2. Error curves showing rate of improvement in discriminating four types of transformation.

Each of the features in the list in Fig. 3 is or is not a characteristic of each of the 26 letters. Regarding each letter one asks, for example, "Is there a curved segment?" and gets a yes or no answer. A filled-in feature chart gives a unique pattern for each letter. However, the number of potential features for letter-shapes is very large, and would vary from one alphabet and type font to another. Whether or not we have the right set can be tested with a confusion matrix. Children should confuse with greatest frequency the letters having the smallest number of feature differences, if the features have been chosen correctly.

We obtained our confusion matrix from 4-year-old children, who made matching judgments of letters, programmed so that every letter had an equal opportunity to be mistaken for any other, without bias from order effects. The "percent feature difference" for any two letters was determined by dividing the total number of

features possessed by either letter, but not both, by the total number possessed by both, whether shared or not. Correlations were then calculated between percent feature difference and number of confusions, one for each letter. The feature list of Fig. 3 yielded 12 out of 26 positive significant correlations. Prediction from this feature list is fairly good, in view of the fact that features were not weighted. A multi-dimensional analysis of the matrix corroborated the choice of the curve-straight and obliqueness variables, suggesting that these features may have priority in the discrimination process and perhaps developmentally. Refinement of the feature list will take these facts into account, and other methods of validation will be tried.

Detecting Distinctive Features

If we are correct in thinking that the child comes to discriminate graphemes by detecting their distinctive features, what is the learning process like? That it is perceptual learning and need not be verbalized is probable (though teachers do often call attention to contrasts between letter shapes.) An experiment by Anne D. Pick (6) was designed to compare two hypotheses about how this type of discrimination develops. One might be called a "schema" or "prototype" hypothesis, and is based on the supposition that the child builds up a kind of model or memory image of each letter by repeated experience of visual presentations of the letter; perceptual theories which propose that discrimination occurs by matching sensory experience to a previously stored concept or categorical model are of this kind. In the other hypothesis it is assumed that the child learns by discover-

Features	A	B	C	E	K	L	N	U	X	Z
Straight segment										
Horizontal	+			+	+					+
Vertical		+		+	+	+	+			
Oblique /	+				+				+	+
Oblique \	+				+		+		+	
Curve										
Closed		+								
Open vertically								+		
Open horizontally			+							
Intersection	+	+		+	+				+	
Redundancy										
Cyclic change		+		+						
Symmetry	+	+	+	+	+			+	+	
Discontinuity										
Vertical	+					+			+	
Horizontal				+			+	+		+

Fig. 3. Example of a "feature chart." Whether the features chosen are actually effective for discriminating letters must be determined by experiment.

ing how the forms differ, and then easily transfers this knowledge to new letter-like figures.

Pick employed a transfer design in which subjects were presented in step 1 with initially confusable stimuli (letter-like forms) and trained to discriminate between them. For step 2 (the transfer stage) the subjects were divided into three groups. One experimental group was given sets of stimuli to discriminate which varied in new dimensions from the *same standards* discriminated in stage 1. A second experimental group was given sets of stimuli which deviated from *new standards*, but in the same dimensions of difference discriminated in stage 1. A control group was given both new standards and new dimensions of difference to discriminate in stage 2. Better performance by the first experimental group would suggest that discrimination learning proceeded by construction of a model or memory image of the standards against which the variants could be matched. Conversely, better performance by the second experimental group would suggest that dimensions of difference had been detected.

The subjects were kindergarten children. The stimuli were letter-like forms of the type described earlier. There were six standard forms and six transformations of each of them. The transformations consisted of two changes of line to curve, a right-left reversal, a 45-degree rotation, a perspective transformation, and a size transformation. Table 1 gives the errors of discrimination for all three groups in stage 2. Both experimental groups performed significantly better than the control group, but the group that had familiar transformations of new standards performed significantly better than the group given new transformations of old standards.

We infer from these results that, while children probably do learn prototypes of letter shapes, the prototypes themselves are not the original basis for differentiation. The most relevant kind of training for discrimination is practice which provides experience with the characteristic differences that distinguish the set of items. Features which are actually distinctive for letters could be emphasized by presenting letters in contrast pairs.

Decoding Letters to Sounds

When the graphemes are reasonably discriminable from one another, the decoding process becomes possible. This process, common sense and many psychologists would tell us, is simply a matter of associating a graphic stimulus with the appropriate spoken response—that is to say, it is the traditional stimulus-response paradigm, a kind of paired-associate learning.

Obvious as this description seems, problems arise when one takes a closer look. Here are just a few. The graphic code is related to the speech code by rules of correspondence. If these rules are known, decoding of new items is predictable. Do we want to build up, one by one, automatically cued responses or do we want to teach with transfer in mind? If we want to teach for transfer, how do we do it? Should the child be aware that this is a code game with rules? Or will induction of the rules be automatic? What units of both codes should we start with? Should we start with single letters, in the hope that knowledge of single-letter-to-sound relationships will yield the most transfer? Or should we start with whole words, in the hope that component relationships will be induced?

Carol Bishop (7) investigated the question of the significance of knowledge of component letter-sound relationships in reading new words. In her experiment, the child's process of learning to read was simulated by teaching adult subjects to read some Arabic words. The purpose was to determine the transfer value of training with individual letters as opposed to whole words, and to investigate the role of component letter-sound associations in transfer to learning new words.

A three-stage transfer design was employed. The letters were 12 Arabic characters, each with a one-to-one letter-sound correspondence. There were eight consonants and four vowels, which were combined to form two sets of eight Arabic words. The 12 letters appeared at least once in both sets of words. A native speaker of the language recorded on tape the 12 letter-sounds and the two sets of words. The graphic form of each letter or word was printed on a card.

The subjects were divided into three groups—the letter training group (L), the whole-word training group (W), and a control group (C). Stage 1 of the experiment was identical for all groups. The subjects learned to pronounce the set of words (transfer set) which would appear in stage 3 by listening to the recording and repeating the words. Stage 2 varied. Group L listened to and repeated the 12 letter-sounds and then learned to associate the individual graphic shapes with their correct sounds. Group W followed the same procedure, except that eight words were given them to learn, rather than letters. Learning time was equal for the two groups. Group C spent the same time-interval on an unrelated task. Stage 3 was the same for the three groups. All subjects learned to read the set of words they had heard in stage 1, responding to the presentation of a word on a card by pronouncing it. This was the transfer stage on which the three groups were compared.

At the close of stage 3, all subjects were tested on their ability to give the correct letter-sound following the presentation of each printed letter. They were asked afterward to explain how they tried to learn the transfer words.

Figure 4 shows that learning took place in fewest trials for the letter group and next fewest for the word group. That is, letter training had more transfer value than word training, but word training did produce some transfer. The subjects of group L also knew, on the average, a greater number of component letter-sound correspondences, but some subjects in group W had learned all 12. Most of the subjects in group L reported that they had tried to learn by using knowledge of component correspondences. But so did 12 of the 20 subjects in group W, and the scores of these 12 subjects on the transfer task were similar to those of the letter-trained group. The subjects who had learned by whole words and had not used individual correspondences performed no better on the task than the control subjects.

It is possible, then, to learn to read words without learning the component letter-sound correspondences. But transfer to new words depends on use of them, whatever the method of original training. Word training was as good as letter training if the subject had analyzed for himself the component relationships.

Learning Variable and Constant Component Correspondences

In Bishop's experiment, the component letter-sound relationships were regular and consistent. It has often been pointed out, especially by advocates of spelling reform and revised alphabets (8), that in English this is not the case. Bloomfield (9) suggested that the beginning reader should, therefore, be presented with material carefully programmed for teaching those orthographic-phonic regularities which exist in English, and should be introduced later and only gradually to the complexities of English spelling and to the fact that single-letter-to-sound relationships are often variable. But actually, there has been no hard evidence to suggest that transfer, later, to reading spelling-patterns with more variable component correspondence will be facilitated by beginning with only constant ones. Although variable ones may be harder to learn in the beginning, the original difficulty may be compensated for by facilitating later learning.

A series of experiments directed by Harry Levin (10) dealt with the effect of learning variable as opposed to constant letter-sound relationships, on transfer to learning new letter-sound relationships. In one experiment, the learning material was short lists of paired-associates, with a word written in artificial characters as stimulus and a triphoneme familiar English word as response. Subjects (third-grade children) in one group were given a list which contained constant graph-to-sound relationships (one-to-one component correspondence) followed by a list in which this correspondence was variable with respect to the medial vowel sound. Another group started with a similarly constructed variable list and followed it with a second one. The group that learned lists with a variable component in both stages was superior to the other group in the second stage. The results suggest that initiating the task with a

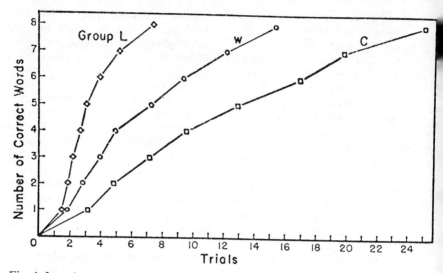

Fig. 4. Learning curves on transfer task for group trained originally with whole words (W), group trained with single letters (L), and control group (C).

variable list created an expectation of learning set for variability of correspondence which was transferred to the second list and facilitated learning it.

In a second experiment, the constant or variable graph-sound relation occurred on the first letter. Again, the group with original variable training performed better on the second, variable list. In a third experiment adult native speakers of English and Spanish were compared. The artificial graphs were paired with nonsense words. Again there was more transfer from a variable first list to a variable second list than from a constant to a variable one. Variable lists were more difficult, on the whole, for the Spanish speakers, perhaps because their native language contains highly regular letter-sound relationships.

A "set for diversity" may, therefore, facilitate transfer to learning of new letter-sound correspondences which contain variable relationships. But many questions about how the code is learned remain to be solved, because

the true units of the graphic code are not necessarily single letters. While single-letter-sound relations in English are indeed variable, at other levels of structure regularity may be discovered.

Lower- and Higher-Order Units

For many years, linguists have been concerned with the question of units in language. That language has a hierarchical structure, with units of different kinds and levels, is generally accepted, though the definition of the units is not easily reached. One criterion of a unit is recodability—consistent mapping or translation to another code. If such a criterion be granted, graphic units must parallel linguistic units. The units of the writing system should be defined, in other words, by mapping rules which link them to the speech code, at all levels of structure.

What then are the true graphic units? What levels of units are there? Exactly

124

...ow are they mapped to linguistic ...its? In what "chunks" are they per-...ived? We must first try to answer ...ese questions by a logical analysis of ...roperties of the writing and speech ...stems and the correspondences be-...veen them. Then we can look at the ...ehavior of skilled readers and see how ...its are processed during reading. If ...e logical analysis of the correspond-...nce rules is correct, we should be able ...) predict what kinds of units are actu-...ly processed and to check our predic-...ons experimentally.

Common sense suggests that the unit ...r reading is the single grapheme, and ...at the reader proceeds sequentially ...rom left to right, letter by letter, across ...he page. But we can assert at once and ...nequivocally that this picture is false. ...or the English language, the single ...raphemes map consistently into speech ...nly as morphemes—that is, the names ...f the letters of the alphabet. It is pos-...ible, of course, to name letters se-...quentially across a line of print ("spell ...ut" a word), but that is not the goal ...f a skilled reader, nor is it what he ...does. Dodge (11) showed, nearly 60 ...years ago, that perception occurs in ...reading only during fixations, and not ...at all during the saccadic jumps from ...one fixation to the next. With a fast ...tachistoscopic exposure, a skilled reader ...can perceive four unconnected letters, ...a very long word, and four or more ...words if they form a sentence (12). ...Even first graders can read three-letter ...words exposed for only 40 milliseconds, ...too short a time for sequential eye-...movements to occur.

Broadbent (13) has pointed out that ...speech, although it consists of a tem-...poral sequence of stimuli, is responded ...to at the end of a sequence. That is, it ...is normal for a whole sequence to be ...delivered before a response is made.

For instance, the sentence "Would you give me your ———— ?" might end with any of a large number of words, such as "name" or "wallet" or "wife." The response depends on the total message. The fact that the component stimuli for speech and reading are spread over time does not means that the phonemes or letters or words are processed one at a time, with each stimulus decoded to a separate response. The fact that o is pronounced differently in BOAT and BOMB is not a hideous peculiarity of English which must consequently be re-formed. The o is read only in context and is never responded to in isolation. It is part of a sequence which contains constraints of two kinds, one morpho-logical and the other the spelling pat-terns which are characteristic of Eng-lish.

If any doubt remains as to the un-likelihood of sequential processing letter by letter, there is recent evidence of Newman (14) and of Kolers (15) on sequential exposure of letters. When letters forming a familiar word are ex-posed sequentially in the same place, it is almost impossible to read the word. With an exposure of 100 milliseconds per letter, words of six letters are read with only 20 percent probability of ac-curacy; and with an exposure of 375 milliseconds per letter, the probability is still well under 100 percent. But that is more than 2 seconds to per-ceive a short, well-known word! We can conclude that, however graphemes are processed perceptually in reading, it is not a letter-by-letter sequence of acts.

If the single grapheme does not map consistently to a phoneme, and further-more, if perception normally takes in bigger "chunks" of graphic stimuli in a single fixation, what are the smallest graphic units consistently coded into phonemic patterns? Must they be whole words? Are there different levels of units? Are they achieved at different stages of development?

Spelling Patterns

It is my belief that the smallest component units in written English are spelling patterns (16). By a spelling pattern, I mean a cluster of graphemes in a given environment which has an invariant pronunciation according to the rules of English. These rules are the regularities which appear when, for instance, any vowel or consonant or cluster is shown to correspond with a given pronunciation in an initial, medial, or final position in the spelling of a word. This kind of regularity is not merely "frequency" (bigram frequency, trigram frequency, and so on), for it implies that frequency counts are relevant for establishing rules only if the right units and the right relationships are counted. The relevant graphic unit is a functional unit of one or more letters, in a given position within the word, which is in correspondence with a specified pronunciation (17).

If potential regularities exist within words—the spelling patterns that occur in regular correspondence with speech patterns—one may hypothesize that these correspondences have been assimilated by the skilled reader of English (whether or not he can verbalize the rules) and have the effect of organizing units for perception. It follows that strings of letters which are generated by the rules will be perceived more easily than ones which are not, even when they are unfamiliar words or not words at all.

Several experiments testing this prediction were performed by Gibson, Pick, Osser, and Hammond (18). The basic design was to compare the perceptibility (with a very short tachistoscopic exposure) of two sets of letterstrings, all nonsense or pseudo words, which differed in their spelling-to-sound correlation. One list, called the "pronounceable" list, contained words with a high spelling-to-sound correlation. Each of them had an initial consonant-spelling with a single, regular pronunciation: a final consonant-spelling having a single regular pronunciation; and a vowel-spelling, placed between them, having a single regular pronunciation when it follows and is followed by the given initial and final consonant spellings, respectively—for example, GL/UR/CK. The words in the second list, called the "unpronounceable" list, had a low spelling-to-sound correlation. They were constructed from the words in the first list by reversing the initial and final consonant spellings. The medial vowel spelling was not changed. For example, GLURCK became CKURGL. There were 25 such pseudo words in each list, varying in length from four to eight letters. The pronunciability of the resulting lists was validated in two ways, first by ratings, and second by obtaining the number of variations when the pseudo words were actually pronounced.

The words were projected on a screen in random order, in five successive presentations with an exposure time beginning at 50 milliseconds and progressing up to 250 milliseconds. The subjects (college students) were instructed to write each word as it was projected. The mean percentage of pronounceable words correctly perceived was consistently and significantly greater at all exposure times.

The experiment was later repeated with the same material but a different judgment. After the pseudo word was exposed, it was followed by a multiple-choice list of four items, one of the correct one and the other three the most common errors produced in the previous experiment. The subject chose the word he thought he had seen from the choice list and recorded a number (its order in the list). Again the mean of pronounceable pseudo words correctly perceived significantly exceeded that of their unpronounceable counterparts. We conclude from these experiments that skilled readers more easily perceive as a unit pseudo words which follow the rules of English spelling-to-sound correspondence; that spelling patterns which have invariant relations to sound patterns function as a unit, thus facilitating the decoding process.

In another experiment, Gibson, Osser, and Pick (*19*) studied the development of perception of grapheme-phoneme correspondences. We wanted to know how early, in learning to read, children begin to respond to spelling-patterns as units. The experiment was designed to compare children at the end of the first grade and at the end of the third grade in ability to recognize familiar three letter words, pronounceable trigrams, and unpronounceable trigrams. The three-letter words were taken from the first-grade reading list; each word chosen could be rearranged into a meaningless but pronounceable trigram and a meaningless and unpronounceable one (for example, RAN, NAR, RNA). Some longer pseudo words (four and five letters) taken from the previous experiments were included as well. The words and pseudo words were exposed tachistoscopically to individual children, who were required to spell them orally. The first-graders read (spelled out) most accurately the familiar three-letter words, but read the pronounceable trigrams significantly better than the unpronounceable ones. The longer pseudo words were seldom read accurately and were not differentiated by pronunciability. The third-grade girls read all three-letter combinations with high and about equal accuracy, but differentiated the longer pseudo words; that is, the pronounceable four- and five-letter pseudo words were more often perceived correctly than their unpronounceable counterparts.

These results suggest that a child in the first stages of reading skill typically reads in short units, but has already generalized certain regularities of spelling-to-sound correspondence, so that three-letter pseudo words which fit the rules are more easily read as units. As skill develops, span increases, and a similar difference can be observed for longer items. The longer items involve more complex conditional rules and longer clusters, so that the generalizations must increase in complexity. The fact that a child can begin very early to perceive regularities of correspondence between the printed and spoken patterns, and transfer them to the reading of unfamiliar items as units, suggests that the opportunities for discovering the correspondences between patterns might well be enhanced in programming reading materials.

I have referred several times to *levels* of units. The last experiment showed that the size and complexity of the spelling patterns which can be perceived as units increase with development of reading skill. That other levels of structure, both syntactic and semantic, contain units as large as and larger than the word, and that perception of skilled readers will be found, in suitable experiments, to be a function of these factors is almost axiomatic. As yet we have little direct evidence better than Cattell's original discovery (*12*) that when words are structured into a sentence, more letters can be accurately perceived "at a glance." Developmental studies of perceptual "chunking" in relation to structural complexity may be very instructive.

Where does meaning come in? Within the immediate span of visual perception, meaning is less effective in structuring written material than good spelling-to-sound correspondence, as Gibson, Bishop, Schiff, and Smith (*20*) have shown. Real words which are both meaningful and, as strings of letters, structured in accordance with English spelling patterns are more easily perceived than nonword pronounceable strings of letters; but the latter are more easily perceived than meaningful but unpronounceable letter-strings (for example, BIM is perceived accurately, with tachistoscopic exposure, faster than IBM). The role of meaning in the visual perception of words probably increases as longer strings of words (more than one) are dealt with. A sentence has two kinds of constraint, semantic and syntactic, which make it intelligible (easily heard) and memorable (*21*). It is important that the child develop reading habits which utilize all the types of constraint present in the stimulus, since they constitute structure and are, therefore, unit-formers. The skills which the child should acquire in reading are habits of utilizing the constraints in letter strings (the spelling and morphemic patterns) and in word strings (the syntactic and semantic patterns). We could go on to consider still superordinate ones, perhaps, but the problem of the unit, of levels of units, and mapping rules from writing to speech has just begun to be explored with experimental techniques. Further research on the definition and processing of units should lead to new insights about the nature of reading skill and its attainment.

Summary

Reading begins with the child's acquisition of spoken language. Later he learns to differentiate the graphic symbols from one another and to decode these to familiar speech sounds. As he learns the code, he must progressively utilize the structural constraints which are built into it in order to attain the skilled performance which is characterized by processing of higher-order units —the spelling and morphological patterns of the language.

Because of my firm conviction that good pedagogy is based on a deep understanding of the discipline to be taught and the nature of the learning process involved, I have tried to show that the psychology of reading can benefit from a program of theoretical analysis and experiment. An analysis of the reading task—its discriminatory and decoding aspects as well as the semantic and syntactical aspects—tells us *what* must be learned. An analysis of the learning process tells us *how*. The consideration of formal instruction comes only after these steps, and its precepts should follow from them.

References and Notes

1. See C. C. Fries, *Linguistics and Reading* (Holt, Rinehart, and Winston, New York, 1963), for an excellent chapter on past practice and theory in the teaching of reading.
2. In 1959, Cornell University was awarded a grant for a Basic Research Project on Reading by the Cooperative Research Program of the Office of Education, U.S. Department of Health, Education, and Welfare. Most of the work reported in this article was supported by this grant. The Office of Education has recently organized "Project Literacy," which will promote research on reading in a number of laboratories, as well as encourage mutual understanding between experimentalists and teachers of reading.
3. E. J. Gibson, J. J. Gibson, A. D. Pick, H. Osser, *J. Comp. Physiol. Psychol.* 55, 897

(1962).

4. E. J. Gibson, H. Osser, W. Schiff, J. Smith, in *A Basic Research Program on Reading*, Final Report on Cooperative Research Project No. 639 to the Office of Education, Department of Health, Education, and Welfare.

5. The method was greatly influenced by the analysis of distinctive features of phonemes by Jakobson and M. Halle, presented in *Fundamentals of Language* (Mouton, The Hague, 1956). A table of 12 features, each in binary opposition, yields a unique pattern for all phonemes, so that any one is distinguishable from any other by its pattern of attributes. A pair of phonemes may differ by any number of features, the minimal distinction being one feature opposition. The features must be invariant under certain transformations and essentially relational, so as to remain distinctive over a wide range of speakers, intonations, and so on.

6. A. D. Pick, *J. Exp. Psychol.*, in press.

7. C. H. Bishop, *J. Verbal Learning Verbal Behav.* 3, 215 (1964).

8. Current advocates of a revised alphabet who emphasize the low letter-sound correspondence in English are Sir James Pitman and John A. Downing. Pitman's revised alphabet, called the Initial Teaching Alphabet, consists of 43 characters, some traditional and some new. It is designed for instruction of the beginning reader, who later transfers to traditional English spelling. See I. J. Pitman, *J. Roy. Soc. Arts* 109, 149 (1961); J. A. Downing, *Brit. J. Educ. Psychol.* 32, 166 (1962); ———, "Experiments with Pitman's initial teaching alphabet in British schools," paper presented at the Eighth Annual Conference of International Reading Association, Miami, Fla., May 1963.

9. L. Bloomfield, *Elem. Engl. Rev.* 19, 125, 183 (1942).

10. See research reports of H. Levin and J. Watson, and H. Levin, E. Baum, and S. Bostwick, in *A Basic Research Program on Reading* (see 4).

11. R. Dodge, *Psychol. Bull.* 2, 193 (1905).

12. J. McK. Cattell, *Phil. Studies* 2, 635 (1885).

13. D. E. Broadbent, *Perception and Communication* (Pergamon, New York, 1958).

14. E. Newman, *Am. J. Psychol.*, in press.

15. P. A. Kolers and M. T. Katzman, paper presented before the Psychonomic Society, Aug. 1963, Bryn Mawr, Pa.

16. Spelling patterns in English have been discussed by C. C. Fries in *Linguistics and Reading* (Holt, Rinehart, and Winston, New York, 1963), p. 169 ff. C. F. Hockett, in *A Basic Research Program on Reading* (see 4), has made an analysis of English graphic monosyllables which presents regularities of spelling patterns in relation to pronunciation. This study was continued by R. Venezky (thesis, Cornell Univ., 1962), who wrote a computer program for obtaining the regularities of English spelling-to-sound correspondence. The data obtained by means of the computer permit one to look up any vowel or consonant cluster of up to five letters and find its pronunciation in initial, medial, and final positions in a word. Letter environments as well have now been included in the analysis. See also R. H. Weir, *Formulation of Grapheme-Phoneme Correspondence Rules to Aid in the Teaching of Reading*, Report on Cooperative Research Project No. 5-039 to the Office of Education, Department of Health, Education and Welfare.

17. For example, the cluster GH may lawfully be pronounced as an F at the end of a word, but never at the beginning. The vowel cluster EIGH, pronounced /ā/ (/ej/), may occur in initial, medial, and final positions, and does so with nearly equal distribution. These cases account for all but two occurrences of the cluster in English orthography. A good example of regularity influenced by environment is [c] in a medial position before *t* plus a vowel. It is always pronounced /S/ (*social, ancient, judicious*).

18. E. J. Gibson, A. D. Pick, H. Osser, M. Hammond, *Am. J. Psychol.* 75, 554 (1962).

19. E. J. Gibson, H. Osser, A. D. Pick, *J. Verbal Learning Verbal Behav.* 2, 142 (1963).

20. E. J. Gibson, C. H. Bishop, W. Schiff, J. Smith, *J. Exp. Psychol.* 67, 173 (1964).

21. G. A. Miller and S. Isard, *J. Verbal Learning Verbal Behav.* 2, 217 (1963); also L. E. Marks and G. A. Miller, *ibid.* 3, 1 (1964).

AUDITORY-VISUAL INTEGRATION IN NORMAL AND RETARDED READERS

HERBERT G. BIRCH, M.D., Ph.D. and LILLIAN BELMONT, Ph.D.

Department of Pediatrics, Albert Einstein College of Medicine, New York, New York

FOR THE STUDENT of behavioral and adaptive organization, an important step in understanding the evolution of the nervous system has been the recognition of mechanisms used by organisms in integrating information arriving as inputs from the different sensory modalities. The capacity to assimilate and organize such multimodal information underlies the higher organism's ability to exhibit behavioral plasticity, as well as to modulate and modify its behavior. Potentially, it frees the organism from the stereotypy and fixity of response that characterizes lower forms of life.[4, 16] The evolutionary process was characterized succinctly by Sir Charles Sherrington[17] when he said:

"The naive would have expected evolution in its course to have supplied us with more various sense organs for ampler perception of the world. . . . The policy has rather been to bring by the nervous system the so-called 'five' into closer touch with one another. . . . A central clearing house of sense has grown up. . . . Not new senses, but better liaison between old senses is what the developing nervous system has in this respect stood for."

When applied to the analysis of mechanisms underlying normal and aberrant behavior, this principle, deriving from comparative neurophysiology and comparative psychology, has in earlier studies led us to explore the development of intermodal equivalence in normal children[7] and to analyze disturbances of intersensory integration in neurologically damaged persons.[5, 6] It is this principle that the present study applies to children with reading disability.

We are in complete accord with the view that children with reading disabil-

---

This report is based on research supported in part by the National Institute of Health, NINDB, Grant No. B3362, and grants from The Association for the Aid of Crippled Children and the National Association for Retarded Children.

We wish to thank the members of Obstetric Medicine Research Unit (MRC) of the University of Aberdeen, Scotland, and the educational authority of that city for their indispensable assistance in making this study possible. The specific investigation is one part of a broader co-operative program for the study of social and biological factors in child development.

AMERICAN JOURNAL OF ORTHOPSYCHIATRY, 1964, Vol. 34., pp. 852-861.

ity do not constitute a single homogeneous group.[14] Different individuals may derive their learning inadequacy from biological, social and emotional circumstances. Nevertheless, we thought it worth-while to test the suggestion previously advanced by one of us[3] that one among the several possible causes for subnormality in learning to read could be a primary inadequacy in the ability to integrate auditory and visual stimuli. We therefore tested the explicit hypothesis that impairment in auditory-visual integration would occur more commonly in a group of children with reading retardation than it would in normal agemate controls.

In the course of an epidemiologic study of Scottish school children, intermodal equivalence between auditory and visual stimuli was examined in children with significant degrees of reading retardation. The child's ability to interrelate auditory and visual stimuli was studied by a method of equivalence.[11,12]

The demand made was the identification of a visual dot pattern that corresponded to the patterning of a rhythmic auditory stimulus. The relationship explored, therefore, was between a temporally structured set of auditory stimuli and a spatially distributed set of visual ones.

The specific task for the subject was an auditory-visual pattern test developed in our laboratories. Auditory test items used and visual stimuli from which selections were made are in FIGURE 1.

Taps were sounded with a half-second pause between short intervals and a one-second pause between long intervals. The visual stimuli were covered during the tapping. The three visual patterns from which the specific selection was to be made were exposed immediately after the presentation of the auditory stimulus. A stencil was used, so that on any exposure only the portions of the sheet containing the specific set of visual dot patterns appropriate to the given auditory presentation were exposed.

AUDITORY TAP PATTERNS	VISUAL STIMULI		
EXAMPLES			
A • •	• •	• •	• • •
B • • •	• • •	• • •	• • •
C • • •	• • •	• • •	• • •
TEST ITEMS			
1 • • • •	• • • •	• • • •	• • • •
2 • • • •	• • • •	• • • •	• • • •
3 • • • • •	• • • • •	• • • • •	• • • • •
4 • • • •	• • • •	• • • • •	• • • •
5 • • • • • •	• • • • • •	• • • • • •	• • • • • •
6 • • • • •	• • • • •	• • • • •	• • • • •
7 • • • • • •	• • • • • •	• • • • • •	• • • • • •
8 • • • • • • •	• • • • • • •	• • • • • • •	• • • • • • •
9 • • • • • •	• • • • • •	• • • • • •	• • • • • •
10 • • • • • •	• • • • • •	• • • • • •	• • • • • •

FIGURE 1. Auditory and visual test stimuli. Large and small spaces represent approximate time intervals of 1 sec. and 0.5 sec., respectively. Correct choices were not underlined on the test forms.

131

The following testing procedure was followed: The subject and examiner were seated at opposite sides of the examining table facing one another. The examiner said: "I am going to tap out some patterns. Listen." Using the edge of the table and a pencil, the Examiner tapped out the examples, a, b, and c (Figure 1), pausing from 3 to 5 seconds between examples.

The subject was then shown the response sheet containing the visual dot patterns and told: "Each pattern you hear is going to be like one of the dot patterns you see here." Examiner points to sheet. "Let me show you, Listen!" The examiner once again tapped out example a and this time showed the subject the visual dot item. The examiner then asked the subject, "Which one of these did you hear?" Simultaneously, and independently of the subject's answer, the examiner pointed to the three items and showed the subject the correct choice, saying, "It's this one."

For the next two examples, b and c, the examiner said, "Listen again, and then you show me which one you heard." In each instance, the examiner tapped the pattern and asked, "Which one is it?" If the subject made the correct choice, he was told, "That's right." If the subject made an incorrect choice, the examiner said, "No, it's this one," and pointed to the correct choice. Following the three examples, the ten test items were given.

The subject was told: "Listen carefully and pick out the dots which look like the taps you hear." Following this, the specific multiple-choice item containing the choice appropriate for the given auditory pattern was shown to the subject. Only first choices were accepted, and no changes in response were permitted.

The subjects were retarded and normal readers drawn from the total population of school children in the city of Aberdeen, Scotland, who had been born in 1953. At the time of the present study all of these children were between 9 years, 4 months and 10 years, 4 months of age. Six months prior to the present study, all children in the city's public, private and parochial schools, representing 99.87 per cent of the total number of children in this birth year, were tested for reading abilities with the co-operation of the educational authority. The tests used for assessing reading skills were a British sentence reading test, Form N.S. 6, published by the National Foundation for Educational Research in England and Wales, and three parts of the American Metropolitan Achievement Test, Elementary Battery, Form B, Test 1, Word Knowledge, Test 2, Word Discrimination, and Test 3, Reading. All tests were given in the classroom by standardized procedures.

To eliminate sex differences, which have been shown to exist in reading retardation,[2] and because reading disturbance is significantly more frequent in boys than in girls, only boys were used in the present study. The distributions from which the children were drawn excluded all mentally subnormal children and consisted of children whose IQ was greater than 80.

The two groups that were compared were as follows:

1. Retarded readers. The retarded reader group was defined as the 173 boys in the 1953 birth year whose raw

scores were at the lowest 10 per cent level on at least three out of four of the reading tests. From these, 150 children were chosen randomly for the auditory-visual equivalence study.

2. *Normal readers.* The comparison group was made up of boys in the same birth year but not in the lowest 10 per cent of readers. Fifty subjects were chosen on a random basis from the 173 children who had been matched to the poor readers on the basis of birth date, sex and school class. Age distributions for both groups are presented in TABLE 1. The groups do not differ significantly in age.

The examiners had no knowledge of the reading group to which the child tested belonged.

The mean reading raw scores on all four tests for both groups are given in TABLE 2. It can be seen that differences in ability between the two groups on each of the four reading tests are significant at better than the .001 level of

confidence. Intelligence test data are available on all subjects and will be considered in connection with the analysis of results.

RESULTS

To test the hypothesis that impairment in auditory-visual integration would be more commonly found in a group of intellectually normal children with reading retardation than in age-mate controls having more adequate reading skill, the number of correct responses on the auditory-visual pattern test made by the subjects in each of the two reading groups were compared. The findings (TABLE 3 and FIGURE 2), indicate that the retarded readers had a lower mean number of correct responses and that the obtained difference between the two groups is statistically significant at better than the .001 level of confidence. This finding suggests that the group of poor readers dealt less effectively with a task requiring judgments of auditory and visual equivalence. In addition to the highly significant difference obtained between mean group performances, the distributions presented in FIGURE 2 indicate, that whereas only 14 per cent of the retarded readers made one error or less on the auditory-visual pattern test (achieved scores of 9 and 10), over 40 per cent of the normal readers did so.

The relationship of auditory-visual test score to reading test performance is expressed for normal readers in TABLE 4 and for retarded readers in TABLE 5. In these tables the mean raw scores on the four reading tests are contrasted for those children who made correct judgments on five or less of the auditory-visual pattern test items (A-V 0-5 Correct; with those who made correct judg-

TABLE 1

AGE DISTRIBUTIONS FOR RETARDED AND NORMAL READERS

Age in years and months	Number of subjects	
	Retarded readers (N=150)	Normal readers (N=50)
10-4	3	0
10-3	11	1
10-2	13	2
10-1	13	8
10-0	15	4
9-11	18	4
9-10	11	7
9-9	11	4
9-8	5	3
9-7	9	3
9-6	13	4
9-5	19	5
9-4	9	5
Mean Age	9 yrs. 10 mos.	9 yrs. 9 mos.
S.D.	0 yrs. 3.6 mos.	0 yrs. 3.3 mos.

ments on six or more of the test items (A-V 6-10 Correct). For both groups of subjects, those who had lower A-V scores also had lower mean reading scores on all four reading tests. On three of the reading tests (Word Knowledge, Word Discrimination and Reading) there were statistically significant differences in mean scores between those *normal* readers who were respectively poor and good on the auditory-visual pattern test. Similarly, when the reading performances of the group of *retarded* readers is exam-

TABLE 2

COMPARISONS BETWEEN RETARDED AND NORMAL READERS ON THE FOUR READING TESTS

		Group	
Reading test		Retarded readers (N=150)	Normal readers (N=50)
British Reading	M	12.8	24.5
	S.D.	4.0	4.3
		t=17.7;	
		p<.001	
Word Knowledge	M	18.4	36.0
	S.D.	7.9	6.1
		t=14.7;	
		p<.001	
Word Discrimination	M	13.9	28.1
	S.D.	5.6	5.0
		t=16.05;	
		p<.001	
Reading	M	12.7	26.6
	S.D.	4.8	7.5
		t=12.30;*	
		p<.001	

*Since there was a significant difference in the variances, the Cochran correction of the *t*-test was applied.

TABLE 3

SCORES ON THE AUDITORY-VISUAL PATTERN TEST FOR THE RETARDED AND NORMAL READERS

	Mean	S.D.	t	p
Retarded readers (N=150)	5.9	2.3		
			3.42	<.001
Normal readers (N=50)	7.2	2.5		

ined (TABLE 5), all four mean reading scores are lower for the poor A-V subjects than for the good A-V subjects, with the difference in mean scores statistically significant for the British Reading Test and for Word Knowledge. Therefore, a low score on the auditory-visual pattern test not only served to distinguish retarded from normal readers, but within each of these groups tended to identify those with lower reading scores.

Since it is well known[10] that retarded readers tend to have lower IQ's than do normal readers, it was considered necessary to analyze the findings with respect to general intellectual level. This analysis could be readily carried out since IQ test scores were available* for the 200 children. The relevant data are presented in TABLES 6 and 7.

The normal readers did in fact achieve a significantly higher mean IQ than did the poor readers (p < .001). However, when the IQ data for each of the reading ability groups are analyzed in relation to auditory-visual test performance, it is found that the relationship is not direct or simple. Those children who functioned poorly on the auditory-

*Results were available on a self-administered group test of intelligence (7+ test) for 198 of the 200 subjects of the present study. This intelligence test is administered routinely to all children in the Aberdeen school system after the seventh but before the eighth birthday. At the time of the present study, individual [Wechsler Intelligence Scale for Children (WISC)] tests of intelligence were given each child and the results of such individual testing did not result in any change in the significance of mean IQ differences between the groups.

visual pattern test had the lower mean IQ's independently of whether they were normal or retarded readers. The difference in man IQ for "poor" and "good" A-V groups is statistically significant within both the retarded and the normal reading groups. Further, the retarded readers who are in the good A-V group are not distinguishable in terms of mean IQ (99.7) from the normal readers who fall into the poor A-V group (IQ 99.5).

Since a general relationship between IQ and reading level was found to exist, but two groups with equivalent mean IQ's showed radically different A-V scores, it seemed necessary to clarify further the relationship between auditory-visual functioning and reading performance. We therefore have analyzed the auditory-visual test performance of both retarded readers and normal readers by studying only those members of both groups whose IQ was 100 or above. At IQ 100 it would be expected that the children had the general intellectual ability necessary for learning to read with normal facility. The data in TABLE 8, on children with IQ's of 100 or more, indicate that the original difference between retarded readers and normal readers in auditory-visual ability is sustained. It is clear, then, that, even when lower normal levels of IQ are eliminated, retarded readers as a group deal less effectively with tasks requiring judgments of auditory-visual equivalence than do normal readers.

This finding is reinforced by two additional analyses. When the frequency of the members of each group making eight or more, or six or less, correct auditory-visual judgments is compared (TABLE 9), it is clear that children with IQ's of 100 and over function differently on the

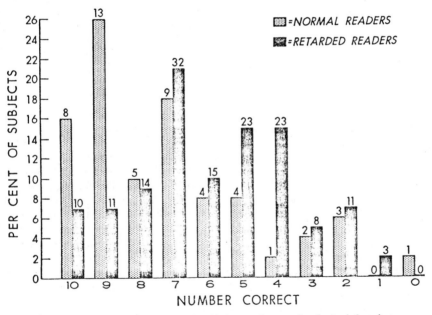

FIGURE 2. Distributions of auditory-visual judgments in normal and retarded readers.

135

auditory-visual pattern test in accordance with their reading skill (chi^2 = 2.893; p < .05, one-tailed).

When the IQ's obtained on the WISC are correlated with auditory-visual test performance for the entire group of both retarded and normal readers (TABLE 10), the correlation coefficients although significant are low and at a maximum account for less than 15 per cent of the variance. These findings make it clear that the relation of auditory-visual test performance to reading cannot be accounted for by IQ differences. Further, when the Full Scale IQ

obtained on the WISC, a nonreading individual test of intelligence, is correlated with auditory-visual test performance in the low A-V portion of the retarded reading group, zero order correlations between auditory-visual test performance and general intelligence are obtained. These findings make it clear that the relation of auditory-visual pattern test performance to reading is not a direct function of IQ differences.*

DISCUSSION

Learning to read as an educational task requires the ability to transform temporally distributed auditory patterns into spatially distributed visual ones. Harris[9] has suggested that for the beginning reader "reading is largely concerned with learning to recognize the symbols which represent spoken words." A primary disturbance in the ability to integrate stimuli from the two critical sense modalities, hearing and vision, may well serve to increase the risk of becoming a poor reader. Consequently, one of the characteristics underlying reading readiness as well as some types of reading retardation may be the development of the ability to make judgments of auditory-visual equivalence.

The major finding of the present study was that judgments of auditory-visual equivalence were significantly worse in a group of retarded readers than in normal readers. The analyses strongly suggest that the ability to treat visual and auditory patterned information as equivalent is one of the factors that differentiates good from poor readers. Further, within the groups of normal and retarded readers, the auditory-visual pattern test performances did, in the

TABLE 4

READING SCORES FOR NORMAL READERS WITH GOOD AND POOR AUDITORY-VISUAL ABILITY*

Reading test		Group	
		A-V 0-5 Correct (N = 11)	A-V 6-10 Correct (N = 39)
British Reading Test	M	23.3	24.8
	S.D.	4.5	4.3
		t = 1.03; p < .15	
Word Knowledge	M	31.5	37.3
	S.D.	7.9	4.8
		t = 2.31;** p < .025	
Word Discrimination	M	26.0	28.9
	S.D.	6.3	4.5
		t = 1.74; p < .05	
Reading	M	21.8	27.9
	S.D.	8.7	6.7
		t = 2.50; p < .01	

*One-tailed tests applied because of the directional nature of the hypothesis.

**Since there was a significant difference in the variances, the Cochran correction of the t-test was applied.

*Full analysis of the relation of intellectual pattern to auditory-visual function and to reading ability will be the subject of a separate report.

present investigation, differentiate subjects with lower from those with higher reading scores. These findings make more specific the suggestion of Rabinovitch,[14] that difficulties in integration are the major kinds of difficulty faced by children with primary reading retardation.

The obtained differences in intersensory performance could occur if deficiencies existed in the functioning of either of the sensory modalities. However, audiometric screening did not result in the finding of any children with a significant degree of hearing impairment, and no child in either group had a significant uncorrected visual disturbance. Consequently, it is unlikely that sensory inadequacy as such can account for the findings, although it is of course possible

TABLE 5

READING SCORES FOR RETARDED READERS WITH GOOD AND POOR AUDITORY-VISUAL ABILITY*

Reading test		Group	
		A-V 0–5 Correct (N = 68)	A-V 6–10 Correct (N = 82)
British	M	12.2	13.3
	S.D.	3.9	4.1
		t = 1.711;	
		p < .05	
Word Knowledge	M	17.0	19.6
	S.D.	6.9	8.5
		t = 2.08;	
		p < .025	
Word Discrimination	M	13.7	14.1
	S.D.	5.6	5.7
		t = 1.38;	
		p < .10	
Reading	M	12.3	13.0
	S.D.	5.0	4.7
		t = 0.882;	
		p < .20	

*One-tailed tests applied because of the directional nature of the hypothesis.

that more subtle types of dysfunction in auditory or visual perception might exist.

Since the child was required to identify an appropriate visual pattern after receiving the auditory stimuli, the test-

TABLE 6

MEAN IQ'S OF THE GROUPS STUDIED

	Mean IQ	S.D.
Retarded readers		
Total Group (N = 149)	96.7	10.3
A-V 0–5 Correct (N = 67)	93.1	8.0
A-V 6–10 Correct (N = 82)	99.7	11.0
Normal readers		
Total Group (N = 49)	110.8	11.6
A-V 0–5 Correct (N = 10)	99.5	7.3
A-V 6–10 Correct (N = 39)	113.7	10.7

ing situation involved auditory memory as well as intersensory equivalence per se. As a consequence, poor intersensory performance could derive from defective immediate auditory memory. In the design of the present experiment, control for such memory factors existed in the evidence available on the Digit Span sub-test of the WISC, in which immediate auditory recall is tested. Since no significant difference in such recall scores existed between high and low A-V performers, it is most unlikely that a simple auditory memory deficit underlay the obtained intersensory differences.

It is of interest that there was a relationship between auditory-visual test performance, reading level and IQ. However, when children with low normal IQ were eliminated from consideration, auditory-visual pattern test performance continued to distinguish adequate from inadequate readers. Nevertheless, the significant general relationship between auditory-visual integrative ability and IQ suggested that this type of intersensory integration in its more complex and general form may be one of the processes that underlies adaptive behavior and thus IQ. In other words, one might hypothesize that those persons who are able to perceive and integrate more of the multimodal inputs are more likely to be the more "intelligent" individuals.

TABLE 7

SIGNIFICANCE LEVELS FOR MEAN IQ COMPARISONS

	t	p
Retarded readers vs. normal readers	8.06	< .001
A-V 0–5 vs. A-V 6–10 (Retarded readers)	4.26*	< .001
A-V 0–5 vs. A-V 6–10 (Normal readers)	3.94	< .001

*Since there was a significant difference in the variances, the Cochran correction of the t-test was applied.

Although our results for the retarded readers and the normal readers on the auditory-visual pattern test clearly distinguished between the two groups, it would be incorrect to assume that the ability adequately to judge auditory-visual equivalences is the sole factor underlying reading incompetence. There was overlap between groups in auditory-visual test performance so that some individuals who were normal readers had difficulty with the auditory-visual task. Also, some individuals who were poor readers had little difficulty in coping with the demand to translate auditory into visual information. Moreover, although, among normal readers, those with the lower auditory-visual test performance had the lower reading scores, they were still significantly better readers than were the poor readers with adequate ability to judge auditory-visual equivalences. Our findings therefore suggest that for certain individuals an incapacity in auditory-visual equivalence is only one factor underlying poor reading.

TABLE 8

AUDITORY-VISUAL FUNCTIONING IN RETARDED AND NORMAL READERS WITH IQ'S OF 100 AND OVER

	A-V Scores			
Group	Mean	S.D.	t	p*
Retarded readers (N=53)	7.1	2.4		
			2.39	< .01
Normal readers (N=35)	8.2	1.7		

*One-tailed test applied because of the directional nature of the hypothesis.

TABLE 9

NUMBER OF SUBJECTS WITH IQ'S OF 100 AND ABOVE IN RELATION TO AUDITORY-VISUAL TEST GROUPS

	Auditory Visual Pattern Test	
	6 or fewer correct	8 or more correct
Poor readers (N=42)	15	27
Normal readers (N=28)	4	24
Chi²=2.893 P*<.05		

*One-tailed test because of the directional nature of the hypothesis.

Other studies have indicated that emotional disturbances,[8] cultural deprivation,[15] disturbances in lateralization of function[13] and other indicators of neurologic dysfunction may also be related to the production of reading retardation. Whether these associations represent mechanisms for reading retardation or represent parallel disturbances is as yet unclear.[1] The inability to integrate auditory and visual stimuli, however, appears to have specific relevance to learning to read and appears to be one of the several factors that contribute to reading disability.

TABLE 10

PRODUCT-MOMENT COEFFICIENTS OF CORRELATION BETWEEN AUDITORY-VISUAL SCORE AND WISC IQ FOR NORMAL AND RETARDED READERS

($N = 200$)

	r
A-V vs. Full Scale IQ	.38
A-V vs. Verbal IQ	.27
A-V vs. Performance IQ	.30

SUMMARY

The relation of auditory-visual integration to reading retardation was studied in 200 children nine and ten years of age. One hundred and fifty were retarded readers and 50 were normal readers. The retarded readers were significantly less able to make judgments of auditory-visual equivalence than were the normal readers. Within the two groups of readers, those children with lower auditory-visual performance tended to have the lower reading scores. When children with low normal IQ were eliminated from consideration, the significant difference in auditory-visual test performance between the retarded and normal readers was sustained. The findings were interpreted to indicate that the development of auditory-visual integration has specific relevance to reading, although it is not the sole factor underlying reading incompetence.

REFERENCES

1. BELMONT, L. AND H. G. BIRCH. 1963. Lateral dominance and right-left awareness in normal children. Child Develop. 34(2): 257-270.
2. BENTZEN, F. 1963. Sex ratios in learning and behavior disorders. Amer. J. Orthopsychiat. 33(1): 92-98.
3. BIRCH, H. G. 1962. Dyslexia and the maturation of visual function. In Reading Disability, J. Money, Ed. The Johns Hopkins Press. Baltimore.
4. ———. 1954. Comparative psychology. In Areas of Psychology, F. L. Marcuse, Ed. Harper & Bros. New York.
5. BIRCH, H. G., I. BELMONT, T. REILLY AND L. BELMONT, 1962. Somesthetic influences on the perception of visual verticality in hemiplegia. Arch. Phys. Med. 43(11): 556-560.
6. ———. 1961. Visual verticality in hemiplegia. Arch. Neurol. 5(4): 444-453.
7. BIRCH, H. G. AND A. LEFFORD. 1963. Intersensory development in children. Monogr. Soc. Res. Child Develop. 28 (5).
8. BLANCHARD, P. 1946. Psychoanalytic contributions to the problem of reading disabilities. In Psychoanal. Stud. Child, Vol. 2. International Universities Press. New York. : 163.
9. HARRIS, A. J. 1948. How to Increase Reading Ability, 2nd ed. Longmans, Green. New York. : 9.
10. KAWI, A. A. AND B. PASAMANICK. 1959. Prenatal and paranatal factors in the development of childhood reading disorders. Monogr. Soc. Res. Child Develop. 24(4).
11. KLÜVER, H. 1933. Behavior Mechanisms in Monkeys. University of Chicago Press. Chicago.
12. ———. 1936. The study of personality and the method of equivalent and nonequivalent stimuli. Character and Personality. 5(2): 91-112.
13. ORTON, S. T. 1937. Reading, Writing and Speech Problems in Children. W. W. Norton & Co. New York.
14. RABINOVITCH, R. D., A. L. DREW, R. DeJONG, W. INGRAM AND L. WITHEY. 1954. A research approach to reading retardation. In Neurology and Psychiatry in Childhood. Williams & Wilkins. Baltimore.
15. RIESSMAN, F. 1962. The Culturally Deprived Child. Harper & Bros. New York.
16. SCHNEIRLA, R. C. 1962. Comparative psychology. Encyclopaedia Britannica. 18: 690Q-703.
17. SHERRINGTON, C. S. 1951. Man on His Nature. Cambridge University Press. Cambridge, Eng. : 287-289.

SECTION VI

CHILD NEUROSIS

SCHOOL PHOBIA:

RAPID TREATMENT OF FIFTY CASES [1]

WALLACE A. KENNEDY

Human Development Clinic, Florida State University

School phobia, a dramatic and puzzling emotional crisis, has attracted considerable attention for a number of years. Phobias in general are the subjects of widely differing theories of dynamics and treatment. The controversy regarding the treatment of children's phobias dates from the earliest case studies presented by Freud (1909), continues through the laboratory demonstrations of Watson and Jones (Jones, 1924) to the more recent experimental treatment of Wolpe (1954). There have been five broad reviews since the earliest paper presented by Johnson et al. in 1941: Klein (1945), Waldfogel, Cooledge, and Hahn (1957), Kahn (1958), Glasser (1959), and Sperling (1961). These reviews in the main support the contention that the major weight of evidence thus far leans toward the psychoanalytic interpretation of phobias, while the work of Wolpe is more consistent with the approach presented herein.

The psychoanalytic theory stresses the role of the mother in the development of school phobia. A close symbiotic relationship, which displays itself in an overdependency, is present between the mother and child. Stemming from an unsatisfactory relationship with her own mother, the mother finds it difficult to cope with her own emotional needs. The father often is in a competing role with the mother, and seems to try to outdo her in little tasks around the home: in trying to strengthen his own image, he depreciates that of the mother. He too overidentifies with the child. Thus, the emotional climate of his family prevents the child from ever finding out whether or not he, of his own volition, can solve problems. Possessive, domineering parents tend to make the child's growth toward independence difficult. His guilt regarding his own impulses is transformed into depression: the anxiety can reach extreme proportions.

On the other hand, Wolpe sees the phobia as a learned reaction, which he treats through direct symptom attack with what he calls reciprocal inhibition, or desensitization.

Interest in the school phobia problem, which occurs at the rate of 17 cases per thousand school-age children per year, has been greatly intensified in the past few years. An extremely significant advance was made by Cooledge and the Judge Baker group in 1957, when they presented evidence that there were not one, but two types of school phobia, which, although sharing a common group of symptoms, differed widely in others. These are referred to as Type 1 School Phobia, or the neurotic crisis, and Type 2 School Phobia, or the way-of-life phobia. The common symptoms are: (*a*) Morbid fears associated with school attendance; a vague dread of disaster; (*b*) Frequent somatic complaints: headaches, nausea, drowsiness; (*c*) Symbiotic relationship with mother, fear of separation: anxiety about many things: darkness, crowds, noises; (*d*) Conflict between parents and the school administration.

At the Human Development Clinic of Florida State University, 10 differential symp-

[1] The research reported herein was supported through the Human Development Clinic of Florida State University, Tallahassee, Florida.

JOURNAL OF ABNORMAL PSYCHOLOGY, 1965, Vol. 70., pp. 285-289.

toms between Type 1 and Type 2 School Phobia have been determined. A differential diagnosis can be made logically and empirically on the basis of any 7 of the 10.

Ten Differential School Phobia Symptoms

Type 1

_1. The present illness is the first episode.
2. Monday onset, following an illness the previous Thursday or Friday.
3. An acute onset.
4. Lower grades most prevalent.
5. Expressed concern about death.
6. Mother's physical health in question: actually ill or child thinks so.
7. Good communication between parents.
8. Mother and father well adjusted in most areas.
9. Father competitive with mother in household management.
10. Parents achieve understanding of dynamics easily.

Type 2

1. Second, third, or fourth episo.ic.
2. Monday onset following minor illness not a prevalent antecedent.
3. Incipient onset.
4. Upper grades most prevalent.
5. Death theme not present.
6. Health of mother not an issue.
7. Poor communication between parents.
8. Mother shows neurotic behavior; father, a character disorder.
9. Father shows little interest in household or children.
10. Parents very difficult to work with.

PROBLEM

In the Fall of 1957 the Clinic embarked upon an experimental procedure for the treatment of Type 1 School Phobia—a procedure similar to that of Rodriguez, Rodriguez, and Eisenberg (1959) with one major exception: whereas Rodriguez made no distinction between types of school phobia and treated in the same manner all cases which came to the clinic, the 50 cases reported herein were selected on the basis of the criteria mentioned above. The Florida State University Human Development Clinic, as a teaching and research clinic, does not generally see deeply disturbed children, but refers them to other agencies.

In the 8-year period covered by the report, there have been 6 cases which would meet the criteria of Type 2 School Phobia. These 6 cases were treated by supportive therapy for the children and parents. None of the 6 Type 2 cases had more than three of the 10 Type 1 criteria, and the results were completely dissimilar to those reported for the 50 Type 1 cases. All of the Type 2 cases were chronic in nature. All had family histories of one or more parents seriously disturbed. Two of the cases were diagnosed as having schizophrenia; 2 were diagnosed as having character disorders with the school phobia being a minor aspect of the case. One of the 6 was hospitalized; 1 was sent to a training school. Of the 4 remaining, 2 were able to go to college, although their records were poor and their symptoms continued. These 6 cases were in treatment for an average of 10 months. In no circumstances was a school phobia case changed from Type 1 to Type 2, or vice versa.

This experimental procedure with Type 1 School Phobia was begun with considerable caution, with only 1 case in 1957 and 2 the following Spring. The treatment involved the application of broad learning theory concepts by blocking the escape of the child and preventing secondary gains from occurring. In addition, the child was reinforced for

TABLE 1

YEAR OF TREATMENT AND SEX OF 50 TYPE ONE SCHOOL PHOBIA CASES

Year	Male	Female	Total
1957	1	0	1
1958	1	1	2
1959	4	2	6
1960	4	8	12
1961	6	3	9
1962	5	4	9
1963	4	5	9
1964	0	2	2
Total	25	25	50

TABLE 2

SYMPTOM CHECKLIST AND SEX OF 50 TYPE ONE SCHOOL PHOBIA CASES

Symptom	Male	Female	Total
1. First attack	25	25	50
2. Monday onset—Thursday illness	24	25	49
3. Acute onset	25	23	48
4. Lower grades	22	18	40
5. Death theme	22	22	44
6. Mother's health an issue	23	21	44
7. Good parental marital harmony	24	23	47
8. Good parental mental health	23	24	47
9. Father helper in the house	21	21	42
10. Parents achieve insight quickly	24	25	49

TABLE 3

AGE AND SEX OF 50 TYPE ONE SCHOOL PHOBIA CASES

Age	Male	Female	Total
4	0	1	1
5	3	1	4
6	2	3	5
7	3	2	5
8	3	1	4
9	3	5	8
10	4	3	7
11	1	2	3
12	3	0	3
13	2	4	6
14	1	2	3
15	0	0	0
16	0	1	1
Total	25	25	50

going to school without complaint. This rapid treatment procedure has now been followed with 50 cases.

Subject Population

Subjects for the 50 cases over an 8-year period were school-age children, all suffering from the first evidence of a phobic attack, from the geographical area served by the Human Development Clinic of Florida State University. The subject distribution by year and sex is illustrated in Table 1, by symptom and sex in Table 2, by age and sex in Table 3, and by grade and sex in Table 4.

The fathers' mean age for the male subjects was 36; the mothers', 35. For the female subjects the fathers' mean age was 38; the mothers', 36. The boys' mean age was 9; that of the girls', 10. There was no definite pattern in birth order of the subjects, or in number of siblings.

Method and Results

During the course of the past 8 years, 50 cases of Type 1 School Phobia have been treated. Five of these cases might be considered semicontrols because they were untreated Type 1 cases of some duration, or they were Type 1 cases unsuccessfully treated elsewhere before they were seen at the clinic. One of these semicontrol cases had been out of school for 1 year, and the other 4 had been out for over 3 months.

All 50 of the cases responded to the treatment program with a complete remission of the school phobia symptoms, and follow-up study indicates no evidence of any outbreaks of substitute symptoms or recurrence of the phobia.

In the follow-up schedule the parents were phoned in about 2 weeks, and again in 6 weeks, to see if the progress had continued. They were then phoned on a yearly basis, except in 1961, when follow-up interviews were conducted reaching 19 of the 21 cases completed at that time. During the course of the 8 years, 6 families were lost because

of moving with no forwarding address. Of these lost cases, none had been followed less than 2 years, 2 were followed 3 years, and 1 for 4 years.

RAPID TREATMENT PROCEDURE

The rapid treatment program for Type 1 school phobia involves six essential components: good professional public relations, avoidance of emphasis on somatic complaints, forced school attendance, structured interview with parents, brief interview with child, and follow-up.

Good Professional Public Relations

It is necessary to establish good communication with schools, physicians, and parent groups, such that the cases are likely referred on the second or third day of the phobic attack. This groundwork involves the typical mental health consultation and case-by-case follow-up with the referring source.

Avoidance of Emphasis on Somatic Complaints

If phobic qualities predominate, that is, if the child conforms to seven of the differential symptoms of Type 1 School Phobia, emphasis on somatic complaints should be avoided. For instance, the child's somatic complaints should be handled matter-of-factly, with an appointment to see the pediatrician after school hours. Abdominal pains will probably require the pediatrician to make a prompt physical examination, but this can probably be done on the way to school.

TABLE 4

GRADE AND SEX OF 50 TYPE ONE SCHOOL PHOBIA CASES

Grade	Male	Female	Total
Nursery School	0	2	2
Kindergarten	4	0	4
First	4	4	8
Second	0	1	1
Third	6	4	10
Fourth	3	4	7
Fifth	2	2	4
Sixth	3	1	4
Seventh	2	2	4
Eighth	0	2	2
Ninth	1	2	3
Tenth	0	1	1
Total	25	25	50

Forced School Attendance

It is essential to be able to require the child to go to school and to be willing to use any force necessary. In all of the present cases, simply convincing the parents of this necessity and having them come to a firm decision, has generally been enough. The ability to be decisive when necessary has been essential.

Have the father take the child to school. These fathers are not unkind, and they can show authority when necessary.

Have the principal or attendance officer take an active part in keeping the child in the room.

Allow the mother to stand in the hall, if she must, or to visit the school during the morning, but not to stay.

Structured Interview with the Parents

Stressing the following points, conduct with the parents a structured interview designed to give them sufficient confidence to carry out the therapeutic program even in the face of considerable resistance from the child.

Lead the interview. The confidence of the parents is greatly increased by the interviewer's verifying the history rather than taking it. Correctly anticipating 7 out of 10 variables within a family structure is well calculated to induce full cooperation.

Be optimistic. Stressing the transient nature, the dependable sequence of a difficult Monday, a somewhat better Tuesday, and a symptom-free Wednesday, tends to lighten the depression of the parents regarding their child's unwillingness to go to school.

Emphasize success. Type 1 cases always recover. Ninety percent of the Type 1 phobics stay at school most of the first day. Along with optimism comes a slight mobilization of hostility which helps the parents to follow the plan.

Present the formula. Simply but directly, with repetition for emphasis, outline a plan for the parents to follow, assuming that it is the end of the school week by the time of the referral and that the interview with the parents is conducted on Thursday or Friday.

Parent Formula

Do not discuss in any way, school attendance over the weekend. There is nothing a phobic child does better than talk about going to school. Don't discuss going to school. Don't discuss phobic symptoms. Simply tell the child Sunday evening, "Well, son, tomorrow you go back to school."

On Monday morning get the child up, dressed, and ready for school. Give the child a light breakfast to reduce the nausea problem. Have the father take the child matter-of-factly off to school. Don't ask him how he feels, or why he is afraid to go to school, or why he doesn't like school. Simply take him to school, turn him over to the school authorities, and go home.

If the child therapist has not seen the child the previous week, he may see him after school on the first day.

On Monday evening, compliment the child on going to school and staying there, no matter how resistant he has been, no matter how many times he has vomited, cried, or started to leave. If he has been at school for 30 minutes on Monday, progress is being made. Tell the child Monday evening that Tuesday will be much better, and make no further mention of the symptom.

Tuesday can be expected to be a repetition of Monday, but with everything toned down considerably. On Tuesday evening, encourage and compliment the child strongly for doing so much better.

Wednesday should be virtually symptom free. Wednesday evening, with considerable fanfare, give a party for the child in honor of his having overcome his problem.

Brief Interview with the Child

The child himself should be seen only briefly by the child therapist and only after school hours. The content of the interview should be stories which stress the advantage of going on in the face of fear: how student pilots need to get back into the air quickly after an accident, and how important it is to get right back on the horse after a fall. In addition the therapist can describe real or imaginary events in his own childhood when he was frightened for awhile but everything turned out all right: all to stress to the child the transitory nature of the phobia.

Follow-Up

Follow-up by phone, being chatty and encouraging and not oversolicitous. In the long-range follow-up, chat with the parents about further school phobia symptoms, incidence of other phobias, school attendance records, academic progress, and the occurrence of other emotional problems in the child.

DISCUSSION

Two legitimate concerns have been expressed regarding preliminary reports at local meetings. The first is a concern about the claim of complete remission for all 50 cases— a claim inconsistent with the usual child guidance clinic success rate—and the consequent belief that the criterion for success is simply too narrow. Only self-report data and reports from school administrations are available regarding the symptom-free nature of these children once this phobic episode has passed. It is true that no diagnostic evaluation has been undertaken with any of these children during follow-up. It must be remembered, however, that the definition of symptom remission is restricted to those obvious symptoms which might conceivably lead the parents or school officials to re-refer the children to the clinic. In this regard, these 50 children in the Type 1 School Phobia group are symptom free.

Because of the nature of the Human Development Clinic and the nature of this project, careful selection has been exercised in accepting cases, as mentioned above. Due to the relationship between the schools and the clinic, and the clear definition of cases suitable for the project, there is reason to believe that the majority of Type 1 School Phobia cases in the five-county area the clinic serves have come to our attention, whereas the local county mental health clinic has received a high percentage of the Type 2 cases. The success of the Type 2 cases of school phobia accepted by the Human Development Clinic for teaching purposes has not been remarkable.

The second concern is that perhaps what is called Type 1 School Phobia is not really a severe phobic attack at all, but borders on malingering of a transient nature which would spontaneously remit in a few days anyway. In fact, because of the apparent sound mental health of the family as a group, its middle-class values which stress school, and the family's good premorbid history, including the academic record of the child, there is little reason to doubt that the majority of the cases would eventually return to school whatever treatment was undertaken. However, our five semicontrol cases and evidence seen from other clinics of Type 1 cases that have been out of school for prolonged periods suggest that this method of treatment may accelerate or facilitate the remission. Recommendation for the use of this technique is, restricted, then, to those cases showing Type 1 symptoms which, in spite of their possible transient nature, present a rather serious problem to teachers, parents, and counselors.

REFERENCES

COOLEDGE, J. C., HAHN, PAULINE B., & PECK, ALICE L. School phobia: Neurotic crisis or way of life. *American Journal of Orthopsychiatry*, 1957, 27, 296–306.

FREUD, S. *Analysis of a phobia in a five-year-old boy*. Std. Ed., New York: W. W. Norton, 1909.

GLASSER, K. Problems in school attendance: School phobia and related conditions. *Pediatrics*, 1959, 55, 758. (Abstract)

JOHNSON, A. M., et al. School phobia: A study of five cases. *American Journal of Orthopsychiatry*, 1941, 11, 702. (Abstract)

JONES, M. C. A laboratory study of fear: The case of Peter. *Journal of Genetic Psychology*, 1924, 31, 308–315.

KAHN, J. H. School refusal—some clinical and cultural aspects. *Medical Officer*, 1958, 100, 337. (Abstract)

KLEIN, E. The reluctance to go to school. *Psychoanalytic Study of the Child*, 1945, 1, 263. (Abstract)

RODRIGUEZ, A., RODRIGUEZ, MARIA, & EISENBERG, L. The outcome of school phobia: A follow-up study based on 41 cases. *American Journal of Psychiatry*, 1959, 116, 540–544.

SPERLING, M. Analytic first aid in school phobias. *Psychoanalytic Quarterly*, 1961, 30, 504. (Abstract)

WALDFOGEL, S., COOLEDGE, J. C., & HAHN, P. B. Development, meaning and management of school phobia. *American Journal of Orthopsychiatry*, 1957, 27, 754. (Abstract)

WOLPE, J. Reciprocal inhibition as the main basis of psychotherapeutic effects. *A.M.A. Archive of Neurology and Psychiatry*, 1954, 72, 204–226.

ETIOLOGY AND COVARIATION OF OBSTINACY, ORDERLINESS, AND PARSIMONY IN YOUNG CHILDREN

E. M. HETHERINGTON

University of Wisconsin

and YVONNE BRACKBILL

University of Colorado Medical School

In a paper first published in 1908, Freud (9) hypothesized a relation between "anal eroticism" and a cluster of personality traits—obstinacy, orderliness, and parsimony. His observations led him to propose that these traits develop as unchanged perpetuations of anal erotic activities, as sublimations of such activities, and as reaction formations against them. Subsequently, Brill (6), Jones (11), Freud (10), Abraham (1), Menninger (12), and other psychoanalytic writers have elaborated and further specified the behavioral manifestations of these basic traits. Orderliness is said to be expressed in bodily cleanliness, propriety, tidiness, punctuality, a preference for symmetry rather than asymmetry, and reliability and conscientiousness in the performance of minor duties. Obstinacy is manifested in stubbornness, passive aggression, and ritualistic persistence. Parsimony is shown through miserliness and irrational attitudes toward money, acquisitiveness, avarice, cupidity, and hoarding.

Even in his earliest account, Freud indicated his belief that the three character traits are not of equal importance in the whole complex. According to him, parsimony and obstinacy are more basic to and closely related

CHILD DEVELOPMENT, 1963, Vol. 34., pp. 919-943.

in the anal character. Orderliness he saw as the least "constant element" in the complex.

Subsequent developments in psychoanalytic theory attempted to account for individual differences in the extent to which these traits developed. It was postulated that the extent of development is determined by libidinal fixation during the anal erotic period, which in turn is determined by the time and method of toilet training. Freud states, "The anal-erotic drives meet in infancy with the training for cleanliness, and the way in which this training is carried out determines whether or not anal fixations result. The training may be too early, too late, too strict, too libidinous" (7, p. 305).

Two basic questions have been investigated by psychologists concerned with the validity of analytic formulations about "anal" character traits. The first is whether the three traits covary. If individual A is more parsimonious than individual B, is he also more obstinate and more orderly? The second question is more difficult to answer than the first and is logically separable from it. It concerns the etiology of these traits. Can toilet training experiences be singled out from all other antecedent events as the one most probable cause of parsimony, obstinacy, and orderliness? If they can, will the degree of these traits be directly related to dimensions of toilet training such as severity?

A few studies have focused on the question of trait covariation. Sears (14) found significant positive intercorrelations among ratings of obstinacy, orderliness, and parsimony in fraternity men. Barnes (2) had male college students rate themselves on a list of adjectives selected to be representative of the oral, anal, and phallic stages. The ratings were then factor analyzed. Two factors were found which could be interpreted in terms of anal traits. The first factor contained loadings on orderliness, cleanliness, reliability, and obedience with respect to the law. A second factor included parsimony, resentfulness, and sadism. Barnes found the remaining six factors impossible to interpret in terms of levels of psychosexual development. Finally, G. M. Rapaport (13), using both self-rating scales and TAT protocols, found intertrait correlations that were in the predicted direction but nonsignificant. A methodological difference of possible importance between this and the preceding two studies—both of which found positive evidence of trait covariation—was Rapaport's use of female as well as male Ss.

Other studies have been primarily concerned with the question of the etiology of obstinacy, orderliness, and parsimony. Bernstein (4) studied the possible relation of coercive toilet training to various personality and behavioral characteristics in 5-year old children. Toilet training data was obtained from medical reports and from an interview with the mother. Information about the child was obtained from observation, a play interview, and the mother's interview. The results offered little empirical support for the psychoanalytic theoretical account of etiology. Coercive toilet training was not related to frequency of constipation, tendency to collect things, finger painting test scores, or to cold cream smearing test scores. It was, however, positively related to negativism, separation anxiety, and lack of spontaneous communication. Beloff (3), using male and female undergraduates, found no relation between anal traits and age of completing bowel training, as reported by the students' mothers. A significant relation was found between anality scores for mothers and offspring on Beloff's 28-item questionnaire.

This finding suggests an alternative explanation of causative factors in the development of obstinacy, orderliness, and parsimony. The processes of identification with the parent and of direct learning via rewards and punishments administered by the parents may be more influential in the formation of these personality traits than are any factors exclusively connected with bowel training. If a correlation should exist between toilet training and the subsequent appearance of certain behaviors in the child, it may be because toilet training is one of many situations in which the child must learn to behave as his parents demand. Such a relation could be due to parental behaviors that are repetitively displayed in a great range of socialization situations. The possibility that toilet training is the first real struggle for dominance may add to its importance, but the fact that it is followed by many other lengthy campaigns of consequence—bedtime, eating, control of aggression, etc.—detracts from the singularity of its influence. A dimension of parental behavior which would be repeatedly manifested in a variety of these socialization situations would be parental dominance, the extent to which the parent demands of the child complete conformity, unconditional surrender in each consecutive struggle.

The present study is concerned with both trait[1] covariation and the etiology of obstinacy, orderliness, and parsimony. Young children were used as Ss, to avoid the distortions that frequently occur when bright, sophisticated college students are asked to reveal themselves on paper and pencil tests. Behavioral situations were used to obtain measures of obstinacy, orderliness, and parsimony. These measures required a minimum of indirect, inferential interpretation and were closely representative of the sorts of behaviors to which the personality constructs refer.

METHOD

Subjects

The study began with 48 5-year old kindergarten children enrolled at a nursery school in Newark, New Jersey. Thirteen Ss were discarded because they did not complete all tasks or because their parents refused to fill out the questionnaire. The final group of Ss consisted of 15 girls, 20 boys, and their mothers and fathers.

No divorced parents or families in which a parent was absent were included in the sample. The Ss were white and from the lower middle

---

[1] By "trait," the present investigators mean a generic term referring to a class of behaviors that are relatively stable in their frequency of occurrence throughout the organism's history and that are traditionally thought of as indices of personality.

socioeconomic class. Of the 15 girls, six were Catholic, seven were Protestant, and two were Jewish. Ten boys were Catholic, nine were Protestant, and one was Jewish.

Experimental Material

The experimental material consisted of 10 behavioral tests for the children and a questionnaire for their parents. The behavioral tests included (a) circle crossing, (b) unsolvable formboard, (c) spool stacking, (d) bear-boy picture series, (e) penny drive, (f) rock collecting, (g) crayon sharing, (h) ink blot preference, (i) locker ratings, and (j) finger painting. Tests a, b, c, and d were designed as measures of obstinacy; e, f, and g, as measures of parsimony; and h, i, and j as measures of orderliness. The questionnaire was designed to measure the frequency of parental behaviors judged as indices of parsimony, orderliness, obstinacy, and dominance in regard to spouse and child and severity of initial as well as current toilet training practices.

Procedure

With one exception, all the behavioral test procedures permitted the use of more than one E, thus allowing sex of E to be counterbalanced against sex of S.

The procedures specific to each test were as follows:

Circle crossing. This test was designed to measure persistence in a tedious task under promise of an insignificant monetary reward upon completion of the task. Each S was tested individually at a desk on which there was a shiny new penny and a pile of 50 sheets of paper with 56 circles on each sheet. The E said,

> See this bright new penny? It will be yours if you can cross out all the circles on these sheets of paper. Just draw a line through each circle like this. You must cross out all the circles on every page to win the penny. If you don't finish all the pages, you won't get anything. Do you understand?

If the child failed to comprehend the directions, they were repeated. The first time S stopped crossing out circles for longer than 1 minute, E said, "You're doing very well, but remember every circle must be crossed out before you win the penny." A time limit of 40 minutes was set for the task. Performance was measured in terms of the number of circles crossed out and the number of minutes the child persisted in the task.

Unsolvable formboard. This test measured the persistence with which S tried to solve an unsolvable task. Subjects were tested individually. Each S was seated before a large formboard with 20 apertures and 20 pieces of cardboard of various colors, shapes, and sizes. The pieces were placed in a predetermined arrangement on the table between S and formboard. Nine of the pieces could be successfully fitted into the holes in the formboard. The remaining 11 pieces did not fit because of slight irregularities in shape or size. Each child was instructed as follows:

You've played at jigsaw puzzles before, haven't you? Well, this is a big jigsaw puzzle. Each of these pieces will fit perfectly into one of these holes, like this. (The E demonstrated with a circle and then removed it.) You are to put all the pieces into their right holes. Remember, they must fit exactly. All right, begin.

At the first error, E said, "That doesn't fit, does it? Remember that it will fit perfectly. Keep trying. You're doing very well."

The time limit was 20 minutes. Performance was recorded as the number of minutes the child persisted with the formboard before announcing that he wished to stop or as the number of minutes preceding a one-minute period of inactivity that was followed by a negative response to E's query about wishing to continue.

Spool stacking. The purpose of this test was to assess extent of perseverance in a ritualistic, stereotyped, endless activity. The test was administered individually. The apparatus was similar in construction and operation to a child's dump truck. It consisted of two oblong containers, 6½ by 5½ inches, one of which was raised 4 inches above the other. The higher box contained 30 spools of 1-inch diameter arranged in six rows of five spools each. These spools could be dumped into the lower container by pulling a lever, which tilted the floor and released the back of the upper container.

The operation of the apparatus was demonstrated by E, who dumped the spools into the lower box and then carefully replaced them systematically in rows in the upper box while saying,

> Here is a new game for you to play. This handle makes all the spools shoot out into this box just like a dump truck, and then all the spools can be put back into the top box again in rows. In this game the spools are always arranged neatly in rows before being dumped. You fill the tray and dump the spools and then fill the tray and dump them again. In this kind of game, you can go on forever filling and dumping, and you can play it as long as you like. When you want to stop playing, just let me know. You can stop anytime you want. Now, begin.

If the child attempted to vary the procedure, E said, "No, the game must always be played in the same way. Arrange the spools so they all fit neatly in rows, then dump them, then arrange them the same way again." A time limit of 40 minutes was imposed, and performance was recorded in terms of the number of spools placed as well as the number of minutes the child continued to play before asking to stop.

Bear-boy picture series. This tested stubbornness in the sense of clinging to an initial position in spite of its increasing inappropriateness and in spite of pressure from E to change. The picture material consisted of a series of nine drawings, each mounted on a separate card. The first picture was clearly that of a bear. In each successive picture a few lines were altered to make the bear appear increasingly like a boy. The final drawing showed a little boy in a sailor suit and hat. Results from a pilot study indicated that the middle picture of the series was called "boy" and "bear" equally often.

Subjects were run individually. They were instructed as follows: "You will be shown some pictures, one at a time, and will be asked to say what you think each picture is. Just name what is in each picture. For example, what do you think this is?" The first picture was then presented. Every S responded, "A bear." The E then said, "A bear? You're sure it's a bear? That's funny. Most people think it's a boy. Are you sure it's a bear? Almost all other children say it's a boy." The remaining pictures were presented in serial order; on each presentation S was asked to name the picture and then was pressured by E to change his response from "bear" to "boy." The score was the last card in the series which S called a bear.

Penny drive. This procedure was a modified version of the pencil drive measure used by Blum and Miller (5) in their study of the oral character. The present procedure measured S's ability to resist strongly aroused internal pressures to donate money for a charitable cause. The test was conducted in the classroom, where, early in the day, every child was given 10 bright new pennies. He was told that the pennies belonged to him and that he could do whatever he wished with them. An hour later, a totally unfamiliar E appeared and told the class the following sad story:

> I'm here to collect money for poor little children who need every cent we can get. Some of these children don't have enough clothes to wear or food to eat. They didn't even have a turkey dinner or get toys at Christmas because their mommies and daddies don't have any money. If you can give these kiddies enough of your pennies we will be able to give them all the things they've missed and need so badly. Every penny you can give will help. Every penny counts. This can will be placed behind a screen at the back of the room so you can put as many pennies for the poor hungry children in it as you want and no one can see you doing it. I will come back at the end of the day to take the can of pennies to the needy children. Remember, every penny will help.

The E was a woman with considerable skill in dramatic presentation. (The fact that sobbing was clearly audible in the classroom toward the end of her exhortation gives an indication of its effectiveness.)

A large container with a slot in the top was placed behind a screen at the rear of the room. The screen was utilized to reduce any direct social pressure to donate. The can was collected four hours later.

Each coin had been previously marked with a tiny dot of colored indelible ink on a specific area of the coin. The pennies given to each child had a unique combination of placement and color of dot. The contributors were identified through this coding. A tally was made of the number of pennies returned by each child. There was no danger of S's contributing coins other than the experimental pennies, because it was a rule of the kindergarten that any money a child brought to school had to be left with the teacher for safekeeping.

Rock collecting. This study measured the hoarding of objects of no intrinsic value. Common coarse gravel was used because of its lack of real value, its ready accessibility outside the experimental situation, and because many psychoanalysts regard rocks as a transition object in the symbolic relating of feces and money. A large crate of gravel was placed at the front of the classroom and shoeboxes were given to each child. The children were told,

> This is a box of little rocks like you find at the beach or on some roads. You can have all the rocks you want and you can keep them as long as you want, but you must leave them at school. If you get tired of your pebbles you can put them back in the big box. If you want to have them you can keep them in the boxes we have given you. Bring your boxes up and pick out as many pebbles as you want, one at a time. Remember, you can have all the rocks you want and keep them as long as you want at school. Don't take them home. When you don't want the rocks anymore, put them back in the big box because we don't want to lose any.

On each successive school day for a week, the children were told, if they wished to return any rocks, they could just put them in the big box. The number of rocks taken in the initial session by each child was surreptitiously tallied. The number of rocks retained one week later was also counted.

Crayon sharing. This test measured Ss' generosity, or lack of it, in sharing objects with classmates who had none. The test was run in two sessions, one month apart. In the first session half the class was given a box of 20 crayons and was told, "We're going to give some of you crayons today. We're sorry we don't have enough boxes for everyone, but if those of you who get crayons want to give some away to the children who don't have any, you may do so."

A month later the procedure was repeated, but this time crayons were given to those Ss who had not received any the first time. No children had any crayons of their own in the classroom in either session. The number of crayons *not* loaned or shared during a one-hour drawing period was recorded.

Ink blot preference. This was a test of the psychoanalytic assumption that anal individuals manifest a preference for symmetry over asymmetry. The stimuli were 10 pairs of ink blots. Each pair was composed of a symmetrical and an asymmetrical blot mounted on separate cards. One pair was presented at a time. The right or left position of the symmetrical or asymmetrical cards was varied randomly. Each pair of cards was exposed for 30 seconds. There was a 5-second interval between pairs. The S was instructed to point to the blot he liked best, the one that "looked prettier" to him in each pair. The number of symmetrical preferences was recorded.

Locker ratings. These ratings measured consistent neatness and orderliness in everyday behavior. Each child in the kindergarten was as a matter of routine assigned a locker in which to keep his belongings, such as coat, hat, scarf, gloves, boots, toys, and the towel on which he lay during rest periods. Three judges independently rated locker orderliness for all children on three different days separated by four-day intervals. The lockers were identified by numbers only, so that the judge did not know which child he was rating. An 8-point Likert-type rating scale was used, ranging from a scale value of 1 for extremely disorderly to 8 for extremely orderly. Although the judges did not receive formal pretraining in rating this dimension, all of them had had previous experience in using Likert scales. The mean interjudge reliability for day 1 ratings was .94. The trait consistency over time, or test-retest reliability, day 1 with day 3 ,was .97.

Finger painting. This test measured the extent to which S attempted to remain clean, neat, and orderly in a situation allowing unlimited messiness and disorder. Each S was tested individually in a small room with an adjoining washroom. Jars containing red, orange, yellow, green, blue, purple, brown, and black paints were arranged in random fashion on a table. The child was given an apron to wear. All Ss had had previous experience in finger painting.

The E demonstrated the use of finger paints to the child and said, "I know you've had fun with finger paints before. A lot of the fun of finger painting is smearing the paint different ways with hands or elbows or arms —or some people like to use their face and feet, too. I want you to paint a picture. Just scoop out as much of as many different colors as you wish and paint any way you like."

A dampened sheet of 22 by 16 inch glazed paper was then placed before the child, and he was permitted to paint for 16 minutes.

The separately recorded measures making up the composite finger painting score were the following: (a) latency before beginning to paint, measured from the time the sheet of paper was placed before S to the time he first applied paint to it; (b) the number of parts of the body—fingers, hands, arms, face, and feet—used in painting; (c) use of warm-bright vs. cool-dark colors; (d) use of the whole sheet of paper as opposed to only part of it; (e) blending vs. carefully separated placement of colors; (f) frequency of comments about dirtying self or objects in the room, or about the feel of the paint; and (g) frequency of washing and of requests to go to the bathroom. Higher composite scores indicated greater orderliness.

Parent questionnaire. The fathers and mothers of all Ss were administered a questionnaire (reproduced in the Appendix) which was designed to measure parental personality characteristics and child training techniques believed to be relevant to the development of anal traits in children. The mother's questionnaire, consisting of 84 items, contained scales for obstinacy, orderliness (including cleanliness), parsimony, dominance in regard to husband and child, and severity of both initial and current toilet training methods. The father's questionnaire consisted of 66 items; it contained the same scales, except for toilet training, and items which were inappropriate for males. The toilet training scale was omitted from the father's questionnaire because, from our own pilot work as well as from the results of others, it appears that in most families the mother is the principal determiner of toilet training practices—or at least is the more reliable source of report about them. The mothers were also asked to note the age at which toilet training was begun and the age at which it was completed.

The questionnaire was constructed on the basis of consensual face validity. A large pool of items was submitted to five experienced clinical psychologists, who independently judged whether each item measured obstinacy, orderliness, parsimony, dominance, severity of toilet training practices, or none of these dimensions. Only those items that were agreed upon unanimously were included in the questionnaire.

Using a pilot sample of 54 mothers, a test-retest reliability coefficient of .89 was obtained for the mother's questionnaire. The two administrations were separated by an interval of one month.

Fifty-two of the 54 mothers gave test-retest information on the age in months at which toilet training was begun and completed. Forty-one mothers gave exactly the same ages for age beginning on test and on retest. For the remaining 11, the mean discrepancy in the two reports was 1.95 months. Forty-one mothers, not necessarily the same as above, gave exactly the same ages for age completed on test and on retest. For the remaining 11, the mean discrepancy in the two reports was 2.72 months.

For the purpose of administering the questionnaire, each item was printed on a separate card, and the cards were stacked in a deck. The order of the cards was randomized, each parent receiving a different random order. The parent was instructed that each card was to be dropped into one of two boxes with slot-tops. One box was marked *true*, the other *false*. Both boxes were sealed so that it was impossible for a card to be removed once it had been dropped through the slot. Parents were asked to answer the items as quickly and accurately as possible.

Results and Discussion

Intercorrelations among all measures were calculated for both sexes together and for boys and girls separately, using Pearson product-moment correlation. Although there had been only chance differences between means and variances for the two sexes on the dependent variables, the correlation matrices revealed marked sex differences in intratrait consistency, intertrait consistency, and parent-child agreement. This result was unanticipated. It was also unwelcome. Where the investigators had planned on one study and a large sample, they found they had acquired two studies and two small samples. Because of the extensive sex differences, the results are tabled and discussed separately for males and females.

Intratrait Correlations

Obstinacy. The intercorrelations among measures of obstinacy are presented for girls in Table 1 and for boys in Table 2. Time and frequency measures on the spool and circle tests were recorded and analyzed separately, since it was thought they might involve slightly different aspects of obstinacy. From the results shown in Tables 1 and 2, this precaution seems not to have

TABLE 1

INTERCORRELATIONS AMONG OBSTINACY MEASURES: GIRLS

	1	2	3	4	5
1. Time spent, circle test					
2. No. of circles, circle test	.79****				
3. Time spent, formboard	.67***	.66***			
4. Time spent, spool test	.52**	.48*	.68***		
5. No. of spools, spool test	.03	.19	.44*	.72****	
6. No. of bear responses, bear-boy test	.36	.38	.48*	.39	.47*

* $p < .10$.
** $p < .05$.
*** $p < .01$.
**** $p < .001$.

been justified. Although the correlation between time and frequency measures for the same task falls short of 1.00, the correlations among these and other measures are roughly of the same magnitude, no matter whether the time or frequency data are used.

The one aberrant measure within the obstinacy complex is the bear-boy test. The number of bear responses on this test is not related to a statistically significant degree with any of the other obstinacy measures for either boys or girls. In the case of the girls, the direction of the relation is consistent with that of the other obstinacy measures. For the boys, however, not only are the correlations between bear-boy and other obstinacy tests nonsignificant, but four of them are negative in sign.

The reason for the discrepancy in results between the bear-boy test and the rest of the obstinacy complex most probably stems from an essential

TABLE 2

INTERCORRELATIONS AMONG OBSTINACY MEASURES: BOYS

	1	2	3	4	5
1. Time spent, circle test					
2. No. of circles, circle test	.50**				
3. Time spent, formboard	.68****	.33			
4. Time spent, spool test	.60***	.50**	.17		
5. No. of spools, spool test	.50**	.53**	.14	.63****	
6. No. of bear responses, bear-boy test	—.29	—.05	—.11	—.18	.14

** $p < .05$.
*** $p < .01$.
**** $p < .001$.

difference in the nature of the behaviors measured. The circle crossing, unsolvable formboard, and spool tests involved persistent behavior the limit of which was determined by the child himself. These activities were self-propelled and relatively free of interference from E. On the other hand, the bear-boy test measured the extent to which S clung to his initial position in the face of increasingly contradictory evidence and in spite of pressure from E to abandon his position. Stubbornness in an interpersonal situation is the important element here, and this can be better understood by illustrating the extent to which Ss' responses were independent of the changes in the visual stimulus. It will be recalled that the picture series had been drawn so that card 5 was perceived by uninstructed pilot Ss equally often as bear and boy. Furthermore, none of the pilot Ss perceived card 3 as a boy nor card 7 as a bear. Yet 15 Ss of the main sample acquiesced on or before presentation of card 3 to E's suggestion that the bear was a boy, while four Ss refused to acknowledge seeing a boy on cards 7 or 8. Indeed, one child—the most consistently "anal" S of the sample—looked at card 9 with its unmistakable little sailor-suited boy and adamantly maintained she saw a bear.

In summary, these considerations, together with the results themselves, suggest that persistence and social stubbornness are not the same trait, particularly in the case of young boys. Stated differently, the implication is that "obstinacy," as it has been used in lay terms and analytic theory alike, does not have a unitary behavioral referent.

Orderliness. Tables 3 and 4 present the intercorrelations among orderliness measures for girls and boys. The only statistically significant relation for either sex is that between ratings of locker orderliness and number of preferences for symmetrical over asymmetrical ink blots. The composite finger painting score does not correlate highly with either of these.

It should be noted that psychoanalytic theory would most probably have predicted some inconsistencies between measures of orderliness. Of the three traits said to figure in the development of anality, obstinacy and parsimony tend to be direct extensions or sublimations of anal erotic activities. Orderliness may also involve sublimation but is frequently a result of reaction formation against anal impulses. Abraham (1) notes that the mechanism of reaction formation is never completely successful and that the repressed

TABLE 3

INTERCORRELATIONS AMONG ORDERLINESS MEASURES: GIRLS

	1	*2*
1. No. of symmetrical choices, ink blots		
2. Locker rating	.96****	
3. Finger painting	.40	.33

**** $p < .001$.

157

TABLE 4

INTERCORRELATIONS AMONG ORDERLINESS MEASURES: BOYS

	I	*2*
1. No. of symmetrical choices, ink blots		
2. Locker rating	.77****	
3. Finger painting	.27	.14

**** $p < .001$.

impulse may emerge in certain situations. He points out that personality trends such as orderliness which are based on this process tend to be characterized by ambivalence and instability. Reaction formation may be more readily maintained in a situation involving routinized behavior than in a situation in which the *E* tempts the child to engage in smearing, albeit socially acceptable smearing, since this is the kind of activity against which the child's still imperfect defense is directed.

There is further evidence to support the interpretation that finger painting was a better measure of the activity being defended against than of the defense. Although finger painting does not correlate to a statistically significant degree with the two other orderliness measures, for girls it does correlate significantly with the composite obstinacy measure ($r = .52$, $p < .05$) and with the composite parsimony measure ($r = .76$, $p < .01$). The same correlations for boys fall short of significance. This is the only case in which a single measure was found to have lower intratrait correlations than inter- or across-trait correlations.

Parsimony. Tables 5 and 6 show the intercorrelations among parsimony measures for girls and for boys. All the intercorrelations are significant for both sexes. If the children were acquisitive, retentive, and selfish in one

TABLE 5

INTERCORRELATIONS AMONG PARSIMONY MEASURES: GIRLS

	I	*2*	*3*
1. No. kept, penny test			
2. No. taken, rock test	.78****		
3. No. retained, rock test	.85****	.89****	
4. No. kept, crayon test	.82****	.56**	.71***

** $p < .05$.
*** $p < .01$.
**** $p < .001$.

TABLE 6

INTERCORRELATIONS AMONG PARSIMONY MEASURES: BOYS

	1	2	3
1. No. kept, penny test			
2. No. taken, rock test	.69****		
3. No. retained, rock test	.58***	.81****	
4. No. kept, crayon test	.86****	.63***	.68****

*** $p < .01$.
**** $p < .001$.

situation, they were predictably acquisitive, retentive, and selfish in the other test situations. The within-trait consistency among measures of parsimony is more striking than it is for either obstinacy or orderliness. Within the range of tasks and subject-characteristics sampled in this study, parsimony appears to be the most influential and stable of the three personality traits, or at least the first of the traits to reach this point in the course of development.

Trait Covariation

Children. Tables 7 and 8 show, separately for girls and boys, the intercorrelations among the composite measures of obstinacy, orderliness, and parsimony. For girls, orderliness is closely related to both obstinacy and parsimony. Obstinacy and parsimony, however, are not related at all. In fact, the difference between the two correlations, parsimony-obstinacy (frequency measure) and orderliness-obstinacy, approaches significance, while the difference between parsimony-obstinacy (either measure) and orderliness-parsimony is significant ($p = .05$), in spite of the small sample size.

TABLE 7

INTERCORRELATIONS AMONG TRAITS: GIRLS

	1	2	3
1. Obstinacy (time measures)			
2. Obstinacy (frequency measures) ..	.83****		
3. Orderliness	.52**	.56**	
4. Parsimony	.13	.06	.78****

** $p < .05$.
**** $p < .001$.

TABLE 8

INTERCORRELATIONS AMONG TRAITS: BOYS

	I	2	3
1. Obstinacy (time measures)			
2. Obstinacy (frequency measures) ..	.72****		
3. Orderliness	—.08	—.23	
4. Parsimony	—.09	—.23	.10

**** $p < .001$.

For these results, the order of magnitude of relation is in direct contradiction to Freud's observation that parsimony and obstinacy are more closely related to each other than either is to orderliness.

In the case of the boys, trait covariation is nonexistent; all the intercorrelations among trait scores are clearly nonsignificant.

For both girls and boys, time and frequency measures of obstinacy are too highly correlated to conclude that they are measuring differentiable aspects of obstinacy of any importance. For that reason, only one is used in subsequent analyses. The time measure was arbitrarily chosen for this purpose.

Altogether, these results yield rather poor confirmation for the hypothesized covariation of obstinacy, orderliness, and parsimony. There is only partial support in the girls' data and no evidence at all for intercorrelation in the boys' data.

Parents. Table 9 presents the intercorrelations among maternal personality traits, as derived from the mothers' questionnaire. The cleanliness and orderliness measures were combined, since these behaviors are usually subsumed under the generic term "orderliness" in psychoanalytic literature and

TABLE 9

INTERCORRELATIONS AMONG TRAITS: MOTHERS

	I	2	3	4
1. Obstinacy				
2. Orderliness (inc. cleanliness)	.52***			
3. Parsimony	.28	.55****		
4. Dominance	.22	.37**	.23	
5. Severity of toilet training	.04	.47***	.03	.37**

** $p < .05$.
*** $p < .01$.
**** $p < .001$.

since there was no empirical difference between them. The pattern of correlations is strikingly similar to the pattern of correlations in the girls' matrix (Table 7). In both cases, orderliness is closely related to obstinacy and to parsimony, whereas obstinacy and parsimony are not related to each other.

The degree to which the mother dominates her husband and child is related to the severity of her toilet training methods and to her emphasis on orderliness and cleanliness, but it is not significantly related to extent of obstinacy and parsimony.

TABLE 10

INTERCORRELATIONS AMONG TRAITS: FATHERS

	1	2	3
1. Obstinacy			
2. Orderliness (incl. cleanliness)	.00		
3. Parsimony	.16	—.02	
4. Dominance	.11	.59****	—.04

**** $p < .001$.

The intercorrelations for fathers' questionnaire measures are shown in Table 10. As was the case for mothers and daughters, there is a remarkable similarity between fathers and sons in the extent of trait covariation or, more precisely, in the absence of it. Also for fathers, as was true for mothers, dominance is related to orderliness.

TABLE 11

CORRELATIONS BETWEEN MOTHER AND DAUGHTER TRAIT SCORES

Mother	DAUGHTER			
	Obstinacy§	Orderliness	Parsimony	Composite Score‡
Obstinacy	.74***	.55**	.16	.58**
Orderliness†	—.05	.44*	.39	.33
Parsimony	.20	.72***	.78****	.72***
Composite Score‡	.34	.73***	.58**	.68***
Dominance	.09	.44*	.54**	.46*

† Including Cleanliness.
‡ Obstinacy + Orderliness + Parsimony.
§ Time measures.
* $p < .10$.
** $p < .05$.
*** $p < .01$.
**** $p < .001$.

On the question of trait covariation, we are led to conclude that, whether the data come from behavioral or questionnaire measures and whether from children or adults, they lend no support to an unqualified statement that obstinacy, orderliness, and parsimony vary together. Furthermore, two of the four sets of data directly contradict the Freudian position that obstinacy and parsimony are the more closely related of the three personality traits.

Parent-Child Similarity in Personality Traits

Girls. Table 11 contains the correlations between personality trait scores for mothers and daughters. In general, it appears that mothers who are orderly, obstinate, and parsimonious have daughters who are orderly, obstinate, and parsimonious. With the borderline exception of orderliness (.10 > p > .05), both the composite and single, like-trait correlations are highly significant.

On the other hand, the same correlations for father and daughter (Table 12) are clearly nonsignificant, with the exception of borderline significance in the case of obstinacy.

TABLE 12

CORRELATIONS BETWEEN FATHER AND DAUGHTER TRAIT SCORES

Father	Obstinacy§	DAUGHTER Orderliness	Parsimony	Composite Score‡
Obstinacy	.60**	.31	.31	.50*
Orderliness†	.00	—.15	.00	—.06
Parsimony	—.22	.17	.38	.16
Composite Score‡	—.14	—.04	.37	.10
Dominance	.01	—.10	.05	—.01

† Including Cleanliness.
‡ Obstinacy + Orderliness + Parsimony.
§ Time measures.
* $p < .10$.
** $p < .05$.

If similarity may be used as an index of identification, then the discrepancy in results between Tables 11 and 12 fulfills the investigators' expectation: the little girl identifies with the like-sexed parent and acquires the mother's salient behavioral-personality characteristics. It is interesting to note, with respect to the girls' identification, that the pattern of father-daughter trait correlations reflects with fair accuracy the pattern of father-mother trait correlations. For this particular sample of 15 parents, the correlations between fathers and mothers on parsimony and obstinacy are positive and moderate in size (.27 and .27 in both cases), while the correlation on orderliness is negative and low (—.15). This suggests that degree of father-daughter similarity is *not* an index of identification, but that it is determined by a third factor—the degree of similarity of *mother* to father.

TABLE 13

CORRELATIONS BETWEEN MOTHER AND SON TRAIT SCORES

Mother	Obstinacy§	Orderliness	Parsimony	Composite Score‡
			S O N	
Obstinacy	.24	.09	—.36	—.09
Orderliness†	.29	.38*	.04	.33
Parsimony	.02	.32	.10	.19
Composite Score‡	.24	.34	.04	.23
Dominance	.08	.06	—.18	—.07

† Including Cleanliness.
‡ Obstinacy + Orderliness + Parsimony.
§ Time measures.
* $p < .10$.

Boys. There are no significant relations between mother and son personality traits (Table 13) or between father and son personality traits (Table 14). These results were surprising, even though the investigators had not expected as much evidence of father-son identification as of mother-daughter identification—given the usual situation during the first five years of 24-hour contact between mother and son but not between father and son. Even more striking than the absence of father-son similarity was the lack of similarity between son and *either* parent.

TABLE 14

CORRELATIONS BETWEEN FATHER AND SON TRAIT SCORES

Father	Obstinacy§	Orderliness	Parsimony	Composite Score‡
			S O N	
Obstinacy	—.06	.20	—.28	—.11
Orderliness†	.00	.35	—.14	.00
Parsimony	—.17	—.04	.26	.08
Composite Score‡	—.06	.31	—.10	—.01
Dominance	—.02	.06	—.34	—.25

† Including Cleanliness.
‡ Obstinacy + Orderliness + Parsimony.
§ Time measures.

A more refined analysis of the mother-son and father-son data was made in an attempt to find some explanation of these strange results. The analysis took into account the relative dominance of the two parents within each family. The reasoning by which we singled out dominance as the suspect variable was as follows. Dominant, aggressive behavior is the appropriate or perhaps the essential characteristic of the masculine role in our society. Since proper sex roles are already quite apparent to 5-year-olds, a 5-year-old boy may admire and be more prone to identify with his father when the father rather than the mother dominates family life. By the same token, it should be the case that the sons of weak fathers simply continue to identify with their first love, the dominant mother. The same conclusion may be drawn by hypothesizing that young boys tend to identify with the aggressor (8).

For the purpose of such an analysis, the raw scores on dominance were first converted to z scores, for both the boys' fathers and for their mothers. Then a difference score for each set of parents was calculated. Of the 20 families, mother proved to be the dominant member in eight, and father in 12. The relation between the composite personality trait scores of father and son was examined, but this time sons in mother-dominated homes were studied separately from those in father-dominated homes. For the 12 boys living in father-dominant homes, there is some evidence of identification with the fathers—in the sense of similarity in the extent to which the father and son are both orderly, obstinate, and parsimonious ($rho = .35$). In striking contrast, for the eight boys living in mother-dominated homes, there is a negative correlation between fathers' and sons' personality trait scores ($rho = -.36$). Neither correlation reaches statistical significance, due to the small size of the samples involved.

Two similar analyses were made for the relation between mother and son according to the sex of the dominant parent. The results are in essential agreement with the first two analyses. In father-dominant homes, there is no hint of a relation between the mother's personality trait scores and her son's ($rho = -.10$). But when mother dominates the home, she also appears to dominate her son's personality development ($rho = .45$). Again, the two correlations are not statistically significant.[2]

Toilet Training and Personality

As reported by the girls' mothers, the mean age at which toilet training was begun was 12.1 months; the mean age by which it was finished was

---

[2] On the parent questionnaire, the total number of dominance items was different for mothers and fathers, being 17 and 14, respectively. The authors thus chose to derive z scores from the two distributions separately. z scores based on a single distribution of fathers' and mothers' scores combined have the disadvantage of being derived from proportions but the advantage of more accurately representing father-mother differences in dominance. For readers who prefer this second approach, it should be noted that the two

22.2 months. The corresponding figures for the boys were 10.5 months and 23.1 months. No relation was found for either sex between age of beginning, time to complete, or age at completion of toilet training and subsequent development of obstinacy, orderliness, or parsimony. Nor was any relation found between age of beginning, time to complete, or age at completion of toilet training and the severity of toilet training.

TABLE 15

CORRELATIONS BETWEEN TOILET TRAINING VARIABLES AND
CHILDREN'S PERSONALITY TRAIT SCORES

	Composite Trait Score‡	
	Girls	Boys
Severity of toilet training (past and current)	—.58**	.22
Age at which toilet training began	.02	.20
Age at which toilet training finished	.12	—.18
No. of months to complete training	.15	—.02

‡ Orderliness + Obstinacy + Parsimony.
** $p < .05$.

The one statistically significant correlation in Table 15 is a suspicious looking negative correlation indicating that the less severe the mother's toilet training methods, the more orderly, obstinate, and parsimonious is her daughter. Both the size and direction of this correlation coefficient are the joint results of small sample size and the possibly false report of two of the 15 mothers regarding severity of toilet training. These two mothers—whose daughters, incidentally, obtained the two highest composite trait scores for girls—professed such leniency in toilet training that their scores on this variable were more than three standard deviations below the mean of the remaining 13 scores. When the scores of these two women and those of their daughters are excluded, the correlation between girls' composite trait score and severity of mothers' toilet training changes from —.58 to +.20, or roughly, to the same figure as obtained for boys.

It makes little difference which correlation coefficient is assumed to be more nearly valid as far as the analytic theory of etiology is concerned. Neither figure supports the postulated relation of severe toilet training to high degrees of obstinacy, orderliness, and parsimony. The same negative conclusion applies to the analytic emphasis on age of toilet training. On the other hand, the low positive correlation between severity of toilet training

methods yield identical results except for the correlation between fathers and boys living in father-dominated homes. This correlation becomes .23 when based on a single z-score distribution.

165

and composite trait score, unequivocal at least in the case of the boys, leads to the conclusion that toilet training itself has no direct causative role in later personality development. Any influence it may appear to have is only an indirect function that is mediated by the stable, salient maternal behaviors, particularly dominance, which figure prominently not only in toilet training but in all subsequent socialization situations as well. The correlation between dominance and severity of toilet training is .37, $p < .05$ (Table 9).

Summary and Conclusions

This study investigated the validity of some hypotheses drawn from psychoanalysis and some derived from behavior theory. Psychoanalysis assumes that the personality traits of obstinacy, orderliness, and parsimony covary. A proposition subsidiary to this is that, of the three traits, obstinacy and parsimony are more closely related than either is to orderliness. The second major analytic hypothesis is that the extent to which the three traits develop is determined by the time and manner of toilet training.

An alternative hypothesis concerning the etiology of these traits whether in single or multiple occurrence was suggested. It was proposed that the extent of development of these or other personality traits are determined through processes of identification with and direct learning from the parent. It was further proposed that if there is any relation between toilet training practices and personality, it is attributable to the sorts of maternal behaviors, particularly dominance, that are displayed again and again in this and each succeeding socialization situation.

To test these hypotheses, 35 5-year-old children (15 girls and 20 boys) were used as Ss in 10 situational tests. The tests were chosen on the basis of their representativeness of the behaviors commonly referred to by the terms, obstinacy, orderliness, and parsimony. The mothers and fathers of these children answered questionnaires designed to measure the extent to which they themselves were obstinate, orderly, and parsimonious as well as the extent to which they dominated the rest of the family. In addition, the mother was questioned regarding the severity of her toilet training methods, the age at which she had started toilet training her child, and the age at which toilet training had been completed.

Intercorrelations among all measures were calculated for both sexes together and for boys and girls separately. Because of extensive sex differences in the correlations, though not in means and standard deviations, the results were discussed separately for males and females.

From the analysis of within-trait consistency of the individual measures, the following conclusions were drawn. In psychoanalytic theory and lay usage alike, *obstinacy* has generally been used to cover both persistence and stubbornness in interpersonal situations—as if these were equivalent behavioral referents. The results of this investigation suggest that persistence and social stubbornness are not at all closely related types of behavior, particularly in the case of young boys. *Orderliness*—at least at age 5—appears as a consistent trait only if the measures used to assess it sample routinized behaviors. When the child is invited to be disorderly without penalty, his behavior cannot be predicted from a trait score derived from orderliness in routinized behavior and well-established preferences. *Parsimony,* on the other hand, is highly predictable from one situation to another for both sexes. If the children in this study were acquisitive, retentive, and selfish in one test situation, they were also acquisitive, retentive, and selfish in other test situations.

The analysis in terms of intercorrelations among the three personality traits yielded poor confirmation for the analytically hypothesized covariation of obstinacy, orderliness, and parsimony. This was true for both children and adults. There was no evidence at all for trait covariation from either the boys' data or their fathers' data. In the girls' and their mothers' data, orderliness was closely related to both obstinacy and parsimony, but obstinacy and parsimony were quite unrelated. Such a pattern of covariation directly contradicts Freud's observation that parsimony and obstinacy are more closely related to each other than either is to orderliness. The remarkable similarity in pattern between boys and fathers and between girls and mothers does increase the tenability of the hypothesis that identification with parents is the principal determiner of the child's personality structure.

The investigators' hypothesis finds more direct support from the results correlating personality trait scores for parent and child. It is clearly the case that little girls' personality trait scores are quite predictable if one knows the mothers' scores, but not at all predictable given the fathers' scores. For boys, identification and the acquiring of paternal personality characteristics is not so straightforward. The results of the study suggest that if the mother is more dominant than the father, identification is apparently interfered with, or at least retarded, so that the boy's personality is like his mother's and unlike his father's. Conversely, boys with dominant fathers resemble their fathers and not their mothers in terms of obstinacy, orderliness, and parsimony. The implication of this finding for methodology is that, at least at early ages, parent-child similarity may be appropriately used as an index of identification in the case of daughters and mothers, but it is not an appropriate measure for the more complex father-son situation.

From the data on toilet training, one can only conclude that analytic theory is not correct in maintaining that too early, too late, or too severe training leads to high degrees of obstinacy, orderliness, and parsimony. Since previous investigations using the scientific method have come to the same conclusion, one might suggest that it is time for psychoanalysis to reconsider its adamant perpetuation of this aspect of its theory. Most certainly it is time to discard the "anal" from "anal personality traits"—a term that has too long accepted as fact an unproved, perhaps untenable, hypothesis.

Parent Questionnaire

Items Measuring Obstinacy

1. When I make a promise, I always keep it. (T)
2. After I have made a decision, even though I may change my mind, I usually stick by the decision. (T)
3. When I start something, I practically always see it through to the end. (T)
4. I generally stick at a job even when I can't see any immediate results. (T)
5. People who know me well sometimes joke about my being "stubborn." (T)
6. I stick up for what I know is right. (T)
7. I frequently buy things from door-to-door salesmen that I don't really need. (F)
8. Many times I do things that everyone else likes to do but I don't. (F)
9. I am easily convinced by other people's arguments. (F)
10. I am usually the one who gives in when my husband (wife) and I disagree about something. (F)
11. I frequently do things with my husband (wife) that he likes but that do not interest me at all. (F)

Items Measuring Orderliness

12. I have my child put his room in order every day. (T)
13. I have my child put his playthings away every night before he goes to bed. (T)
14. I have definite rules about what my child can and cannot do in the living room. (T)
15. I usually plan things out before I start to do something. (T)
16. I generally weigh all the alternatives I can think of before coming to a decision. (T)
17. In training my child, I have emphasized the importance of neatness and orderliness. (T)
18. I sometimes permit my child to play with his food. (F)
19. I allow my child to rearrange the living room or dining room furniture when he is playing there. (F)
20. Sometimes I drop by to see friends that live outside my immediate neighborhood without knowing whether they're at home or not. (F)
21. We sometimes leave dirty dishes over night. (F)
22. My linen closet is rather untidy. (F) (omitted on father's scale)
23. I don't have the time to bother keeping the things in my bureau drawers arranged neatly and in order. (F)

Items Measuring Cleanliness (Note: In the text, these items were considered jointly with the orderliness items.)

24. During the summer, I frequently take two or more baths or showers a day. (T)

25. Except for the most unusual circumstances, I always take a shower or bath every day. (T)
26. When something drops on the floor, I don't leave it there—I pick it up. (T)
27. I never sit on an unprotected public toilet seat. (T)
28. I have instructed my child never to eat food that has fallen on the floor. (T)
29. I do some cleaning (vacuuming, mopping, or dusting) at least every other day. (T) (omitted on father's scale)
30. When making a salad, I wash each leaf of lettuce separately. (T) (omitted on father's scale)
31. When mopping floors, I use a germicide or bleach in addition to soap. (T) (omitted from father's scale)
32. My child gets a bath or shower every day. (T)
33. I have tried to teach my child to stay out of dirt and mud when he plays outside. (T)
34. I have definitely tried to teach my child the value of cleanliness. (T)
35. I often wear my good clothes around the house. (F)
36. I seldom bother to clean house before company comes. (F) (omitted from father's scale)
37. I often sit or lie on the floor. (F)
38. I have never disciplined my child for getting dirty or muddy. (F)

Items Measuring Parsimony

39. I keep a budget. (T)
40. I keep a list of who has borrowed what and when. (T)
41. When going out with other people, I practically always "go Dutch." (T)
42. When someone borrows something from me and does not return it soon, I usually remind him to return it. (T)
43. One of my hobbies is collecting things. (T)
44. Whenever possible, I buy things during sales. (T)
45. I usually do not throw things away, since even though I have no use for them at present, I might sometime in the future. (T)
46. I usually try not to waste time. (T)
47. I have encouraged my child to collect things as a hobby. (T)
48. I plan to encourage (or already have encouraged) my child to save money in a piggy bank or regular bank account. (T)
49. I have developed a routine for doing housework that is fairly efficient and time saving. (T)
50. I urge my child to get rid of old or worn out toys. (F)
51. In training my child, I have emphasized sharing things with other children (over and above his brothers and sisters). (F)
52. I am frequently late for appointments. (F)
53. I sometimes buy my husband (wife) a present even when it is not a special occasion. (F)
54. When someone comes to the house asking for contributions to a cause, I always donate something. (F)
55. I frequently offer to lend things even if I have not been asked. (F)

56. I never put off writing a thank-you letter. (F)
57. When someone asks to borrow something from me, I never refuse them. (F)

Items Measuring Dominance

58. My child has learned that when I tell him to do something *now*, I mean it. (T)
59. I practically always see to it that my child eats everything on his plate. (T)
60. I go with my husband when he buys a suit or overcoat. (T) (omitted on father's scale)
61. When there is a difference of opinion in our house, my point of view is often the one that is accepted in the end. (T)
62. I open all the mail that comes to the house. (T)
63. I try to know something about the other children my child plays with. (T)
64. I have disciplined my child more than once for not telling me where he was going when he played outside. (T)
65. I have disciplined my child more than once for going too far away from home. (T)
66. Once I have made a decision, I do not let my child argue with me about it. (T)
67. My husband (wife) makes more of the decisions about child raising than I do. (F)
68. I very rarely fix foods for my child that I know he dislikes. (F) (omitted from father's scale)
69. I frequently ask my husband what he would like to eat for dinner. (F) (omitted from father's scale)
70. In order to avoid an argument with my husband (wife), I often give in even though I know I'm right. (F)
71. In order to avoid an argument with my child, I often let him have his own way. (F)
72. I always ask my husband (wife) if he (she) is free on a particular night before I make a social date. (F)
73. If my child interrupts me when I'm in the middle of something, I generally drop what I'm doing to attend to him. (F)
74. As far as I am concerned, my child is free to play with whomever he wishes around the neighborhood, even if I don't know the other child. (F)

Items Measuring Severity of Toilet Training (omitted on father's scale)

75. During the time I was toilet training my child, I had to discipline him occasionally for not moving his bowels when he was supposed to (or moving them when he wasn't supposed to). (T)
76. Occasionally I have to give my child something to prevent loose stools or diarrhea. (T)
77. Occasionally I have to give my child a laxative. (T)
78. When I was toilet training my child, I would put him on the toilet at least five times a day. (T)
79. When I was toilet training my child, unless he did something before then, I would leave him on the toilet for at least 20 minutes. (T)

80. I once had to punish my child for putting his hands in the toilet bowl. (T)

81. I never let my child sit on an unprotected public toilet seat. (T)

82. I have never given my child an enema. (F)

83. I generally don't keep track of my child's bowel movements. (F)

84. I have never disciplined my child for soiling his pants right after getting up off the toilet. (F)

REFERENCES

1. ABRAHAM, K. Contributions to the theory of the anal character. In *Selected papers*. Hogarth Press, 1927. Pp. 370-392.

2. BARNES, C. A. A statistical study of Freudian theory of levels of psychosexual development. *Genet. Psychol. Monogr.*, 1952, 45, 105-175.

3. BELOFF, H. The structure and origin of the anal character. *Genet. Psychol. Monogr.*, 1957, 55, 141-172.

4. BERNSTEIN, A. Some relations between techniques of feeding and training during infancy and certain behavior in childhood. *Gent. Psychol. Monogr.*, 1955, 51, 3-44.

5. BLUM, G. S., & MILLER, D. R. Exploring the psychoanalytic theory of the oral character. *J. Pers.*, 1952, 31, 287-304.

6. BRILL, A. A. Anal eroticism and character. *J. abnorm. Psychol.*, 1912, 7, 176-203.

7. FENICHEL, O. *The psychoanalytic theory of neuroses*. Norton, 1945.

8. FREUD, A. *The ego and the mechanisms of defense*. Hogarth Press, 1948.

9. FREUD, S. Character and anal eroticism. In *Collected papers*. Vol. II. Hogarth Press, 1924. Pp. 45-50.

10. FREUD, S. On the transformation of instincts with special reference to anal eroticism. In *Collected papers*. Vol. II. Hogarth Press, 1924. Pp. 164-171.

11. JONES, E. Anal erotic character traints. In *Papers on psychoanalysis* (1st Ed.). Wood, 1913. Pp. 531-555.

12. MENNINGER, W. C. Characterologic and symptomatic expressions related to the anal phase of psychosexual development. *Psychoanal. Quart.*, 1943, 12, 161-195.

13. RAPAPORT, G. M. A study of the psychoanalytic theory of the anal character. Unpublished doctoral dissertation, Northwestern Univer., 1955.

14. SEARS, R. R. Experimental studies of projection: I. Attribution of traits. *J. soc. Psychol.*, 1936, 7, 151-163.

SECTION VII

CHILD PSYCHOSIS

ESTABLISHING FUNCTIONAL SPEECH
IN ECHOLALIC CHILDREN

Todd Risley and Montrose Wolf

University of Kansas, U.S.A.

INTRODUCTION

Echolalia

". . . autistic children usually do learn to talk, sometimes very well, but their speech fails to follow the normal patterns. Often prominent in their speech is a compulsive parroting of what they hear called echolalia. They pick up a phrase, a name, a snatch of song, or even a long verse, and repeat it endlessly" (Stone and Church, 1957).

The sporadic and usually inappropriate imitation of words, phrases and snatches of song, is observed in many deviant children. Although this behavior pattern is generally associated with the diagnosis of emotional disturbance or autism, it is also a frequently observed behavior pattern of children diagnosed as retarded or brain-damaged. The procedures described in this paper have been developed from work with echolalic children with almost every conceivable diagnosis. Indeed, the records of each of these children usually contained diagnoses of retardation and brain-damage as well as autism, each label applied to the same child by a different diagnostician. For our procedures, the diagnostic classification of the child is largely irrelevant. The presence or absence of echolalia is the important predictor of the ease of establishing more normal speech in a deviant child.

In alleviating any deficit in behavior, the most time-consuming task is the teaching of new topographies of behavior. When a child's repertoire does not include a particular behavior and the child cannot be taught by conventional means, training can be carried out by the behavior modification technique called *shaping*. This procedure involves the long and intricate process of reinforcing behaviors which resemble (although, perhaps only remotely) the desired terminal behavior, and then, in successive steps, shifting the reinforcement to behaviors which more and more closely resemble the terminal behavior. When the terminal response is obtained, the response can then be shifted to imitative control by *imitation training*.

BEHAVIOR RESEARCH AND THERAPY, 1967, Vol. 5. No. 1., pp. 73–88.

174

Imitation training involves reinforcing a response made by the child only when it immediately follows the same response made by the therapist. The child's response may already have existed in his echolalic repertoire or it may have been shaped into a high probability response. The therapist can shift the response to imitative control by reinforcing it when it occurs after the presentation of an identical modeled stimulus or *prompt*. In this manner large units of previously randomly occurring behavior can be brought under imitative control. Once a child accurately imitates most words, phrases, and sentences, then any topography of verbal behavior (i.e. any word, phrase, or sentence) can be produced when desired by presenting the child with the prompt to be imitated.

Echolalia, then, is of significance to the therapist, for, since the echolalic child already has verbal responses, the arduous task of shaping them is unnecessary. Once the child's responses are brought under imitative control, so that, for example, he says "that's a cow" when the therapist has just said "that's a cow," the only remaining step is to shift the control of his responses to the appropriate stimuli, so that, for example, he says "that's a cow" to a picture of a cow. This shift to naming is made by *fading out* the imitative prompt in gradual steps as described in detail below. In this manner the responses acquire their appropriate "meanings." Thus, the procedures for establishing functional speech in echolalic children are relatively simple and produce appropriate speech rapidly, in contrast to the procedures which have been used in establishing speech in non-echolalic, speech-deficient children (e.g. Lovaas, 1966: Risley, 1966).

GENERAL PROCEDURES

The authors developed the procedures summarized in this paper while working with children with echolalic speech. The general methodology was initially developed in the course of dealing with the behavior problems of an autistic child named Dicky (Wolf, Risley and Mees, 1964). We will review his case before describing the more refined procedures which evolved from it.

Our contact with Dicky began 4 yr ago when he was 3½ yr old. He had been diagnosed as autistic and had been institutionalized previously for a 3-month period. Prior to this he had been diagnosed variously as psychotic, mentally retarded, and brain-damaged. Dicky had a variety of severe problem behaviors, and lacked almost all normal social and verbal behavior. His verbal repertoire was quite bizarre though not atypical of children diagnosed as autistic. He was echolalic, occasionally exactly mimicking in form and intonation bits of conversation of the staff. He sang songs, "Chicago," for example. He emitted a variety of phrases during tantrums, such as "Want a spanking," and "Want to go bye-bye" but none of his verbal behavior was socially appropriate. He never made requests, asked questions, or made comments. Although he mimicked occasionally, he would not mimic when asked to do so.

Our training began with the attendant presenting, one at a time, five pictures approximately 3 × 4 in. in size, of a Santa Claus, a cat, etc. The attendant would prompt, for example, "This is a cat. Now say cat." After she had gone through all five pictures, she would mix their order and go through them again. Just as Dicky occasionally mimicked the speech of other people, he would occasionally mimic the attendant by saying "This is a cat," or "Now say cat." On those occasions the attendant would say, "Good boy" or "That's right," and give him a bite of his meal. As a result Dicky began mimicking more frequently, until after about a week he was mimicking practically every prompt in addition to almost everything else the attendant said during the session.

However, during this time Dicky was not looking particularly closely at the pictures. Instead, he twisted and turned in his seat. So an *anticipation procedure* was introduced, where anticipating the correct response would result in a reinforcer sooner than if he waited for the prompt. The attendant would present the picture for a period of several seconds before giving the prompt. Gradually, Dicky began looking at the pictures and saying the phrases in the presence of the pictures without the prompts. In 3 weeks he did this in the presence of about ten pictures. We then introduced picture books and common household objects which he learned with increasing ease. At the same time temporally remote events were taught in the following manner. Dicky would be taken outside and swung or allowed to slide and then brought back inside and asked: "What did you do outside?" and then after a few seconds given a prompt. Imitations and finally the correct answers were followed by a reinforcer.

He was taught the answers to other questions such as, "What is your name?" and, "Where do you live?". The question would be asked and, if after a pause he had not answered, the prompt would be given and the correct response reinforced.

After several weeks of training, Dick's verbal repertoire was markedly expanded, although he still had several verbal anomalies, such as imitating the question before answering and reversing his pronouns, e.g. he would ask for a drink by saying, "You want some water." Dicky was released from hospital 7 months after our contact began. The training was continued by his parents, and after about 6 months he was using pronouns appropriately and was initiating many requests and comments, although he still was making frequent inappropriate imitating responses. After attending the Laboratory Preschool at the University of Washington for 2 yr, his verbal skills had developed to the point that he was ready for special education in the public school.

Dicky's verbal behavior now resembles that of a skilled 5-yr old. This means that since his operant training his rate of language development has been approximately normal. This probably has been the result of the diligent efforts of his parents and teachers to provide an environment which reinforced his verbal behavior. However, now the naturally occurring rewards of verbal behavior (see Skinner, 1957, for a discussion of these) appear to be the most important factors in maintaining and expanding his verbal repertoire.

These procedures for developing speech were subsequently refined in the course of working with the following echolalic children

Pat was a blind 12-yr-old boy who has been recently institutionalized with the diagnosis of childhood autism. He had previously been enrolled in a school for the blind, but had been dropped from the program due to his disruptive behavior and general lack of progress.

Billy was a 10-yr-old boy who had been institutionalized for several years with the diagnosis of childhood autism.

Carey was a 7-yr-old boy who lived at home although he had been diagnosed variously as autistic, retarded, and brain-damaged, and institutionalization had been recommended. He had attended a day-school for special children during the previous 2 yr, but had been dropped due to a general lack of progress.

Will was an 8-yr-old boy who had been institutionalized for 2 yr with the diagnosis of severe retardation and brain-damage. He was not considered to be trainable and had been placed on a custodial ward.

The physical arrangement

To work most efficiently with a deviant child, particularly one with disruptive behaviors, the speech training should be carried out in a room containing as few distractions as possible. In our training room, we usually have only chairs for the child and teacher, a desk or table between them, and a small table or chair next to the teacher on which to place the food tray.

In a room where the child may reach for, throw, or destroy many items, turn on and off light switches and climb on furniture, the therapist may inadvertently train the child to engage in these behaviors, since they must be attended to by the therapist. For some children with high rates of tantrums and disruptive behavior, the rooms have been entirely cleared except for the chairs and tables which have been secured to the floor.

The reinforcer

Certain consequences of a behavior will increase the frequency of that behavior. Those consequences, which are technically termed reinforcers, are usually events which are commonly described as important, significant, or meaningful for the particular child. With normal children, attention and praise can be used as consequences to strengthen behavior (Harris *et al.*, 1964). Such sophisticated social consequences often are only weak positive reinforcers for a severely abnormal child. For this reason food must often be relied upon as a reinforcing consequence for modifying speech and other behaviors of deviant children.

The ideal food reinforcer is one which the child particularly "likes", many bites of which can be eaten, and which cannot be readily "played with". We have found that the food reinforcer which best satisfies these criteria is ice cream or sherbet. It is generally a favorite food of children, it can be eaten in quantity, and it disappears rapidly from the mouth. Many other foods have been used, such as sugar coated cereals (Captain Crunch, Fruit Loops), TV dinners, peanut butter sandwiches, and regular meals. Bites of food are given to a child on a spoon or fork. Each bite is small, which allows large numbers of responses to be reinforced before the child becomes satiated.

A small portion of the food (e.g. $\frac{1}{4}$ teaspoon of ice cream) is placed on the spoon. The spoon is held directly in front of the therapist's face. As a child will tend to look at the food, this procedure ensures that he will be looking toward the therapist's face. The therapist then waits until the child's glance shifts from the spoon to his face and reinforces this by quickly presenting the stimulus for the child to imitate. As the sessions progress, a child will tend to look at the food less and at the therapist's face more, and the position of the spoon can then gradually be varied to suit the convenience of the therapist. The same procedure is used later in the program to train a child to attend to pictures or objects, except that, in that case, the spoon is held behind the items.

When the child responds appropriately, the therapist *immediately* says "Good" or "That's right," while extending the spoon of food to the child. This verbal statement serves to bridge the time between the appropriate response and the presentation of the food, and makes the reinforcement contingencies more precise. To save time, the food on the spoon is placed directly in the child's mouth by the therapist.

The effectiveness of the food reinforcer can be increased by mild food deprivation of about half a day. For example, when training sessions are held around noon, the mother or institutional staff are told to provide the child with only a very light breakfast, such as a glass of juice and a vitamin pill. Similar instructions involving lunch are given to caretakers of children for sessions later in the day.

For the most rapid and significant changes in deviant children the necessity of using powerful extrinsic reinforcers, made more effective by sufficient deprivation, *cannot be overemphasized*. (Examples showing the importance of the food reinforcers in the treatment of two children will be presented later.)

The elimination of disruptive behavior

Most deviant children exhibit behavior which is incompatible with the behavior involved in speech training. With echolalic children the most usual disruptive behavior is repetitive chanting of songs or TV commercials, inappropriate imitation of the experimenters, comments, and, frequently, temper tantrums whenever the reinforcer is withheld. The frequency of this behavior must be reduced before notable progress can be made in establishing functional speech. Systematic extinction procedures, in conjunction with reinforcement of appropriate responses incompatible with the disruptive behaviors, have usually been sufficient to eliminate these behaviors.

Mild disruptive behavior in the therapy situation (such as leaving the chair, autistic mannerisms, mild temper tantrums, repetitive chanting, or inappropriate imitation) can usually be eliminated by removing all possible positive reinforcers for these behaviors.

Once the child spends at least some of the session sitting quietly in the chair and has come into contact with the reinforcers, the experimenter should simply look away from the child whenever mild disruptive behavior occurs   When the child is again sitting silently in his chair, the experimenter reinforces this by attending to him and proceeding with the session. (This procedure is technically termed *time-out from positive reinforcement*.)

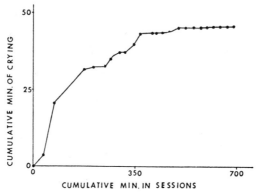

FIG. 1 The elimination of temper tantrums (crying) of Carey. (Each dot represents the end of a session.)

The temper tantrums of a child (Carey) were eliminated as a consequence of these procedures (Fig. 1). The duration of crying systematically declined from an average of 16 min/hr in the first three sessions to an average of 20 sec/hr in the twenty-fourth to twenty-sixth sessions of these conditions.

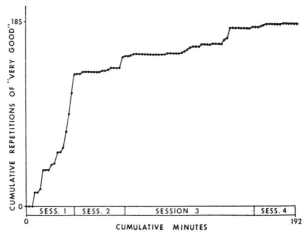

FIG. 2. The elimination of Carey's inappropriate repeating the statement "very good", which accompanied the food reinforcer. Whenever the child would say "very good" the therapist would look away for approximately 5 sec. Each dot corresponds to the 2 min of session time.

178

The procedures were also effective in reducing the frequency with which a child (Carey) inappropriately imitated and repeatedly chanted the verbal statement "Very good" which accompanied the food reinforcer (Fig. 2). During the four sessions in which this behavior was recorded, the rate declined from 3.4 to 0.12/min. By the eighth session this behavior was almost totally absent.

Where disruptive behaviors are at high strength or experimental conditions are such that these behaviors are inadvertently reinforced, a more rigorous time-out procedure may be necessary. This procedure involves both extinction of the undesirable behavior and the removal, for a period of time, of the possibility of *any* behavior being reinforced. Whenever an instance of disruptive behavior occurs, either the therapist leaves the room (with the food tray), or the child is removed to an adjacent room. The therapist re-enters or the child is allowed back in the therapy room only after both (1) a set time period had elapsed (e.g. 10 min) and (2) the child had not engaged in the disruptive behavior for a short period of time (e.g. 30 sec).

Dick's severe temper tantrums accompanied by self-destructive behavior were eliminated by this procedure (Fig. 3). The severity of the tantrums, which necessitated their rapid elimination, also made the tantrums difficult for observers to ignore. It appeared highly likely that the attendants who were working with the child, while attempting to simply ignore (extinguish) the tantrums, would feel compelled to "stop the child from hurting himself" whenever the self-destructive behavior became severe. If this had occurred, they would have been, in effect, differentially reinforcing the more extreme forms of self-destructive behavior thereby increasing the problem.

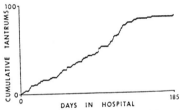

FIG. 3. The elimination of Dick's temper tantrums. The child was isolated in his room for 10 min contingent upon each tantrum, after which time he was allowed to leave the room following 30 sec of silence, each dot represents one day.

To avoid this, the child was isolated in a room whenever temper tantrums occurred. This *time-out* procedure resulted in a gradual decline in the severity of the tantrums (which is not reflected in Fig. 3, as only the frequency of tantrums was recorded) and finally a complete cessation of tantrums.

The effectiveness of either of these procedures is dependent upon the strength of the positive reinforcer which is being withheld. This is another important reason for using the strongest reinforcers possible. When only weak positive reinforcers (such as M&M's with a non-food-deprived child) are used, not only will the progress in speech be slow, but disruptive behavior will be persistent.

The establishment of control over imitation

Although echolalic children do imitate words and phrases, usually this imitation is sporadic and cannot be consistently evoked. Imitation must reliably occur immediately after a word or phrase prompt is presented before significant advances in speech can be made.

179

Reliable and immediate imitation can be obtained by systematic reinforcement of imitation. The therapist presents a given word every 4–5 sec. Whenever the child says this word he is reinforced. Initially the probability of imitation can be somewhat increased by varying the intonation, pitch level and loudness of the word presented; however, this procedure should be deleted as soon as the child is reliably repeating the word.

Systematically reinforcing an imitated word will increase the frequency with which the child imitates that word, but it may also increase the frequency of non-imitative repetitions of the word. Other verbal utterances such as phrases or snatches of song may also increase and should be extinguished. The therpist should wait until the child is silent before again presenting the word to be imitated. In this manner only *imitation* is being reinforced.

When the child is frequently imitating the word (5–6 times/min), extraneous behavior should be extinguished and attending to the therapist reinforced by presenting the word to be imitated only when the child is sitting quietly, looking at the therapist. As the probability of immediate imitation is greater when the child is looking at the therapist, this procedure, which increases the proportion of attending, increases the number of immediate imitations.

When the child is reliably and immediately imitating the first word, a new word is introduced, and the above procedure is repeated. The two words are then alternately presented. When the child is reliably imitating both words, new words are presented interpersed with the two original words. Usually by the second or third word, a general imitative response class will have been established, i.e. the child will then reliably and immediately imitate any new word.

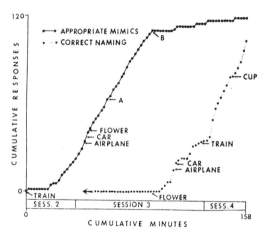

Fig. 4. A record of the initial rate of appropriate imitations (mimics) and correct naming of objects by Carey (see text). Each dot represents 2 min of session time.

Figure 4 shows the establishment of control over a child's (Carey) imitation. From the start of session 2 the word "train" was repeated by the experimenter. The child imitated this word once early in the session, and was reinforced. Sixteen minutes later, during which time he was intermittently having tantrums, he again imitated "train" and was reinforced. After this the rate of imitating the word rapidly increased. Three other words, "flower," "car" and "airplane," were then introduced, and the child imitated each of them on the first presentation as well as on each subsequent presentation. Thus, in approximately 30 min, control was established over the child's imitative speech.

The transition from imitation to naming

Naming involves the emission of the appropriate verbal response in the presence of some stimulus object. After imitative responses occur with high probability and short latency following each verbal prompt, stimulus control is shifted from the verbal prompts (imitation) to appropriate objects and pictures (naming).

Once reinforcement for imitation has produced a high probability of successful imitation of the verbal prompt alone, a picture or object is presented together with the verbal prompt, and the child is reinforced for imitating the name. Then the imitative prompt is faded out, while the child continues to receive reinforcement for saying the object's name.

The therapist holds up an object (if necessary holding the spoonful of food behind it) and says, "What is this?". When the child looks at it, the therapist immediately prompts with the object's name. The child is reinforced for imitating the prompt. When the child is reliably looking at the object without the food being held behind it, the time between the question "What is this?" and the prompt is gradually lengthened to more than 5 sec. If after several trials the child continues to wait for the presentation of the verbal prompt, a *partial prompt* is given, for example, "Trr" for train. If the correct response does not occur within about 5 sec more, the complete prompt is then presented. A correct response is followed by a social consequence such as "right" or "good", and the partial prompt is immediately repeated. A correct response to the partial prompt results in a bite of food.

When the child begins saying the name when only the partial prompt is presented, the therapist continues the above procedure but begins to say the partial prompt more softly. The loudness of the partial prompt is varied according to the child's behavior. When the child fails to respond to a partial prompt and the complete prompt is presented, the next partial prompt is given more loudly. When the child correctly responds to the partial prompt, the next partial prompt is given more softly. This continues until the therapist only "mouths" the partial prompt and then, finally, discontinues it altogether as the child responds to the object and the question "What is this?" with the name of the object.

Throughout this procedure, whenever the child inappropriately imitates the question "What is this?", a time-out is programmed, i.e. the object is withdrawn and the therapist looks down at the table. After 2 or 3 sec of silence by the child, the therapist looks up and continues the procedure.

The transition from imitation to naming with one child (Carey) is illustrated in Fig. 4. From point A in Fig. 4, the pictures of the four objects were held out one at a time, and the child was required to look at them before the therapist said the name. The child quickly began attending to the pictures. The therapist's presentation of the words had been discriminative for the child to imitate and be reinforced. The increased proportion of attending indicated that the word presentations themselves had become reinforcers.

Just before B in Fig. 4, the therapist began delaying naming the picture, requiring a longer period of attending by the child, so that he would be more likely to name the picture instead of imitating the therapist. At B the child began to tantrum during an especially long delay. The therapist merely sat quietly looking down at the table. The tantrum gradually subsided and the therapist again held up the picture (the flower). The child attended to the picture and promptly named it. After this he named the picture with increasing speed with each presentation.

The picture of the airplane was re-introduced. The child immediately said "Car." The therapist said, "No, airplane." The child mimicked this and correctly named the picture when it was immediately re-presented. The remaining two pictures were then re-introduced, and the child correctly named each after a single prompt. After this he correctly named the four pictures when each was presented. Next, a new object, a cup, was presented. After imitating only two prompts, the child correctly named it and continued to name it correctly when it was presented interspersed with the original four pictures. Thus, by the end of the third session a small naming vocabulary had been established.

The following two examples demonstrate the role of food reinforcers in the maintenance of appropriate naming behavior. During the first five training sessions with Will, reliable imitation and then appropriate naming had been developed. The reinforcer involved a variety of edibles, such as ice cream, Coke, and M&M's.

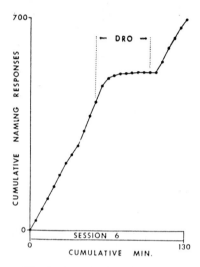

FIG. 5. A cumulative record showing the results of changing the food reinforcement contingency on Wills' rate of correct naming. During the sixth session a DRO contingency (see text) was introduced for 9 min and Will's rate of naming decreased to zero. When the original food reinforcement contingency was reinstated the behavior increased to its pre-DRO rate.

The contribution of the food reinforcer was investigated by reversing the relationship between the naming behavior and the reinforcer. About a third of the way through the sixth session, the procedure was changed so that the child was reinforced only when he *did not* correctly name a picture for 10 sec. This procedure is technically termed *differential reinforcement of other behavior* (DRO) because any behavior except one particular response, in this case naming, is reinforced. As can be seen in Fig. 5, the naming responses dropped from about 8/min to zero. After 45 min, when no naming responses were being made, the procedure was changed back so that naming responses were again the only responses being reinforced. The rate of naming quickly increased to approximately the same rate as during the first part of the session. These results show the power of the reinforcer over the occurrence and accuracy of Will's naming behavior.

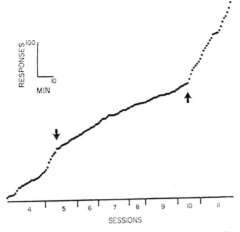

Fɪɢ. 6. A cumulative record showing the effects of Carey receiving bites of ice cream independent of his picture naming responses. For the first session and a half in Fig. 8 Carey was fed a bite of ice cream after each correct response. At the first arrow Carey was allowed to feed himself ice cream independent of his naming responses. At the second arrow the food reinforcers were again made contingent upon correctly naming the pictures. Each dot represents a 1-min period.

Once a reliable rate of naming had been developed with Carey the procedure was changed in that ice cream was given on a non-contingent basis. Instead of giving him bites of ice cream after each correct response, he was given the spoon and the bowl of ice cream and allowed to eat at his own rate. Pictures continued to be presented. he was still asked to name them, and when he named them correctly he was praised. The rate of correct naming dropped immediately from approximately 8 to 3/min and then stabilized at about 2/min (Fig. 6). When the ice cream was again presented only after correct naming responses, the rate immediately increased to approximately 10 responses/min.

To summarize, Carey's results show that after naming responses have been acquired, it may be possible to maintain them (although at a lower rate) with a weak reinforcer such as praise alone, but, as shown in the case of both the children the more powerful food reinforcer maintained a much higher and more steady rate of appropriate behavior.

The expansion of the naming vocabulary

After the child has been taught to name several pictures or objects, naming any new picture or object can be quickly established. However, the child often will not correctly name an item at the beginning of the next daily session or subsequent to learning other new items in the same session. A new response cannot be considered to be added to a child's naming vocabulary until he can name an item when it is presented again after other items have been learned, and following a passage of time. This is accomplished by gradually changing the context in which the item is presented. After a child is consistently naming new items on repeated presentations, a previously learned item is presented. When the child names the old item he is reinforced and the new item is presented again. When the child is reliably naming a new item when it follows one presentation of any of several previously taught items, two, then three, then four old items are presented between each presentation of the new item. (The well-established naming of old items need be reinforced only intermittently with food to maintain accuracy and short latencies.) When the child is reliably naming a new item under these conditions, another new item is introduced. When an item is reliably named the first time it is presented in several subsequent sessions, it can be considered to be a member of the child's naming vocabulary; only occasional reviews in subsequent sessions are needed to maintain it.

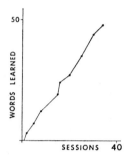

FIG. 7. A cumulative record of Pat's learning to name objects correctly. The name of an object was recorded as "learned" when Pat named it correctly the first time it was presented in three successive sessions.

Figure 7 shows the increasing naming vocabulary of Pat, a blind echolalic boy, who was taught to name common household objects which were placed in his hands. An item was considered to be "learned" when the child correctly named it on its first presentation in three successive sessions.

Carey's naming vocabulary was expanded under two reinforcement conditions. The items to be named were pictures (line drawings) of various objects. Two 10-min sessions a day were held, with separate pictures for each session. In one of the sessions each day, the reinforcer was praise ("That's right, very good") and a bite of ice cream, whereas praise alone was used in the other session. Several pictures were repeatedly presented in a random order during each session. New pictures were added when the child was consistently naming all the pictures used during a session. A picture was considered to be learned when the child correctly named it the first time it was presented, three sessions in a row. It would then be retired until ten subsequent pictures had been learned, at which time it would be presented again to test for recall.

While the child learned to name 50 per cent more pictures when both praise and ice cream were used as reinforcers (——, Fig. 8), his naming vocabulary was significantly expanded when praise was the only reinforcer (- - - -, Fig. 8). Furthermore, items were recalled equally well whether they had been reinforced with praise only or with both praise and ice cream (histogram, Fig. 8). However, following this evaluation, since only one session per day could be held, the more effective reinforcer, a combination of ice cream and praise, was used throughout the remaining sessions. Approximately one new word per session was established with this reinforcer (. . . . ., Fig. 8).

184

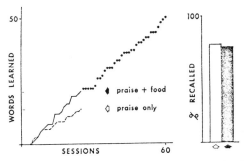

FIG. 8. Records of the number of pictures which Carey learned to name and later recalled in daily sessions under two reinforcement conditions, praise alone ("that's right" or "very good") and both praise and food (bites of ice cream). A picture was considered to be learned when the child named it when it was first presented in three successive sessions. A picture was considered to be recalled when the child correctly named it when it was re-presented after ten subsequent pictures had been learned.

Just as Fig. 7 demonstrates that established naming can be maintained (although at a lower rate) with praise as the only reinforcer, Fig. 9. shows that when a child can readily be taught to name new items with food reinforcers his naming vocabulary can then be significantly expanded (although at a lower rate) when only social reinforcers of the type available in a "normal" environment are used.

The authors consider it necessary to use strong reinforcers such as food to establish the initial instances of appropriate mimicking and naming behavior and to eliminate disruptive behavior in a reasonable period of time. However, it appears that once disruptive behaviors have been eliminated and some appropriate mimicking and naming have been established, these appropriate behaviors can be maintained and expanded by the systematic use of social reinforcers. This does *not* imply that food deprivation and food reinforcers should then be discontinued. The magnitude of a child's speech deficits and the value of a therapist's and of a child's time require the utilization of those procedures which will produce the greatest gains in the shortest time. The strongest reinforcers or combination of reinforcers available should be used in the therapy sessions so long as large behavioral deficits exist. However, social reinforcers outside the therapy sessions can generally be relied upon to maintain and expand the behaviors established in the sessions.

The establishment of phrases

Once naming is established, the response units can be expanded to phrases and sentences. In most cases this expansion occurs without explicit training. In those instances where multiple word units have to be taught, the procedure is the same as in teaching individual words, i.e. mimics of the phrases are reinforced until the phrases are consistently imitated. Then the control is shifted to the appropriate circumstance itself, by introducing partial prompts which are gradually faded out. In this case, the partial prompts are the first word or words of the phrase.

At first, phrases such as "That's a- ——," or "I want——" are taught, using the child's newly acquired naming vocabulary. Then more varied phrases are taught, such as answering the appropriate questions with "My name is——," "I live at——." "I am————years old," "My sisters' names are————and——."

185

Food reinforcers are used to build the initial responses, but, once established, the opportunity to obtain some natural consequence can usually maintain the behavior. For example, for Carey the comment, "Out (or in) the door," was maintained by opening the doors to and from the therapy room. The therapist would say, "Out the door," and when the child would mimic this, the door would be opened.

After several trials on succeeding days, the therapist began introducing a partial prompt, saying only, "Out," and the child continued to say, "Out the door." The partial prompt was then gradually faded out until the therapist put his hand on the door knob and looked at the child, and the child said, "Out the door." The therapist gradually faded in the appropriate controlling stimulus—the question, "Where are you going?" This was presented by at first mumbling it softly as they approached the door and then increasing the volume on succeeding trials. Whenever the child inappropriately imitated the question "Where are you going?" the therapist repeated the question at a lower volume and followed it with a loud partial prompt: "Where are you going? OUT." On succeeding trials the partial prompt, "Out," was then decreased in volume until the child responded to the closed door and the question, "Where are you going?" with the response "Out the door."

The same procedure was used to establish appropriate answers to the question, "Where are you going?", such as "Up the stairs," "Down the hall" or "In the car." In each case, the reinforcer which maintained appropriate answering was simply being allowed to proceed up the stairs, down the hall, and so on. In this manner the child came to make appropriate verbal comments about his environment. Once such simple comments have been learned, the child tends to generalize the grammatical form with appropriate substitutions. One example of such establishment and generalization, which could be termed "generative speech," resulted from a procedure used with Carey. On many occasions at home, this child would chant a word or short phrase over and over, with gradually increasing volume which terminated in piercing shrieks and crying. For example, while standing by the couch, he would repeat "Sit down, sit down." His parents could terminate this by responding in any way, e.g. "Yes, Carey" "O.K., sit down," "You can sit down if you want to," "Be quiet." The parents were requested to record these instances of stereotyped chanting, and also to send him to his room for 5 min whenever the chanting developed into shrieking and crying. This decreased the occurrences of the shrieking   , but did not decrease the frequency of the stereotyped chanting episodes .   The therapist decided to change the form of this behavior, rather than attempt to eliminate it, as it contained elements of appropriate social behavior.

The parents were instructed to turn away from the child when he chanted. One parent (e.g. the father) would then call out the name of the other parent ("Mommy"), and when the child would mimic this the mother would attend to him and "Yes, Carey." The first parent would then say a complete sentence ("I want to sit down, please."). When the child would mimic this, the other parent would respond accordingly ("Oh, you want to sit down. Well, you can sit down right here."). On subsequent occasions the verbal prompts were faded out. Finally, the parents withheld reinforcement by looking away until the child called their names, and they would wait while looking at him until he gave the complete sentence before responding to his request. This procedure was begun at the arrow in Fig. 9 . The stereotyped chanting soon decreased to zero as the child began to indicate more appropriate requests such as "Mommy, I want to sit down, please", or Daddy, I want a drink of water, please."

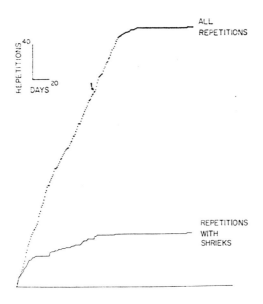

FIG. 9. A cumulative record of episodes of repetitious chanting by Carey at home. From the onset, he was sent to his room for 5 min whenever he began shrieking during one of those episodes. At the arrow his parents began establishing appropriate speech behavior which was incompatible with chanting. Each dot represents one day.

The grammatical structure of "(name), I want———, please," after being established with several people's names and many different requests in the home began to generalize to new people and new requests. One recorded instance of this occurred in the therapy sessions. Prior to the start of each session, when Carey was seated in the room, the therapist would spend some time setting up the tape recorder. During this time the child would usually start chanting "Ice cream, ice cream" softly. When the therapist was ready, he would turn to the child and say, "What do you want?" to which the child had been taught to answer "I want some ice cream." Prior to one session, after the grammatical form of requests mentioned above had been established at home, the child was, as usual, chanting "Ice cream, ice cream" while the therapist threaded the tape recorder. He suddenly stopped and after a pause, said "Mr. (therapist's name), I want some ice cream, please." Most of the elements of this sentence had been established in the therapy sessions, e.g. "Hello, Mr. (therapist's name)," and "I want some ice cream," "but they had always been given as responses to specific stimuli, (e.g. "Hello, Carey" and "What do you want?") However, the particular grammatical structure of "(Name), I want———, please," had only been taught in the home.

Carey's extension of his home training exemplifies our general observation that once rudimentary generative speech and grammatical structure have been established they will tend to generalize broadly, often with appropriate substitutions.

The generalization of appropriate speech

The term "generalization" can refer to the *phenomenon* of the occurrence of appropriate behavior under other than the original training conditions or it can refer to the *procedure* used to establish this occurrence.

While newly acquired appropriate speech often will "spontaneously" generalize widely, the therapist need not passively rely on this phenomenon. He can, instead, set out to extend the occurrence of the behavior to other situations by systematically reinforcing appropriate speech under a variety of conditions. The child can be systematically trained to respond appropriately to a variety of individuals, including members of his family and other caretakers, and in a variety of situations, such as at home, in the family car, and in the therapist's office. Once appropriate speech has been established in the therapy sessions, the child's parents can be present during occasional sessions and the child reinforced for responding appropriately to their questions. Whenever a new word has been established in a therapy session, the therapist can continue to ask for, and reinforce the appropriate use of this word after the formal session, for instance, while walking around the building. The therapist can also conduct therapy sessions in the child's home, teaching the child to name household objects.

Generalization training can be facilitated by initially selecting words and phrases to be taught which can be appropriately asked for frequently during the day, e.g. "car" is better than "zebra," and which are immediately functional in the child's environment, e.g. "I want a cookie."

Perhaps the most effective means of generalizing the appropriate use of speech is to train the parents or caretakers to use the therapeutic procedures. They can then take advantage of naturally-occurring events during the day to generalize appropriate speech to a wide variety of situations, as well as to establish new speech in appropriate contexts.

The usefulness of data in therapy

The gathering of continuous data throughout the course of therapy can be valuable in many ways. For example, it can provide objective information about the long term course of therapy. Behaviors followed over a long period of time, as described in this paper, often reveal an orderliness which is not clear from the day-by-day observations. Gradual changes can be discerned in spite of large daily fluctuations, as in the instance of the rate of Carey's shrieking. The frequency of the shrieks decreased in a manner which was orderly overall even though some of the individual days (sometimes several consecutive days) showed considerable variability.

A second use of data is in the analysis of the functions of therapeutic procedures. An *experimental probe* is usually necessary if the therapist wants to isolate the variables responsible for a behavioral change. Isolation is accomplished by keeping all of the therapeutic conditions the same except one. If varying this condition produces a reliable change in the data, which disappears when the condition is reversed to its pre-experimental value, then the importance of the variable has been established. Sidman (1960) has discussed in detail strategies and considerations for research with individual subjects. Probe experiments of the above type were described in this paper. For example, the role of the food reinforcement contingency in Will's progress in naming was evaluated (Fig. 5). Its importance was dramatically demonstrated when the DRO procedure was interjected into a session. A similar probe experiment, in a slightly different manner and over a longer period of time, demonstrated the function of the food reinforcement in Carey's rate of naming pictures (Fig. 6).

The easiest of data-gathering methods is to use a tape recorder to record all of the sessions. The therapist or an assistant can replay tapes from previous sessions and count the frequencies of various responses (e.g. correct imitations) or the durations of certain behaviors (e.g. temper tantrums, inappropriate chanting). Tapes of earlier sessions are particularly useful for gathering data about behavior that was not originally thought to be of interest.

A multi-pen event recorder can be used if the therapist is certain in advance of the classes of behavior that he will want to record. A bank of push-button switches can be wired from the therapist's table to the recorder so that durations and frequencies of responses can be recorded by the therapist and/or by an independent observer.

A pencil and paper can always be used to take simple frequencies. Duration of a specific behavior can be recorded during each session with a stop watch.

Such data and probe experiments enable the therapist to give a more complete and objective description of his procedures and their effects to others, including colleagues who are also interested in developing a more effective technology of speech modification through a systematic analysis of speech modification procedures.

CONCLUSIONS

This paper indicates that functional verbal behavior can be developed from rudimentary imitative behavior by established behavioral techniques. We have outlined procedures which were effective in establishing functional speech in echolalic children. However, the procedures as they are described here should not be taken as fixed and unchanging. The developing strength of behavioral technology lies in the continued refinement of its procedures.

Acknowledgements—The teachers who played particularly important roles in Dicky's speech development were FLORENCE HARRIS, MARGARET JOHNSTON, EILEEN ALLEN, NANCY REYNOLDS and THELMA TURBITT. Will's data was collected by JACQULYN RAULERSON and THOMAS DILLON under the senior author's supervision. We are indebted to STEPHANIE STOLZ, NANCY REYNOLDS and BETTY HART for critical readings of the manuscript.

REFERENCES

HARRIS F. R., WOLF M. M. and BAER D. M. (1964) Effects of adult social reinforcement on child behavior. *Young Child.* 20, 8–17.
LOVAAS O. I. (1966) A program for the establishment of speech in psychotic children. In (Ed. WING J. K.) *Childhood Autism.* Pergamon Press, Oxford.
RISLEY T. R. (1966) The establishment of verbal behavior in deviant children. Unpublished dissertation, University of Washington.
SIDMAN M. (1960) *Tactics of Scientific Research.* Basic Books, New York.
SKINNER B. F. (1957) *Verbal Behavior.* Appleton-Century-Crofts, New York.
STONE J. L. and CHURCH J. (1957) *Childhood and Adolescence.* Random House, New York.
WOLF M. M., RISLEY T. R. and MEES H. I. (1964) Application of operant conditioning procedures to the behavior problems of an autistic child. *Behav. Res. & Therapy* 1, 305–312.

Epidemiology of Autistic Conditions in Young Children

II. Some Characteristics of the Parents and Children

Victor Lotter, B.A.

Medical Research Council, Social Psychiatry Research Unit, Institute of Psychiatry, London

Introduction

A survey to estimate the prevalence of autistic disorders in all 8—10 year-old children in the County of Middlesex was conducted in 1963/64. Methods used to screen the population and collect data were described in an earlier report (Lotter, 1966 a), in which the prevalence, sex ratio, distribution of intelligence and patterns of onset were discussed. Only a brief description of the survey procedures is therefore presented here.

Using a modified version of Creak's (1961) criteria for the selection of cases, the 78,000 children SOCIAL PSYCHIATRY, 1967, Vol. 1., pp. 163–173.

in the selected age-range were screened in several stages. From behaviour questionnaires completed by nearly all ordinary and special schools, hospitals and institutions containing Middlesex children, and from local authority case records of handicapped children, 135 children were chosen; each child was given intelligence tests, and behaviour descriptions were obtained from an informant who knew him well. 61 children were retained in the series at the end of this stage, and their parents were then interviewed where possible. Both parents were tested on two intelligence scales, a detailed developmental and behaviour description was obtained from the mother, and standard family data were recorded.

After 7 of the 61 children were excluded because of incomplete data, all information, including hospital reports, for the remaining 54 were combined for each child and analysed. Ratings on 24 behaviour items were made and 3 groups were formed on the basis of the resulting "scores":

Group A (Austistic). $N = 15$, cases 1—15. Children showing a combination of marked impairment in personal relationships as well as marked repetitive-ritualistic behaviour. This group included most with the highest over-all scores.

Group B (Autistic). $N = 17$, cases 16—32. Those without the above *combination* of behaviours, who had lower scores and more heterogeneous symptoms.

Group C (Non-autistic, handicapped). $N = 22$, cases 33—54. The remaining children with the lowest scores, many of whom nevertheless had certain behaviours similar to groups A and B. These children were retained as a comparison group.

As used in this report, the term "autistic" is intended to denote any child who met the criteria for inclusion in groups A or B, or the kinds of behaviour used to define these groups, and should be understood here in that sense only.

Ninety-seven per cent of the estimated population were screened. The 35 autistic children found, including 3 excluded from the rating because of incomplete data but who were considered on the basis of available descriptions to be autistic, represent a prevalence rate of 4.5 per 10,000 for autistic disorders at age 8—10 in Middlesex. About half this number had the symptom combination defining group A.

In this report, the results of further analyses of certain epidemiological data are presented.

The Families

1. Fathers' Occupation

Probands were classified according to their fathers' occupations into the 5 social class categories for which there were published national figures. The social class distributions of the autistic probands, the non-autistic comparison group, and the general population are compared in Table 1. The distribution in the non-autistic group is very similar to that expected, while there is a marked over-representation in social classes I and II in the autistic group. The behaviour subgroup A was significantly different from groups B and C combined. (Social classes I and II combined: $X^2 = 3.68$, d.f. 1, $p = <.05$ — One tail test.) The difference between the observed and expected frequencies in the autistic group was statistically significant ($X^2 = 8.07$, d.f. 2, $p = <.02$ — Social classes I and II combined).

There were differences in social class within the whole group of autistic probands. Thus, amongst the 15 group A cases, 9 (60%) were in social classes I and II, compared with 5 (31%) of 16 group B cases. Similarly, of the 16 cases whose early development was not retarded (see LOTTER, 1966 a), 9 (56%) were in social classes I and II, compared with 5 (33%) of 15 retarded probands. Likewise, 8 (80%) of the 10 probands with a setback at onset (see LOTTER, ibid) were in social classes I and II, compared with 6 (28%) of 21 without a setback. A group of 22 probands including all the cases in group A, and all those without early developmental retardation, and all with an onset involving a setback in development, contained 13 of the 14 cases from social classes I and II.

Examination of the social class of the maternal and paternal grandfathers showed few differences between the parents' present social status and the social status of the homes in which they grew up.

2. Parents' Education

The mothers and fathers of the probands were divided into 3 categories according to their educational level (Table 2). Parents of children in group A had significantly more education after the age of 15 years, than the parents of the non-autistic children. Of the fathers in groups A, B and C, 43%, 12$^1/_2$%, and 5% respectively had professional occupations or were university graduates.

Table 1. *Observed and Expected Social Class Distribution of the Survey Probands*

Social class	Autistic probands				Non-autistic probands		General population %
	Group A	Group B	Groups A & B O	E	Group C O	E	
I	5	2	7	1.6	0	1.1	5.0
II	4	3	7	5.7	5	3.9	18.5
III	4	9	13	17.7	12	12.0	57.2
IV—V	2	2	4	6.0	4	4.0	19.3
Totals:	15	16	31	31.0	21	21.0	100.0
Not known:	—	1	1		1		

Note: 1. Proportions in general population of the County of Middlesex based on a 1% sample, National Census, 1951.
2. One illegitimate proband was classified according to the occupation (social class I) of the adoptive father.

Table 2. *Actual and Percentage Distribution of Parents (Mothers and Fathers Combined) According to Educational Level Reached, for the Three Survey Groups*

Educational level	Group A N %		Group B N %		Group C N %	
School up to 15 years only	7	(25)	19	(59)	34	(81)
School after 15, or technical or other further formal training	12	(43)	9	(28)	7	(17)
Professional education or university graduate	9	(32)	4	(13)	1	(2)
Totals:	28	(100)	32	(100)	42	(100)

Data were not known for 2 parents in each group.
Including adoptive parents (father — graduate, mother — school after 15) for 1 child in group A.
Significance: A vs. B vs. C: $X^2 = 24.15$, d.f. $= 4$, $p = < .001$.

3. Parents' Intelligence

Two tests were used to estimate parents' intelligence: the Standard Progressive Matrices, and the Mill Hill Vocabulary Scale (form 1, senior) (RAVEN, 1962). The norms for both tests are expressed in percentile ranges. Score distributions on the two tests are shown in Tables 3 and 4.

Scores could not be obtained for substantial proportions of parents in each subgroup. The social class distribution of the untested parents was in each group similar to that of the whole group (see Appendix A). It is likely therefore that the scores of the untested parents would have resembled those of the tested parents and that their exclusion did not seriously distort the distributions shown.

When the available test scores were examined statistically, the following results were obtained:
a) *The autistic group AB.* All parents: observed

Table 3. *Score Distributions of Mothers and Fathers in Groups A, B and C on the Mill Hill Vocabulary Scale*

Percentile range		Autistic probands							Non-autistic probands			
		Group A		Group B		Group A & B				Group C		
								Mothers		Fathers		
		M	F	M	F	Mothers N %		Fathers N %		Mothers N %		Fathers N %
I	96—100	4	3	2	1	6	(24)	4	(17.4)	1	(5.9)	0	(0.0)
II + 91— 95		1	0	0	1	1	(4)	1	(4.3)	0	(0.0)	1	(6.3)
II 76— 90		0	2	1	1	1	(4)	3	(13.0)	1	(5.9)	0	(0.0)
III + 51— 75		4	5	3	4	7	(28)	9	(39.2)	1	(5.9)	6	(37.5)
III − 26— 50		2	1	5	4	7	(28)	5	(21.8)	9	(52.9)	6	(37.5)
IV 0— 25		1	0	2	1	3	(12)	1	(4.3)	5	(29.4)	3	(18.7)
Totals:		12	11	13	12	25	(100)	23	(100.0)	17	(100.0)	16	(100.0)
Not tested		3	4	4	5	7		9		5		6	
All parents:		15	15	17	17	32		32		22		22	

Table 4. *Score Distributions of Mothers and Fathers in Groups A, B, and C on the Standard Progressive Matrices Scale*

Percentile range		Autistic probands							Non-autistic probands			
		Group A		Group B		Group A & B				Group C		
								Mothers		Fathers		
		M	F	M	F	Mothers N %		Fathers N %		Mothers N %		Fathers N %
I	96—100	4	6	2	3	6	(25.0)	9	(37.4)	3	(17.6)	6	(33.3)
II + 91— 95		1	3	6	0	7	(29.2)	3	(12.5)	1	(5.9)	2	(11.0)
II 76— 90		3	0	0	4	3	(12.5)	4	(16.7)	3	(17.6)	7	(38.9)
III + 51— 75		1	2	3	4	4	(16.7)	6	(25.0)	2	(11.8)	1	(5.6)
III − 26— 50		2	0	0	1	2	(8.3)	1	(4.2)	7	(41.2)	1	(5.6)
IV 0— 25		0	0	2	1	2	(8.3)	1	(4.2)	1	(5.9)	1	(5.6)
Totals:		11	11	13	13	24	(100.0)	24	(100.0)	17	(100.0)	18	(100.0)
Not tested:		4	4	4	4	8		8		5		4	
All parents:		15	15	17	17	32		32		22		22	

vs. expected frequencies, score classes I, II + vs. II, III + vs. III −, IV.

Mill Hill: $X^2 = 13.43$, d.f. 2, $p = <.01$.

Matrices: $X^2 = 98.75$, d.f. 2, $p = <.001$.

b) *The non-autistic group C.* All parents: observed vs. expected frequencies, score classes I, II + vs. II, III + vs. III −, IV.

Mill Hill: $X^2 = 5.12$, d.f. 2, $p = <.10$ (not significant).

Matrices: $X^2 = 23.87$, d.f. 2, $p = <.001$.

c) *The behaviour subgroups.* All parents: groups A vs. B vs. C, score classes I, II + vs. II, III + vs. III −, IV.

Mill Hill: $X^2 = 21.2$, d.f. 4, $p = <.001$.

Matrices: $X^2 = 6,42$, d.f. 4, $p = <.20$ (not significant).

It can be seen that the parents in the autistic group AB were significantly superior to the general population on both tests. Parents in the non-autistic group were inferior to the general population on the Mill Hill Scale, but the difference was not statistically significant. They were, however, significantly superior to the general population on the Matrices test. The results of the intergroup comparisons were consistent with these findings.

According to RAVEN (1941) the Matrices Scale discriminates occupation classes. The high scores in the occupationally inferior group C were therefore unexpected. He also states, however (RAVEN, 1962), that scores tend to cluster into the upper percentile ranges. Further examination of the test scores within social class groupings showed that, for the mothers in social classes III—V, there was a significant difference between the autistic and non-autistic groups (FISHER test, $p = <.01$). Moreover, amongst social class III—V parents in the autistic group, the mother most often obtained a higher score than her husband. Out of 11 cases in the autistic group, 7 mothers had scores equal to, or higher than, their husbands. Out of 11 cases in the non-autistic groups, all mothers were inferior to their husbands and in 4 cases the difference was more than two score classes. This difference between the mothers and fathers in group C was statistically significant (FISHER test, $p = <.005$).

No significant differences were found on the Matrices Scale between the parents of the autistic and non-autistic groups in social classes I—II. However, the greater number of social classes I—II fathers in the autistic group with high scores compared with the non-autistic group approached the 5% level of significance.

The difference between the groups of mothers in social classes III—V may be associated with education. A significantly greater number of social class III—V mothers in the autistic group had some education after age 15 years of age than in the non-autistic group ($p = <.025$, FISHER test). However, amongst social class III—V mothers who attended school up to 15 years of age only, a significantly greater number in the autistic group had scores above the 90th percentile than in the non-autistic group ($p = <.05$, FISHER test). The mothers of the autistic children were, therefore, more intelligent than the mothers of similar social class and educational level in the non-autistic group. There was some further evidence of this in the kinds of work the social class III-V mothers had done before they married. While similar proportions in the autistic and non-autistic groups had clerical or other jobs involving some skill, several in the autistic group had jobs which required special training, such as nurse, post office telegraphist, shorthand-typist, and bank clerk. In the non-autistic group, the jobs tended to involve simpler skills.

Subjects should achieve approximately equivalent percentile rankings on both the Mill Hill and Matrices scales (RAVEN, 1962). For most parents in the survey, scores were within one, or at the most two, percentile ranks on the two tests. However, out of 11 social class III—V fathers in group C, 6 had Matrices scores three or more score classes above their vocabulary scores.

4. Mental Health

a) The parents. Data could be obtained for 28 out of the 30 parents in group A, 32 out of the 34 in group B, and 42 out of the 44 in the comparison group C. Of all these 102 parents, 12 had some "mental disturbance". In 2 cases, both parents were affected. Because of the difficulty of obtaining reliable details of milder problems not requiring hospital admission, only those parents who at some time were admitted to a psychiatric hospital will be described in any detail.

Of the 12 affected parents, 6 at some time were admitted to hospital for psychiatric treatment. Case notes could be obtained for 4 of them, and were examined by a psychiatrist (J. W.). Brief details of the illnesses and the psychiatrist's diagnoses are:

The Autistic Group AB

Case 3 (Mother): Recurrent affective disturbances since thyroidectomy at age 32 years. Admitted to hospital at 32 years of age for 1 month. Treated with E.C.T. Diagnosis: cyclothymic personality with recurrent depressions.

Case 15 (Mother): Four previous suicidal attempts. Admitted to hospital at age 35 years for 3 months with depression following problems with a subnormal child (the proband). Treated with E.C.T. Diagnosis: non-psychotic reactive depression.

Case 18 (Mother): Admitted to hospital for 1 month. Delusions and visual hallucinations not specific for schizophrenia. Original hospital diagnosis: hypomania. Final diagnosis: amphetamine psychosis.

Case 23 (Father): Case notes could not be obtained. Reported by his wife (divorced) to have had in-patient psychiatric treatment. Discharged from army as "neurotic"; has tried several different occupations. Reported to have been called a "paranoid psychopath".

Case 11 (Father): Case notes could not be obtained. Reported by his widow to have received in-patient psychiatric treatment. Deserted family and subsequently died in an accident abroad. No details of the nature of the illness could be obtained.

The Non-autistic Group

Case 46 (Father): Several admissions to psychiatric hospitals. Hospital diagnoses varied from presenile dementia to hysteria or schizophrenia. Most recent notes indicated hallucinations controlled by phenothiazines, but earlier evidence of organic impairment not mentioned. Suggested diagnosis: psychosis of unspecified type, possibly schizophrenia.

Details for the remaining 6 parents cannot be considered reliable nor can it be assumed all the parents with milder disturbances are included. Brief details as reported are:

Case 5 (Mother): Said to be "afraid to go outside".

Case 11 (Mother): Widow of father described above. Reports having a "nervous breakdown" when she was 14 years old, as well as after the birth of one of her children.

Case 18 (Father): Husband of mother described above. Receives out-patient group psychotherapy. Said to be an "inadequate psychopath".

Case 24 (Mother): Reported to have had a recent "nervous breakdown" and to be frequently depressed.

Case 27 (Mother): Under medication for long-standing epilepsy.

Case 30 (Mother): Reports having a "breakdown" when she was 15 years old.

There were no reports of similar mild disorders amongst the parents of the non-autistic group.

Thus, in the autistic group, of 60 parents for whom data could be obtained, only 1 was known to have had a psychotic illness, while 4 others had some mental illness requiring in-patient treatment. One out of 42 parents in the non-autistic group had a psychotic illness. The incidence of milder disorders was greater amongst the parents of the autistic group than in the group C parents.

b) The parents' siblings. Data could be obtained about the siblings of altogether 97 parents. These parents had 281 siblings — 62 in group A, 68 in group B, and 151 in group C. Only one of these relatives had a serious mental illness requiring hospital treatment: a sister of the mother in case 3 had a leucotomy and is institutionalised in the U.S.A.

c) The probands' siblings. The 86 living siblings of all the probands (29 in group A, 33 in group B, 24 in group C) ranged in age from 1 to 35 years. Nearly half of them in groups A and B, and a quarter in group C, were under 10 years old.

Five of these 86 siblings had required help at some time from medical or social service agencies on account of their behaviour. In 2 cases, the reason was relatively minor: one was a delinquent, and one was thought to be slightly retarded (one other sibling not included here was epileptic, but otherwise normal). The remaining 3 siblings had more serious disorders; all were in the autistic group.

Case 13: An elder brother, said to have been "difficult" since age 3 when younger sib (the proband) was born. First referred at age 6 years for behaviour difficulties at school. No reliable I.Q. could be obtained at this time, but he attended regularly at a child guidance clinic. By age 7, he had a Binet I.Q. of 65; he was "very anxious, and tended to be afraid of new arrangements". His behaviour was ritualised, and he tended to speak reluctantly. Attendance at the clinic continued until age 11 years. I.Q. remains E.S.N. range. Socially, he is much improved, and attends a boarding school. He was thought at the clinic to be a "very autistic-like child". Present age 12 years.

Case 19: Sister, oldest of 3 children. She was seen at a children's hospital when 3 years old, because of speech and general retardation and temper tantrums. The hospital notes described her at that time as "considerably retarded ... but not ineducable. She seemed a very disturbed little girl unable to make relationships". Further testing at age 5 years suggested she was "above average" intelligence. A recent psychologist's report (at age 10½ years) includes this summary: "She appears to be performing at the E.S.N. level at the moment, but one's strong impression was that this is an average child with a severe personality disorder. Given three wishes, she wanted to go to school, dream about the pixies and have a party with them, and go out with her mummy and daddy. Much of her verbal material was of this bizarre nature, suggesting a psychotic condition." The present writer saw the girl at her home; she was on holiday from a boarding school for E.S.N. children. A large, ordinary looking child, she readily showed her skill at knitting, and with a little encouragement from her family, recited her "tables" up to 25×25 and the names of all the English sovereigns since 1066 to the present day. Once started, she tended to perseverate, and it was difficult to interrupt her recitations. She was friendly and could answer questions sensibly. Her present age is 12 years.

Case 30: Sister, 10th in a family of 12. Speech development was very slow. She was first examined soon after entering ordinary school, and reports were available from a child guidance clinic covering the next 3 years of her life. No physical abnormality was found; she was enuretic, negativistic, easily upset and difficult to examine. I.Q. about 56 at age 8 years, when she was described as "anxious and chaotic". From about age 10 years, she was placed in various special schools, but persistently ran away and was difficult to manage. Short stays in mental hospitals followed, when she was treated with chlorpromazine. At the present time (age 14 years), she is in a mental hospital, I.Q. "in the E.S.N. range", and with a suggested diagnosis of "depressive psychosis".

Thus, of 190 parents, uncles and aunts of the autistic probands, 6 (3.2%) were known to have had a serious mental illness. In no case was the illness known to be schizophrenia. Three (4.8%) of the autistic probands' 62 siblings had a serious mental disorder; all were retarded or disturbed before school age. Amongst the non-autistic probands, 1 parent was known to be psychotic, and no uncles, aunts or siblings had a serious mental illness.

Looked at differently, 8 of the 32 autistic probands had a parent, sibling, uncle or aunt with some serious mental disorder. Only one of the non-autistic probands had a mentally ill relative.

The Children

1. Birth Order and Maternal Age

a) Birth order. The null hypothesis is that all children in a sibship have an equal chance of developing an autistic disorder. The expected frequency of affected children in any ordinal position may thus be calculated for any sibship of a given size. The observed and expected frequencies in each

Table 5. *Observed and Expected Birth Order Frequencies for the Autistic Children in the Survey (Groups A and B Combined)*

Ordinal position	1		2		3		4		5		6+*		Observed	Totals Expected
1	6	(6)	5	(4.5)	5	(3.3)	1	(.75)	—	(.4)	—	(.33)	17	15.3
2			4	(4.5)	3	(3.3)	—	(.75)	1	(.4)	—	(.33)	8	9.3
3					2	(3.3)	2	(.75)	—	(.4)	—	(.33)	4	4.8
4							—	(.75)	1	(.4)	—	(.33)	1	1.5
5									—	(.4)	—	(.33)	—	.73
6+*											2	(.33)	2	.33
Totals:	6	(6)	9	(9)	10	(9.9)	3	(3)	2	(2)	2	(2)	32	31.96

Two illegitimate children born to young mothers were assumed to be first-born, and included in the table.
Two half-sibs (same mother) were included.
* One was 12th out of 12, one 7th out of approximately 8 (data not reliable).

Table 6. *Observed and Expected Birth Order Distribution Compared for the 3 Groups*

Ordinal position	Group A		Group B		Group C	
	O	E	O	E	O	E
1	7	7.15	10	8.17	9	12.92
2	4	4.15	4	5.17	10	5.92
3	2	2.15	2	2.67	3	2.92
4	1	0.82	0	0.67	0	0.25
5	0	0.57	0	0.17	0	0
6+	1	0.17	1	0.17	0	0
Totals:	15	15.01	17	17.02	22	22.01

Including 2 illegitimate children (groups A and B) assumed to be first-born.
Two 1/2 sibs included (group A). Same mother.

sibship among the 32 autistic children discovered in the survey were very similar (Table 5).

There were no marked discrepancies within the subgroups A and B; among the non-autistic handicapped children in group C, there were rather fewer first-born and more second-born than expected (Table 6).

These figures provide no evidence of any birth order effect in the whole group of autistic children or in the behaviourally distinguished subgroups amongst them; the numbers, however, are too small to be conclusive.

b) Maternal age. The survey was limited to children aged 8—10 years on 1st January, 1964, and thus born in the years 1953—1955. National figures (Table 7) for the maternal age distribution in these years were used to calculate a percentage distribution with which the survey data could be compared (Table 8).

Table 7. *Percentage of Births at Various Maternal Ages in the General Population* *

Maternal age	—19	20—24	25—29	30—34	35—39	40—44	45+
Percentage births	4.5	27.6	31.8	22.5	10.0	3.2	0.2

* Source: Registrar-General (1962) Statistical Review, part II. All live births in London and the South-east of England for the years 1953—5.

Table 8. *Maternal Age: Observed and Expected Frequencies for all Probands by Groups*

Maternal age at birth of proband	Group A		Group B		Group C	
	O	E	O	E	O	E
—19	2	.7	—	.8	—	1.0
20—24	1	4.1	6	4.7	6	5.8
25—29	4	4.8	9	5.4	2	6.7
30—34	4	3.4	1	3.8	11	4.7
35—39	3	1.5	—	1.7	2	2.1
40—44	1	.48	1	.54	—	.7
45—49	—	.03	—	.03	—	.04
Totals:	15	15.01	17	16.97	21	21.04

Note: Maternal age was not known for 1 proband in group C. Including 2 illegitimate probands. (Group A, maternal age 19 years; Group B, maternal age 20 years.)

In neither autistic group was there a significant discrepancy from the expected frequencies. There was a slight tendency for maternal age to be higher in group A and lower in group B; these differences cancelled out when the two autistic subgroups were combined, so that in the whole group of autistic children the maternal age distribution corresponded very closely with that expected. In the non-autistic group C, there was an excess of mothers in the 30 to 35 year age group but no excess over 35 years.

Examination of the relationship between maternal age and birth order showed that in group A, of 4 children born to mothers over 35, 2 were first-born and one was a second-birth. These cases were largely reponsible for the higher frequency of older mothers in group A.

Table 9. *Distribution of Birth Weights of 51 Survey Probands Compared with a National Sample*

| Birth weight (lbs/ounces) | Group A | | Group B | | Total A+B | | Group C | | Expected |
	N	%	N	%	N	%	N	%	% frequency
under 2.3	—		—		—				.3
2.3 —3.4	—		—		—		1	(4.8)	.6
3.5 —4.6	—		—		—		1	(4.8)	1.0
4.7 —5.8	1	(7.1)	1	(6.2)	2	(6.7)	4	(19.0)	4.3
5.9 —6.9	2	(14.3)	1	(6.2)	3	(10.0)	3	(14.3)	18.0
6.10—7.11	6	(42.9)	8	(50.0)	14	(46.7)	4	(19.0)	35.9
7.12—8.13	2	(14.3)	5	(31.4)	7	(23.3)	7	(33.3)	27.0
over 8.13	3	(21.4)	1	(6.2)	4	(13.3)	1	(4.8)	9.3
Totals:	14	(100.0)	16	(100.0)	30	(100.0)	21	(100.0)	96.4

Notes: 1. Data were not available for 1 case in each survey subgroup.
2. In 28 cases where maternity hospital records were available, the recorded birthweight was used.
3. Source of expected frequencies: BUTLER and BONHAM (1963), Table 43. Expected frequencies do not add to 100% because of unavailable data in the original study.

2. Birth Weight

Birth weight is accurately reported retrospectively by mothers (ROBBINS, 1963; LOTTER, 1966 a).

Comparisons were made amongst the survey subgroups, between the probands and the general population (Table 9), and between the probands and their siblings.

An immature birth may be defined as less than 5½ lbs. (DRILLIEN, 1964). There was no excess of immaturity at birth amongst the autistic probands, but over a quarter of the non-autistic probands had birth weights under 5½ lbs. The median weight for the autistic probands (Group A = 127.5 ounces, Group B = 121 ounces) was higher than in group C (109.5 ounces), but the differences were not statistically significant (Median test: SIEGEL, 1956).

Birth weights for the siblings are not listed here. It may be said, however, that the distribution amongst the siblings showed similar differences between the groups as were found amongst the probands. The median birth weights for probands and siblings were very similar in all the groups, except C where the probands were relatively smaller at birth than their siblings. In group C, there was an excess of immaturity in both probands and siblings.

Birth weight varies with the sex of the child, boys tending to be heavier than girls (BUTLER and BONHAM, 1963, Table 42). About 11.5% of boys have birth weights over 8 lbs. 13 ounces, compared with 7% of girls (op. cit.). All 5 survey probands who weighed over 8 lbs. 13 ounces were boys; the number of boys in group A who weighed over 8 lbs. 13 ounces (3 out of 10) was thus raised above the expected 11.5%. Out of 4 siblings who were as heavy as this, 3 (2 boys, 1 girl) were in group A, and 1 (a girl) was in group B.

3. Complications During Pregnancy and Birth

Birth histories could be obtained for 49 of the 54 probands, and 67 of the 87 siblings. Seventeen of the siblings for whom data could not be obtained belonged to two large families. Maternity hospital records were available for 29 of the probands and 38 of the siblings.

Some hospital reports were more detailed than others. Because of this and the obvious difficulty of comparing hospital reports with data provided retrospectively by mothers, detailed analysis of the data was not attempted. Information was recorded on a 63 item schedule similar to that used by TAFT and GOLDFARB (1964), but excluding several of the "historical" items. Randomly arranged and identified only by number, protocols were rated by a physician.

For each case a score was allocated for each of 3 periods (pregnancy, delivery, and neonatal) on a 0—3 scale, according to the judged severity of the complication. The total possible score for each case was 9.

A significantly greater number of protocols based on hospital reports had total ratings of 3 or more ($X^2 = 7$, d.f. 1, $p = <.01$). SPEARMAN rank correlations between ratings based on hospital and mothers' reports for the same children were .59 for probands and .38 for siblings. Various explanations are possible for these results: the most important were considered to be selective referral of potentially complicated cases to hospital, and relatively better recall by mothers for handicapped children. It was assumed, however, that *major* complications would not be under-reported by mothers for the siblings born at home, and that where complications were relatively serious (total score 3 or more) scores based on different sources of data would be comparable. Comparisons were, therefore, made according to whether total scores were less than 3, or 3 and over (Table 10). Amongst the group C probands, 33% were rated 3 or more; similar lower proportions of the autistic probands and group C siblings (22%) were rated 3 or more, but only 7% of the group AB siblings. The differences between the various groups were not statistically significant.

Table 10. *Birth Complications — Summary of Ratings for Probands and Sibs in Groups A, B, and C*

Rating	No. of probands/groups			No. of siblings/group		
	A	B	C	A	B	C
0—2	10	12	14	22	19	18
3+	3	3	7	1	2	5
Totals:	13	15	21	23	21	23

There was, therefore, a slight but statistically insignificant tendency for the non-autistic probands to have more complications, and the group AB siblings fewer, than the autistic probands.

4. Other Abnormal Conditions Amongst the Probands

Forty-eight (89%) of all the 54 probands, and 28 (88%) of the 32 autistic children had been examined at some time (many frequently) in hospital departments, whose case notes were available to us. These notes as well as all other available data were examined for any evidence of neurological or serious physical abnormalities, or any situation or incident in early life which might have resulted in serious trauma to the child. A wide range of abnormalities was noted which are listed in Table 11. Some of the children had more than one abnormality. Only three "incidents" were excluded from the table as insignificant: one child had an operation for hernia at age 2½, one was admitted to hospital for 24 hours at age 3—3 for urinary retention, and one underwent an operation to her hip at age 5, long after she was recognised to be abnormal.

All the abnormal conditions included were noted

Table 11. *Evidence for Various Associated Abnormalities in the Survey Probands*

Abnormality noted	Case number	No. of children and groups			
		A	B	C	Total
Diagnosed infantile fits (incl. 1 "Bell's palsy" at 2 yrs.)	25, 26, 28, 34, 40, 50	—	3	3	6
Later fits (status epilepticus at 8 yrs.)	32	—	1	—	1
Abnormal E.E.G. (definite abnormality)	13, 25, 46, 50	1	1	2	4
Abnormal E.E.G. (some suspicion of abnormality)	11, 27	1	1	—	2
Skull X-ray suggests left hemiatrophy	28	—	1	—	1
Congenital protrusion of eye + exploratory operation (age 2)	15	1	—	—	1
Squint. Several corrective operations from 18 months to 4 years	7	1	—	—	1
Deaf — rubella in first 3 months	29, 46	—	1	1	2
Diagnosed hypertelorism	45	—	—	1	1
Coal gas poisoning (12 months)	15	1	—	—	1
Lengthy early institutional care (from before 12 months)	15, 32, 39	1	1	1	3
Severe early illnesses (pneumonia,? meningismus at 18 months)	34	—	—	1	1
Severe early illnesses (oesophagitis, severe tonsillitis, many hospitalisations from 12/12)	35	—	—	1	1
Child blind in first 10 months, registered as "partially sighted"	43	—	—	1	1
Foster care since 12 months, involving episodes of gross neglect	51	—	—	1	1
Epiloia	50	—	—	1	1
Asymmetry of head, query dorsal scoliosis	41	—	—	1	1
"Numerous soft signs indicating brain damage"	42	—	—	1	1
Slight torticollis up to 2nd year	31	—	1	—	1

directly from hospital case-notes without interpretation or selection other than that mentioned above. Mothers' reports added nothing to those available from hospitals; reports of the usual childhood illnesses were not included even where these were described by mothers as "severe".

None of the group A children had fits, and only one (case 15) had severe multiple handicaps. In group B, of 4 children who had fits, 2 also had other signs suggesting some cerebral abnormality (cases 25, 28). A smaller proportion (27%) of children in group A had any of the listed abnormalities than either the behaviourally more heterogeneous autistic group B (41%) or the non-autistic group C (50%).

5. Factors Related to Outcome (at Age 8—10 Years)

In a previous report (LOTTER, 1966 a), it was shown that of the autistic probands (groups A and B) with I.Q. below 55, those who were retarded in early development were more severely handicapped when they were seen than those without early developmental retardation.

When the autistic probands were divided into 3 groups according to functioning I.Q. and whether or not early developmental was retarded, it was found:

a) Of 10 with I.Q.'s above 55, none showed any of the complicating factors listed in Table 10;

b) of 9 with I.Q.'s below 55, but no marked early development retardation, only one (case 7) showed some complicating factor;

c) of 13 with I.Q.'s below 55 and retarded early development, 10 had some complicating factor included in the table.

The difference between the two groups below I.Q. 55 (b and c above) is statistically significant ($p = <.01$, FISHER test).

Thus amongst children with marked autistic behaviour there is a group with low I.Q.'s and retarded early development, who are relatively more severely handicapped by the age of 8 to 10 years, and in whom a relatively greater incidence of neurological and other abnormalities may be found. The presence of additional abnormal conditions of various kinds would thus appear to be related to generally poorer outcome. The kinds of abnormalities noted above are, however, diverse, and the relationship between them and autistic patterns of behaviour is obscure.

Discussion

The selection of cases in the present survey was made on behavioural criteria which include most of the characteristics described by KANNER (1943) as typical of "early infantile autism". The survey subgroup A, defined by KANNER's two major criteria (autism and insistance on sameness), nevertheless included cases in which the early development and age of onset would exclude them from classification as "*infantile* autism". However, because the group of children were chosen for their homogeneity on these two typical aspects of behaviour, no further subdivision has been made for the purpose of comparing the survey data with those available for KANNER's syndrome. The term "autistic" was used to describe all cases meeting the survey selection criteria, and not as a synonym for KANNER's Syndrome (see LOTTER, 1966 a).

A raised socio-economic status amongst parents of autistic children has been observed in several previous studies. The phenomenon was originally pointed out by KANNER (1943) in cases of "infantile autism" and subsequently confirmed by him in a greatly increased number of cases (KANNER, 1949; KANNER and LESSER, 1958). Although observed also in less rigidly defined groups (e.g. CREAK and INI, 1960), the finding has usually been ascribed to referral or diagnostic bias (BENDER, 1959; BRUCH, 1959; CREAK and INI, 1960).

The present survey findings must be taken as evidence that the parents of autistic children are in some respects not representative of the general population, and that the social class differences previously reported by other investigators are not the result only of selection bias. Behaviour ratings made in the present survey of observed and reported contemporary behaviour *before* the mothers were interviewed, were highest for children subsequently allocated to group A, ruling out the possibility that case selection was determined by the more detailed reporting of behaviour by articulate, better educated mothers. For the social class distribution of the autistic probands (group AB) to be made similar to that of the general population, a further 29 autistic children would be needed in social classes III—V. That anything like this number could have been missed is extremely unlikely.

Although there is some agreement between different reports that the socio-economic status of autistic groups is unexpectedly high, no other study has found a frequency (in the equivalent of the English social classes I—II) as high as that observed by KANNER. Ninety per cent of the occupations listed by him (KANNER and LESSER, 1958) would be classified in this way. More usually, 50—60 per cent are reported in social classes I—II (CREAK and INI, 1960; RUTTER, 1966, personal communication).

It is clear from the results of the present survey that amongst autistic children, the proportion in social classes I—II may vary according to how criteria are applied. Amongst the severely subnormal developmentally "retarded" probands in group B who had an onset without a "setback", there were no cases in social classes I—II. The difference between the proportion reported by KANNER and those found by other workers may, therefore, be partly the result of the inclusion in the latter series of severely subnormal children who were retarded in early development. Available case descriptions (KANNER, 1943; KANNER and LESSER, 1958) suggest that few such cases were included in KANNER's series.

The intelligence of the parents of autistic children has been infrequently investigated. In the only two studies known to the present writer (ALANEN et al., 1964; DAVIDS, 1958), mothers of "schizophrenic" children were found to have higher scores on the W.A.I.S. than the mothers in comparison groups of children with "other chronic" or "reactive" psychoses, or who were "emotionally disturbed". In neither study was socio-economic status taken into account.

The excess of intelligent parents in the autistic group was consistent with their socio-economic and educational superiority. Thn non-autistic group C, consisting of children with behaviour not dissimilar to that of the autistic probands (see LOTTER, 1966 a), provided a useful comparison group for the investigation of the parents' intelligence *within* social class groupings. The Matrices scale is relatively less influenced by educational differences (see BURKE, 1958) and was, therefore, the more suitable test for this purpose.

The results of these comparisons suggest that mothers in the autistic group are intellectually superior, independently of social class or level of education. The fathers' scores are more difficult to interpret. VERNON (quoted by BURKE, 1958) has stated that on the Matrices scale individual differences within occupation groups are much larger than differences between these groups. Nevertheless, the unexpected results in group C suggest that further investigation is needed into the relation between parents' scores on these tests and patterns of behaviour in their children.

The present survey findings provide no evidence of a raised incidence of schizophrenia or other psychotic illnesses amongst the parents or other relatives of the autistic probands. They are, thus, in agreement with the results reported in several other studies (EISENBERG and KANNER, 1956; CREAK and INI, 1960; ALANEN, 1964; RUTTER, 1964; WOLFF and CHESS, 1964). Of 574 parents included in these investigations, only 4 ($< 1\%$) had a psychotic illness. In the studies reporting a raised incidence of schizophrenia amongst parents (KALLMAN and ROTH, 1956; BENDER, 1963), the diagnostic criteria used to select cases were very different from those employed in the studies cited above, or in the present survey.

Other mental illness was, however, more frequent in the parents of the autistic probands than in the comparison group C, and more frequent also than in the 5 studies cited above. In those, of the 574 parents, altogether 7 (1.2%) had some serious mental illness, compared with 8% in the present survey.

The value of mental health data about the siblings of the survey probands is limited because many are still very young. However, all 3 seriously abnormal siblings were found in the autistic group. None was severely subnormal and all had at some time been referred to as "psychotic". This proportion of abnormal siblings (4.8%) is higher than the proportion (0—2%) reported in several previous studies to be mentally ill (but not severely subnormal) (KANNER, 1954; CREAK and INI, 1960; BIRCH and GITTELMAN, quoted by POLLACK and GITTELMAN, 1964; RUTTER, 1964).

The comparison of reported abnormalities in siblings is subject to even greater uncertainties than in index cases. Diagnostic criteria, available data and examination procedures may not be similar between cases and siblings (see POLLACK and GITTELMAN, 1964). In siblings, evidence of "brain damage" and mental subnormality is more frequently reported than mental illness. However, if all seriously abnormal siblings are taken together, then the number found in the present survey (4.8%) is similar to the numbers found in the studies cited above (2—5%).

The results of comparing the incidence of mental abnormalities in the immediate families of the survey probands with previous reports are, therefore, equivocal. Comparison, on the other hand, between the autistic and non-autistic probands in the present survey suggests there is a relatively raised incidence of non-schizophrenic mental disorders in the immediate relatives of the autistic children.

Reports of a preponderance of first-born children (KANNER, 1954; PHILLIPS, 1957; BENDER and GRUGGET, 1956; DESPERT, 1951; RIMLAND, 1964) were not confirmed. It has not been suggested that autistic children are born to older mothers and no evidence of a generally raised maternal age was found. A few probands early in a sibship had older mothers; both CREAK and INI (1960) and ALANEN et al. (1964) reported a few mothers over 40 but do not specify the ordinal position of their "psychotic" offspring. The excess of higher social class parents tends to raise the average maternal age; it would, however, be of some interest if a consistent proportion of autistic children were found to be first-

or second-born to mothers over 35 or 40 years old.

The reported incidence of abnormal neurological signs amongst autistic children varies widely. Although data are not uniformly presented, a comparison of the survey findings with previous studies illustrates the considerable differences between reported groups:

Author and date	Classification of group
KANNER (1954)	Infantile autism
CREAK (1963)	Psychotic
BROWN (1963)	Infantile psychosis
RUTTER (1964)	Psychotic
Present study	Autistic syndrome

Several of CREAK's and RUTTER's cases developed fits only in late childhood or adolescence, long after the onset of the autistic disorder; RUTTER (1964) states that evidence of neurological abnormalities increases with increasing age. While only 1 of KANNER's cases had fits, about the same proportion in CREAK's series and in the present survey (12%) had this symptom; in RUTTER's series 24% had fits. It is possible, therefore, that the incidence of fits in the survey probands may rise as they grow older.

Fits are not uncommon in "retarded" children. ILLINGWORTH (1960) reported fits in 16% of "moderately retarded" and 46.8% of "severely retarded" children (excluding mongols and the cerebral palsied). Since neurological abnormalities were found only in the low grade (under I.Q. 55) survey probands with early developmental retardation, it is possible that the relatively low incidence of these signs reported by KANNER may be the result of differences in case selection. Unlike KANNER's group, CREAK's series contained a similar proportion (about 50%) of cases with "retarded milestones" to that found in the survey probands. It seems probable that a similar proportion in RUTTER's series may have been "retarded" in this sense. These differences also suggest an explanation for the relatively greater proportion in KANNER's series with a better outcome (see RUTTER, 1966).

Of the studies cited above, only in that of BROWN were neurological findings related to follow-up status. She found a significant relationship between abnormal EEG patterns and placement at follow-up. The present survey findings also indicate a poorer outcome for autistic probands with evidence of neurological and other abnormalities. It seems probable that in the other groups referred to, cases with such abnormalities also had the poorest outcome.

Previous reports of a high incidence of prenatal or perinatal complications in the histories of "schizophrenic" children (VORSTER, 1960; TAFT and GOLDFARB, 1964) were not confirmed for the autistic probands in the present survey. However, certainly in VORSTER's study, and probably also in TAFT and GOLDFARB's group, case selection was made according to criteria very different from those used in the present survey.

Because of the small numbers of cases involved and the absence of uniform diagnostic criteria, confident conclusions cannot be drawn from the comparison of reported findings about autistic children.

N	Abnormalities reported
100	{ 7 of 28 available EEG's abnormal { 1 had convulsions
100	12 had epilepsy
136	6 had some neurological abnormality 36 (additional) had abnormal EEG
63	16 unquestionable CNS abnormality 18 strong suggestion brain damage
32	7 had fits or abnormal EEG 4 had other abnormal conditions

There is, however, much evidence to suggest that subdivision of autistic conditions according to severity of the resulting handicaps (see also WOLFF and CHESS, 1964) may be useful for several purposes. There are great differences between autistic children least and most severely affected. The differences in outcome are important for the planning of educational and other services. Differences in early development and the incidence of neurological and other abnormalities are of obvious relevance to the investigation of etiological factors. It is essential, therefore, that in addition to explicit criteria for case selection, reports about groups of "autistic", "psychotic", or "schizophrenic" children should include detailed descriptive data to allow the more reliable recognition and comparison of subgroups amongst them.

Acknowledgements. The survey was supported by the Health Department of the Middlesex County Council. The writer wishes to acknowledge help received by Dr. N. O'CONNOR and Dr. J. K. WING, under whose supervision the work was carried out, and Dr. P. GRAHAM who rated the birth histories.

References

ALANEN, Y. O., T. ARAJÄRVI, and R. O. VIITAMÄKI: Psychoses in childhood. Acta Psychiat. Scand. 40, Suppl. 174 (1964).

BENDER, L.: Mental illness in childhood and heredity. Eugenics Quart. 10, 1—11 (1963).

—, and A. E. GRUGETT: A study of certain epidemiological factors in a group of children with childhood schizophrenia. Amer. J. Orthopsychiat. 26, 131—144 (1956).

BROWN, J. L.: Follow-up of children with atypical development (infantile psychosis). Amer. J. Orthopsychiat. 33, 855 to 861 (1963).

BURKE, H. R.: Raven's progressive matrices: a review and critical evaluation. J. genet. Psychol. 93, 199—228 (1958).

BUTLER, N., and D. BONHAM: Perinatal mortality. London: Livingstone 1963.

CREAK, M.: Childhood psychosis: a review of 100 cases. Brit. J. Psychiat. 109, 84—89 (1963).

—, and S. INI: Families of psychotic children. J. Child. Psychol. Psychiat. 1, 156—175 (1960).

— Schizophrenic syndrome in childhood. Dev. Med. Child Neurol. 3, 501—504 (1961).

DAVIDS, A.: Intelligence in childhood schizophrenics, other emotionally disturbed children and their mothers. J. cons. Psychol. 22, 159—163 (1958).

DESPERT, J. L.: Some considerations relating to the genesis of autistic behaviour in children. Amer. J. Orthopsychiat. 21, 335—350 (1951).

DRILLIEN, C. M.: The growth and development of the prematurely born infant. London: Livingstone 1964.

EISENBERG, L., and L. KANNER: Early infantile autism, 1943 to 1955. Amer. J. Orthopsychiat. 26, 556—566 (1956).

GILLIES, S., M. A. MITTLER, and G. B. SIMON: Some characteristics of a group of psychotic children and their families. Bull. Br. Psychol. Soc. 16, 19 (abstract) (1963).

ILLINGWORTH, R. S.: The development of the infant and the young child. London: Livingstone 1960.

KALLMAN, F. J., and B. ROTH: Genetic aspects of preadolescent schizophrenia. Amer. J. Psychiat. 112, 599—606 (1956).

KANNER, L.: Autistic disturbances of affective contact. Nerv. Child. 2, 217—250 (1943).

— Problems of nosology and psychodynamics of early infantile autism. Amer. J. Orthopsychiat. 19, 416—426 (1949).

— To what extent is early infantile autism determined by constitutional inadequacies. Res. Publ. Ass. nerv. ment. Dis. 33, 378—385 (1954).

—, and L. I. LESSER: Early infantile autism. Ped. Clin. N. Amer. 5, 711—730 (1958).

LOTTER, V.: Epidemiology of autistic conditions in young children. Part I: Prevalence. Soc. Psychiat. 1, 24 (1966 a).

— Services for autistic children in Middlesex. In J. K. WING (Ed.): Early childhood autism: Clinical, educational and social aspects. Oxford: Pergamon 1966 b.

PHILLIPS, E. L.: Contributions to a learning theory account of childhood autism. J. Psychol. 43, 117—124 (1957).

POLLACK, M., and R. K. GITTELMAN: Siblings of childhood schizophrenics: a review. Amer. J. Orthopsychiat. 34, 868 to 874 (1964).

RAVEN, J. C.: Standardisation of progressive matrices. Brit. J. Med. Psychol. 19, 137—150 (1941).

— Guide to using the Mill Hill Vocabulary Scale with the Progressive Matrices Scales. London: H. K. Lewis, 1962.

RIMLAND, B.: Infantile autism. New York: Appleton-Century-Crofts 1964.

ROBBINS, L. C.: The accuracy of parental recall of aspects of child development and of child rearing practices. J. abnorm. soc. Psychol. **66**, 261—270 (1963).

RUTTER, M.: Diagnosis and general aspects of child psychosis. Address to the conference on the needs of psychotic children, at Hove. London: Ministry of Education, 1964.

RUTTER, M.: Prognosis: Psychotic children in adolescence and early adult life. In early childhood autism: Clinical, educational and social aspects. (Ed. J. K. WING.) London: Pergamon 1966.

SIEGEL, S.: Nonparametric statistics for the behavioural sciences. London: McGraw-Hill 1956.

TAFT, L. T., and W. GOLDFARB: Prenatal and perinatal factors in childhood schizophrenia. Dev. Med. Child Neurol. **6**, 32—43 (1964).

VORSTER, D.: An investigation into the part played by organic factors in childhood schizophrenia. J. ment. Sci. **106**, 494 to 522 (1960).

WOLFF, S., and S. CHESS: A behavioural study of schizophrenic children. Acta Psychiat. Scand. **40**, 438—466 (1964).

Appendix A

Summary of the social class of parents for whom test scores could not be obtained: by sex of parent and behaviour subgroup

Social class	Vocabulary Scale						Matrices Scale					
	Group A		Group B		Group C		Group A		Group B		Group C	
	M	F	M	F	M	F	M	F	M	F	M	F
I	1	1	—	—	—	—	1	1	—	—	—	—
II	1	2	—	1	—	—	2	2	—	1	—	—
III	1	1	1	2	2	2	1	1	2	2	2	1
IV—V	—	—	2	1	2	3	—	—	1	—	2	2
Not known:	—	—	1	1	1	1	—	—	1	1	1	1
Totals:	3	4	4	5	5	6	4	4	4	4	5	4

Note: M = Mother, F = Father

212

Perceptual Inconstancy in Early Infantile Autism

The Syndrome of Early Infant Autism and Its Variants

Including Certain Cases of Childhood Schizophrenia

Edward M. Ornitz, MD, and Edward R. Ritvo, MD, Los Angeles

WITHIN the decade since the syndrome of early infantile autism was first described by Kanner,[1,2] terms such as childhood schizophrenia,[3] atypical children,[4] children with unusual sensitivities,[5] and symbiotic psychosis[6] were used to conceptualize similar, yet apparently distinctive clinical entities. The tendency to create separate entities was reinforced by a desire for diagnostic specificity and accuracy and etiologic preference. As the symptomatology in these children varies both with the severity of the illness and age, it has been possible to emphasize distinctive clusters of symptoms and relate these to particular theories of causation. For instance, the predominance of disturbances of relating coupled with the prevailing belief in the 1940's and 1950's that specific syndromes in children must be outgrowths of specific parental behaviors or attitudes[7] led to attempts to implicate the parents in the development of early infantile autism. The notion that something noxious was done to the children, presumably by the parents, led to a teleological view of the disturbed behavior. Thus, disturbances of relating, perception, and motility have been described as defensive or protective, as a warding off or withdrawal

ARCHIVES OF GENERAL PSYCHIATRY, 1968, Vol. 18, pp. 76-98.

213

from adverse stimulation or as compensatory self-stimulation.

The purpose of this paper is to describe a single pathologic process common to early infantile autism, certain cases of childhood schizophrenia, the atypical child, symbiotic psychosis, and children with unusual sensitivities. It will be shown that these descriptive categories are variants of a unitary disease. First, we shall describe a specific syndrome of abnormal development which is defined by observable behavior patterns that occur as clusters of symptoms. These clusters of symptoms involve the areas of: (1) perceptual integration, (2) motility patterns, (3) capacity to relate, (4) language, and (5) developmental rate. Secondly, we shall show that a pathologic mechanism underlying the syndrome can be inferred from the nature of the symptom clusters. While this pathologic mechanism may be associated with multivariant etiologic factors, it is operative at birth and makes it impossible for the child to utilize external and internal stimuli to properly organize further development. If maturational or as yet unknown self-corrective factors do not mitigate the influence of this pathologic process, a relatively complete clinical picture of the syndrome develops and persists. If maturational or self-corrective factors do mitigate the influence of this pathologic process, symptoms may wane or shift in predominance resulting in a varying clinical picture. In all such cases the child's later development will show residuals of varying severity. The relationship of these residuals to the primary pathology common to all the symptom clusters will be elaborated.

It will also be emphasized that while early infantile autism must be defined as a behavioral syndrome, it is at the same time a disease. The symptomatology will, therefore, be interpreted as primarily expressive of the underlying pathophysiology rather than being purposeful in the intrapsychic life of the child.

Diagnostic Terminology

The different diagnostic labels which have been used to characterize the large group of young children whose symptomatology has varied from Kanner's criteria for early infantile autism have included pseudoretardation, atypical development, symbiotic psychosis, childhood schizophrenia, and infantile psychosis.

The major criteria for the diagnosis of early infantile autism were the inability to relate to people in the expected manner, failure to use language for communication, an apparent desire to be alone and to preserve sameness in the environment, and preoccupation with certain objects.[1-2]

The term pseudoretardation has been used because many of these children appear retarded while showing intellectual potential which differentiates them from the general group of retarded children.

The term atypical development was originally used to describe children[8] with histories and behavior indicative of grossly uneven ego development. Later, when it became apparent that these children shared some of the features of early infantile autism, the term atypical development became used to denote children in whom relatedness was not quite so disturbed as to make the term autistic appropriate.

The term symbiotic psychosis[6] was used to describe children whose behavior appeared to be the opposite of those with autism. That is, the child rather than being aloof, remote, and emotionally isolated was found to be emotionally fused and physically clinging to the mother.

The term childhood schizophrenia has been used by some authors as a synonym for early infantile autism,[9] by others to describe a presumed separate syndrome,[10] and by some to describe symptoms which others accept as those of early infantile autism without reference to that terminology.[11-12] While some authors[11] describe a continuum of abnormality in which infants and very young children with the symptoms of the autistic child represent the earliest manifestations of schizophrenia, others[10,13] attempt to maintain a distinction between the two conditions wherein the term childhood schizophrenia is reserved for those cases in which the pathologic process appears to begin after the age of 4 to 5. They postulate that in childhood schizophrenia, a prior stage of intact psychic organization has decompensated, whereas in the autistic child, psychic organization failed to develop. However, in our experience, follow-up of some children who were diagnosed autistic prior to the age of 5 reveals the development over the years of a picture indistinguishable from schizophrenia. Brown and Reiser,[14] apparently observing similar changes, reported eight different clinical outcomes (after 9 years of age) of atypical children and included a "schizophrenic" group. Also, in some cases, if detailed retrospective histories of children diagnosed as being schizophrenic after the age of 5 are taken, previously overlooked but diagnostically significant behavioral deviancies can often be elicited. For example, behaviors such as hand-flapping, hypersensitivity to noise, and the failure to adapt to solid foods may be overlooked in ordinary history taking.

Although neither Eisenberg[15] nor Rutter[10] observed paranoid ideas, hallucinations, or delusions in follow-up studies of autistic children, one would not necessarily expect to see these classical symptoms of adult schizophrenia in children. However, in our clinical experience with children, we have observed clear transitions from early infantile autism to the thought disorder characteristic of adult schizophrenia. Similarly, Eisenberg[15] found "peculiarities of language and thought" possibly characteristic of schizophrenia. The case reported by Darr and Worden[16] illustrates an acute schizophrenic reaction in a marginally adjusted adult who had been autistic as a child. When 4 years old, this patient had been examined (Dr. Adolph Meyer) and the classic symptoms of early infantile autism were recorded. At 32 years of age, this woman complained that people would be killed by the poison that was in her, that she would die because she was urinating cider, etc. Tolor and Rafferty[17] found that adolescents diagnosed as schizophrenic scored high on a checklist of symptoms of early infantile autism. While the delineation of early infantile autism from childhood schizophrenia may have prognostic and therapeutic value, available evidence suggests that the former condition can develop into the latter and that so many transitional states occur as to imply a fundamentally similar underlying mechanism in many of the cases. Difference in age of manifest onset rather than separating the two conditions, demonstrates the effect of maturational and developmental level on the way the disease process is expressed.

Reiser[13] has suggested the term infantile psychosis to describe the period from birth to 5 years of age in which the pathologic process develops. He suggests this term as encompassing and, therefore, replacing all of the other terminology just discussed. He feels that the designation "psychotic" is merited by virtue of impairment in perception, failure to test reality, social isolation and withdrawal, impaired control of instinctual energies, and disturbances of feeling, thinking, and behavior. This description overlaps the syndrome and subclusters of symptoms which will be described in the following sections of this paper. However, the terms psychosis and psychotic are also commonly used in a broader sense than is applicable to these conditions. Therefore, the terms early infantile autism and autistic child will be used in this paper as representative of the group of clinical states under study. Early infantile autism and the other conditions will be further considered as variants or sequelae of a basic disease.

Natural History

Family.—When the syndrome of early infantile autism was first described by Kanner,[1] it was thought that these children came from highly intellectual families in the upper socioeconomic levels. In fact, the parents were from the academic and professional communities and their family life was characterized by obsessive meticulousness and intellectualism. The corollary of these attributes was an emotional coldness often described as "refrigeration."[2] In the subsequent two decades a broader clinical experience with autistic children and their families has revealed that these children come from every socioeconomic class and that the parents may, or may not, be professionally employed. The fathers may indeed be university professors, psychiatrists, electronic engineers, or mathematicians. We have observed, however, that they may be common laborers or artists. Wolff and Chess[9] have made similar observations. While some of the parents are reported to be cold, isolated, or refrigerated individuals, others have proven to be warm, loving, and quite capable of raising normally affectionate siblings of their autistic child. A condition of family disruption and emotional turmoil may surround the infancy or childhood of autistic children[13] or the disease process may develop in a normal emotional climate.[10]

A relative sparcity of schizophrenic parents has been noted by some observers. However, Rutter's[10] failure to find a single schizophrenic parent in his population of autistic children was not confirmed by Goldfarb,[12] Wolff and Chess,[9] or O'Gorman.[18]

It is rare to find more than one nontwin sibling with the disease,[13] and we have seen only one such case. However, J. Simmons (oral communication, June 1967) has followed five families with two nontwin autistic siblings. Dizygotic twins are discordant for early infantile autism. With one exception,[19] all reported cases of monozygotic twins are concordant for the disease when monozygocity has been adequately demonstrated and the disease is not associated with perinatal trauma to one twin.[20-21]

Pregnancy and Delivery.—Available surveys provide conflicting evidence as to the relative incidence of complications during pregnancy and delivery in the mothers of these children as compared to other diagnostic groups. Schain and Yannet[22] and Kanner[23] reported no increase in prenatal and perinatal complications. However, in a well-controlled study, Taft and Goldfarb[24] reviewed hospital charts of autistic children, their siblings, and normal controls. They reported a significantly greater incidence of prenatal and perinatal difficulties in the autistic group.

Postnatal.—In the immediate postnatal period, some autistic children have been described as unusually quiet, motorically inactive, and emotionally unresponsive or, conversely, as ususualy irritable and extremely sensitive to auditory, tactile, and visual stimuli. The same infant may alternately manifest both types of disturbance.

Following the immediate postnatal period two general courses of development may be reported. In the first, the baby shows early signs of deviant development. In the second, relatively normal development is described by the parents until the age of 18 to 26 months, at which time an apparent regression in all areas of behavior rapidly occurs. These children then look identical to the children whose development has been deviant from birth. In many cases, parents report that the "regression" is associated with some concurrent event such as the birth of a sibling, marital rift, economic reversal, or a move to a new home. In other cases, the behavioral changes are associated with factors influencing the child directly, such as illness, hospitalization, or separation from a parent. We have found in several cases where "normal" development was reported during the first 18 months, detailed history taking revealed evidence of deviant development which had gone unnoticed.

Neonatal Period.—Most frequently it is reported that the autistic infant was: "a good baby"; "he never cried"; "he seemed not to need companionship or stimulation"; and "he did not want to be held." Concomitant with being "good," he may have shown a reduced activity level, torpor, and a tendency to cry rarely, if at all. When picked up, he may have been limp with peculiar posturing and flaccid muscle tone. This data obtained from retrospective questioning of parents of autistic children has been confirmed by one prospective study.[25]

First Six Months.—During the early months of development the mothers often report being perplexed by the baby's lack of crying or by their difficulty in relating crying to hunger or to discomfort from other specific needs. These babies seem content to be left alone a great deal. In some family constellations these factors are very disturbing to the mothers, resulting in anxiety and bewilderment which then leads to either compensatory overinvolvement or withdrawal. Either response may result in the mother's loss of self-esteem in her role as mother. In other families, the advent of such an "undemanding" baby is welcomed by a harrassed mother who then leaves the baby alone.

The first definite signs of deviant development may be the baby's failure to notice the coming and going of the mother, a lack or delay of the smiling response, or the lack of the anticipatory response to being picked up. Concomitantly, underreactivity (failure to play with the crib gym or show an interest in toys) and paradoxical overreactivity to stimulation (panic at the sound of a vacuum cleaner or telephone) may occur. Finally, failure to vocalize during the first half year may also be noted.

Second Six Months.—An ominous sign of later pathology may appear when solid foods are introduced. A baby who had fed well at breast or bottle and adapted easily to strained foods may show severe distress when rough textured "junior" and table foods are introduced. Several types of response occur, including refusal to hold food in mouth, refusal to chew or swallow, or intense gagging. After dentition appears, it may become apparent that the infant avoids chewing food. Some of these children actually remain on pureed baby foods and the bottle until their 6th or 7th year.

The disinterest in toys noted during the first six months may precede the active casting or flicking away of toys. Objects placed in the hand may be simply dropped. This behavior may contrast markedly with an alternate tendency to hold an object such as a piece of string, a broken pencil, or a marble. Such a child often is panicked and upset if the object disappears. He may persist in holding onto it for years.

The sequence of motor development may be precocious or retarded or may be characterized by accelerated achievement of one motor skill followed by a lag before development of the next. Also characteristic is the tendency to give up a previously acquired motor skill; the parents often describe the child as not wanting to use an acquired ability.

Mothers frequently describe their autistic children as being unaffectionate. When picked up and held, they may either go limp or stiffen. When put down by the mother, they do not seem to notice. At this point the busy or bewildered mother may leave the baby alone because her feeling that he does not need her is reinforced. By the age of 10 or 11 months these babies do not play "peek-a-boo" and "patty-cake" games and do not imitate waving "bye-bye." The mother's bewilderment at her baby's lack of responsiveness may be further reinforced by his failure to develop communicative speech. The baby who did not "coo" or "babble" earlier may now show a crucial failure to imitate sounds and words. As with motor function, speech development may be retarded or may show precocious advances followed by failure to use words previously learned. Nonverbal communication also lags: the child does not point toward what he wants and does not look toward a desired object.

At this stage of development and later, these children are frequently thought to be deaf. This possibility is often belied by unusual sensitivity to and awareness of certain unexpected or loud sounds. A similar type of sensitivity may also be observed in the visual modality. Sudden changes in illumination may evoke panic. Often the earlier tendency of babies to regard their own writhing hand and finger movements becomes a consuming preoccupation. Other sensory modalities may also be affected. For example, unusual tactile discrimination with adverse reactions to rough wool fabrics and preference for smooth surfaces occurs. Proprioceptive and antigravity responses may be similarly involved and come to attention when the father who enjoys tossing the child in the air is rebuffed by the baby's distress.

Second and Third Years.—After 12 months, unusual sensitivity to auditory, visual, tactile, and labyrinthine stimulation is often accompanied paradoxically by peculiar and bizarrely expressed pursuit of sensations in these modalities. Noisy, vigorous, and sustained tooth grinding occurs. Some of the children scratch surfaces and listen intently to the sounds they have created. They may pass their eyes along surfaces apparently attending to patterns. They may rub surfaces with their hands, apparently reacting to textural differences. Contrasting with these behaviors, they seem to ignore more meaningful, environmentally determined stimuli.

Between 1 and 3 years of age, repetitive habits, mannerisms, and gestures may begin to develop. They suddenly cease activity, posture, and stare off into space. Frequently, this posturing involves hyperextension of the neck. Such children may begin to whirl themselves and characteristically flutter or flap their arms, hands, or fingers. The fingers may flick against stable objects or in the air. A variant of flapping is an oscillatory motion of the hand and forearm. As the child learns to walk and run, he frequently does so almost exclusively on his toes. Toe walking, whirling, and flapping may be seen as slow, consistent, repetitive mannerisms which may be suddenly interrupted by peculiar darting or lunging movements accompanied by excited gesticulation of the arms. Certain external stimuli, such as spinning objects (children's tops), may set off these explosive, yet organized patterns of activity. Continuous body rocking and head rolling are also frequently observed. These behaviors may become organized into complex repetitive sequences. Long hours may be spent spinning tops, wheels, jar lids, coins, or any available object, running back and forth across a room, switching the overhead lights repetitively on and off, and dancing around an object while flapping the hands.

By this age, it may become apparent that there is a lack of eye contact. They seem to look beyond or through people as if looking through a window. Other people can be used as extensions of the child's self, eg, taking the arm of the adult and placing it on a doorknob. In doing this, they do not look at the adult but only at the desired object. Although they may seek out objects for repetitive stereotyped activity, eg, light switches or tops, they usually show an utter lack of interest in toys offered to them.

Fourth and Fifth Years.—By the time the child is between 3 and 5 years old, the unusual sensitivities to external stimulation noted above may decrease. Motor retardation, when it has occurred, is usually overcome and the child becomes capable of physical activities appropriate to his age. Yet, he may not actually engage in such activities as jungle-gym climbing or riding a tricycle because of his lack of social awareness of the activity itself. The tendency to walk on toes, flap arms, and whirl may decrease but in some cases continues for many years.

A major problem in the 3 to 5-year-old child is found in the area of language development. Speech may not have developed at all or if present may be characterized by parroting (echolalia), the parroted phrase being repeated completely out of the social context in which it had been heard. This is called delayed echolalia.[26] These children often make requests by repeating what has been said to them in the interrogative form. For example, the child will say "you want to walk" rather than saying that he wants to go for a walk. Pronoun reversals using "you" or "he" for "I" or "me" are noted,

and the object and subject of discourse are confused. The voice may sound atonal, arhythmic, and hollow.

Syndrome and Subclusters of Symptoms

The symptoms of early infantile autism and its variants have been described in the previous section in terms of their onset of occurrence. This multitude of symptoms will now be classified into certain related subclusters in order that a unified disease process can be delineated.

It is to be emphasized that the subclusters of symptoms are defined on the basis of observable behaviors. There is no a priori assumption that one subcluster of symptoms stands independently of another. In fact, it is one purpose of this paper to show that one of the subclusters (disturbances of perception) may underlie most of the other groups of symptoms which together make up the syndrome.

The subclusters are: (1) disturbances of perception, (2) disturbances of motor behavior, (3) disturbances of relating, (4) disturbances of language, and (5) disturbances of developmental rate and sequence.

It should be emphasized that the total syndrome characterized by these five subclusters of symptoms is based upon detailed observation of over 150 cases by us. It is not implied that in any particular case all symptoms will be seen nor will every subcluster of symptoms achieve full expression. In fact, we have observed individual autistic children who show primarily disturbances of relating and only minimal suggestion of the other subclusters. In contrast, we have seen an occasional child who shows primarily disturbances of perception, with minimal expression of the other subclusters and relatively intact ability to relate.

Disturbances of Perception.—Heightened awareness, hyperirritability, and obliviousness to external stimulation all may occur in the same child. All modalities of sensation may be involved. While auditory changes are most often noted, unusual perceptual aberrations may be seen in the visual, tactile, gustatory, olfactory, proprioceptive, and vestibular senses.

Heightened Awareness of Sensory Stimuli.—*Auditory.*—Attention to self-induced sounds (eg, scratching of surfaces), attention to background stimuli, ear-banging, ear-rubbing, and flicking of the ear are observed.

Visual.—Prolonged regarding of writhing movements of the hands and fingers, brief but intense staring, and scrutiny of visual detail are noted.

Tactile.—The auditory and visual scrutiny is paralleled by passing the hands over surfaces of varying textures.

Olfactory and Gustatory.—Specific food preferences, according to taste and smell, and repetitive sniffing occur.

Vestibular.—The children are unusually aware of things that spin and can become preoccupied with car wheels, phonograph records, or washing machines—far beyond the interest expressed transiently by normal children.

Heightened Sensitivity and Irritability.—*Auditory.*—Unusual fearfulness of sirens, vacuum cleaners, barking dogs, and the tendency to cover the ears in anticipation of such sounds are observed.

Visual.—Change in illumination will occasionally precipitate fearful reactions.

Tactile.—There may be intolerance for certain fabrics. The children often do not accept wool blankets or clothing against the skin, and show a preference for smooth surfaces.

Gustatory.—A specific intolerance toward rough textured "junior" or table foods is observed.

Vestibular.—A marked aversion to being tossed in the air or to ride in elevators occurs. Intense interest and pleasure in spinning objects may alternate with fearful, disturbed, and excited reactions to them.

Nonresponsiveness.—*Auditory.*—Most notable is the disregard of speech and the lack of detectable behavioral response to loud sounds.

Visual.—These children ignore new persons or features in their environment. They may walk into or through things or people as if they did not exist.

Tactile.—Early in the first year of life, they may let objects placed in the hand fall away, as if they had no tactile representation.

Pain.—These children may not react with evidence of pain to bumps, falls, or cuts.

Disturbances of Motor Behavior.—Motor behaviors can be divided into two groups, those that seem to be associated with sensory input and those that seem to be associated with discharge.

Motor Behaviors Apparently Associated With Sensory Input.—*Auditory.*—Scratching at surfaces is often accompanied by bringing the ear down as if to listen to the sound created. Banging of the ear or head may induce intense repetitive auditory and vibratory stimulation. Tooth grinding may have a similar effect.

Visual.—Both the regarding of the slow writhing movements of the hands and fingers and the more vigorous flapping of the hands within the visual field may provide visual input to the child.

Tactile.—Scratching at or rubbing of surfaces provides tactile sensation.

Vestibular.—Autistic children tend to whirl themselves or spend long hours spinning objects, such as tops, can lids, and coins. These activities may provide increased vestibular input. The children may whirl themselves in many ways, for example, while standing up or frequently while sitting on a smooth floor, swiveling around and around on their buttocks. They spin objects in many ways too and will become excited and preoccupied with spinning metal tops or take toys completely unrelated to spinning and find ways of spinning them. They seem to be able to make tops out of almost anything. Often bizarre ritualistic activities accompany the preoccupation with spinning. They will flap their hands and engage in excited, repetitive movements, lunging at the top as if to push against it and then pulling away from it only to repeat the activity again and again. At other times, the same child will appear frightened and run away from the top. The diagnosis was clarified in the case of a 3-year-old child with relatively intact capacity to relate when he was offered a top. He reacted with increasing tension and fearfulness, gesticulating as the top was spun faster. He stared at his hands and then ritualistically patted the floor while engaging in a stereotyped dance around the top. As his excitement increased, he became oblivious to reassurance, stared at the ceiling, and then began to flap his fingers while fixing his gaze intently on the top. When told that he could stop the spinning if he did not like it, he responded by making a "stop" gesture with his hand from a distance. Then he shot at the top with a toy gun, lay down to play "dead" and finally put the top in a cupboard out of sight.

Proprioceptive.—Hand-flapping deserves special mention, as it is an activity that is characteristic and almost pathognomic of the autistic child, although it may be seen occasionally in other syndromes. It may occur only transiently or may become a fixed behavior. It may be associated with states of excitement or occur over prolonged periods unassociated with external stimuli. The flapping of the arms has many modifications, such as wiggling of the fingers, flicking at surfaces, or oscillating of the hand while empty or while holding small toys. Flapping behavior often has an interesting evolution in individual children. In one case it was first noted at 11 months of age that while mouthing a small plastic airplane, the child would rhythmically flick at the wing with one hand while holding it to his mouth with the other. At the age of 5 years, this behavior evolved into a repetitive gesticulation wherein the child would start to put one hand and thumb into his mouth while flicking that hand away with the other. By 8 years of age, he had given up this activity, attempting to follow directions to suppress it; he was observed instead to repetitively flex his extended fingers at the metacarpophalangeal joints over long periods of time. Another child, 4 years old, whose variant of hand-flapping was a rapid oscillation (alternate pronation and supination) of the hand and forearm, developed a pruritic dermatitis and began scratching. As the dermatitis increased, the scratching took on the oscillatory nature of his hand-flapping, and for a period of time substituted in part for the hand movements. As the pruritus abated, he gave up the scratching and again oscillated. In some of the children hand-flapping does not occur spontaneously during examination, although a history of it may be elicited by detailed questioning. It may at times be elicited by specific stimulation, eg, presentation of a top. However, under controlled conditions of observations, it is found to be a remarkably persistent behavior, neither increasing nor decreasing with time (Sorosky, A.; Ornitz, E.; Brown, M.; and Rituo, E., unpublished data).

Other Motor Phenomena.—Toe walking and periodic bursts of excited lunging, gesticulating, and darting movements do not seem especially related to sensory input. The lunging and darting may appear almost seizure-like. Toe walking may occur intermittently or may be the only mode of walking.

Disturbances of Relating.—Poor eye contact, delayed or absent social smile, delayed or absent anticipatory response to being picked up, apparent aversion to physical contact, limpness or stiffening when held, disinterest in looking at, casting away, or bizarre use of toys, a lack of active response to the "peek-a-boo," "pat-a-cake," and "bye-bye" games, and the general preference to being alone are all characteristic. The use of people as an extension of the self, and the more pervasive lack of emotional responsiveness are additional manifestations of disturbed relating.

Disturbances of Language.—Frequently, there is a complete failure of speech to develop. When and if speech does develop, it is often poorly modulated, atonal, arhythmic, and hollow sounding without communicative or affective content. The most prominent specific type of pathologic language is called echolalia.[26] Also, characteristic is pronoun reversal.

Disturbances of Developmental Rate.—The rate of development may be disturbed, leading to discontinuities in the normal sequence. Altered rates of development involving motor and speech areas occur. The child may roll over precociously early and then may not sit without support until 11 months, or he may sit up without support at 5 months and not pull to a stand until 13 months. In the language area he may use a few words at 10 months and fail to use words again until 2 years old, or the early use of words may be followed by a long delay in joining them into phrases. Further, he may successfully perform some skill such as crawling and then may not ever do it again. Some of the children have been described on the one hand as slow and on the other hand as showing precocious motor and language development. The most characteristic finding on infant developmental testing is a marked scatter both between and within sectors of tests such as the Gesell.[27]

Other attempts to group the many symptoms of this disease have been made. Closest to our approach is the work of Creak.[28] She abstracted nine criteria from the descriptive literature on childhood schizophrenia and early infantile autism. These nine points overlap the five subclusters of symptoms described here. Impairment of emotional relations with people and preoccupation with objects have been included here with the other disturbances of relating. Speech disturbance, distortion in motility, and retardation are synonymous with the disturbances of language, motor expression, and developmental rate. Along with abnormal perceptual experience, we consider the unawareness of self-identity, the maintenance of sameness, and anxiety precipitated by change as derivatives of the disturbances of perception.

Change in Syndrome After Early Childhood

One of the most confusing aspects of this disease is that after the age of 5 or 6 years, symptom-complexes of early infantile autism and its variants tend to merge with other clinical entities, eg, childhood schizophrenia (see above). The manifestations of the subclusters of symptoms as they appear past the age of 5 or 6 years will now be discussed.

Relationship to the Environment and Language.—Disturbances of relating and disturbances of language are best considered together; as with increasing age, the capacity to relate depends markedly on the capacity to communicate with others. It has been observed that speech may not develop by the age of 5, in which case the autistic child becomes less and less distinguishable from the large group of severely retarded children.[15] Absence of speech has been correlated with low intelligence.[19] Those autistic children who develop noncommunicative speech and progress no further, when seen again at 10 to 15 years of age, tend to look much as they did when younger.

If they develop communicative speech by 5 years of age, then several possible courses of development are open. First, language

capacity may be quite rudimentary. Communications are literal and concrete, with minimal capacity for abstract thought. Affect tends to be flat, and they do not become emotionally involved with others.

In a second course of development, characteristics typical of organic brain disease become manifest. There may be an impulsiveness, a lack of emotional control, hyperactivity, restlessness, and irritability accompanied by some degree of mental retardation and concrete thinking.

A third developmental course seen during the school years and in early adolescence is identical to that described by others as schizophrenia. This is often an insidious process wherein the child who is diagnosed earlier in life as being autistic becomes harder and harder to distinguish from those children who are called schizophrenic. Language is characterized by loose, free, or fragmented associations leading away from social contact and communication through tangles of irrelevancy and tangential thinking. Bizarre, illusory, or hallucinatory thinking may be present. A distorted fantasy life may be elaborated around some of the earlier behaviors which have been grouped as disturbances of perception or motor expression. For example, the child who evolved hand-flapping into a complex gesticulation wherein one hand and thumb was pushed back from the mouth by a flicking action of the other hand, elaborated the fantasy that his thoughts were falling out of his mouth and that he was pushing them back into his head.

A fourth course of development may evolve either from the schizophrenic stage or follow directly from the autistic syndrome itself. Such children superficially appear to have a relatively normal personality structure or neurotic or characterologic defects. However, careful attention to behavior and a detailed history of earlier development will reveal a clinical picture suggestive of residuals of an earlier autistic syndrome. Particularly, one sees a certain oddness in character and impaired empathy coupled with a lack of social judgment and discrimination. There may be excessive preoccupying interests in mechanical things coupled with a lack of interest in human relationships.

Perceptual and Motor Phenomena.—The disturbances of perception and motor be-

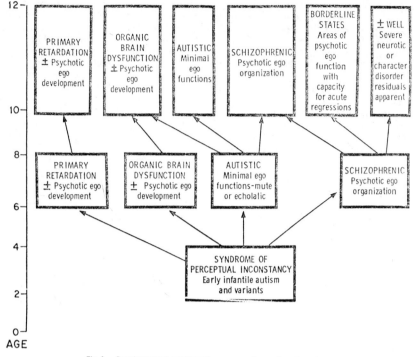

Fig 1.—Developmental relationships among diagnostic categories.

havior may persist during the school years but usually dropout. Some of the children who suffer a schizophrenic outcome still toe-walk, tend to whirl, and also may hand-flap. In the children who develop neurotic or personality disorders, one may under certain circumstances see hand-flapping or one of its variants. For example, one 10-year-old child was examined and purposely presented with a noisy spinning top; he commented that he used to get excited when he saw a top spin. While there was no overt hand-flapping, observation of his crossed hands, one pressing down on the other, revealed a rhythmic contraction of the tendons in the dorsum of the hand. It appeared that he was consciously suppressing the tendency to flap.

These relationships among diagnostic categories are illustrated in Fig 1. Increasing diagnostic specificity as the child gets older is evident.

Differential Diagnosis

The differential diagnosis of early infantile autism and childhood schizophrenia has been thoroughly reviewed by Reiser,[13] Rutter,[10] and Ekstein.[29] Discussion of differential diagnosis here will be limited to those syndromes wherein certain common symptoms suggest etiologic consideration.

In the syndrome of institutionalism,[30] not only are a certain limited number of symptoms common to early infantile autism, but certain aspects of the history may be common to both conditions, making differential diagnosis initially difficult. The child raised in an institution may suffer sensory, emotional, and maternal deprivation, resulting in a developing state of apathy during the first year of life accompanied by a tendency to excessive rocking, transient preoccupation with looking at objects, and athetoid-like movements of the extremities. When followed later, some of these children showed unstable and particularly indiscriminate relating to others, failing to develop a meaningful one-to-one relationship with a mother figure. They also may show deficiencies in abstract thinking. Institutionalism can occur in home settings[31] and we have observed infants with this syndrome, particularly when the mother has suffered a prolonged but inadequately recognized postpartum depression. These infants, although at home, tend to be left alone and are therefore understimulated. The autistic child may also be left alone a great deal, and this can be in response to the mother's bewilderment at his lack of interest in her presence. Thus, the isolation of the autistic child follows rather than precedes the pathologic process. The apathy of the primarily understimulated child can superficially resemble the emotional deficiency of the autistic child, and the prolonged rocking, preoccupation with objects, and peculiar athetoid-like movements can mimic transiently some of their motor expressions. The indiscriminate relating superficially suggests the disturbed type of relating seen in early infantile autism. However, the children who suffer institutionalism either in the institution or at home do not develop the complete autistic syndrome. The myriad ways in which the autistic child expresses deviant development are not seen.

Loss of a maternal figure who has already become significant during the first year also leads to disturbed development. This has been referred to as anaclitic depression.[32] Here profound withdrawal is not accompanied by the other facets of the syndrome of early infantile autism or its variants.

The absence of development of early infantile autism in children suffering from institutionalism (S. Provence, MD, oral communication, November 1966) and following loss suggest that although early infantile autism is in part a profound disturbance of relating, etiologic factors must be looked for within the child. Such factors must lie within the central nervous system; sensory deprivation may at the most be a secondary component in the etiology of this condition.

Reiser[13] has commented on the variety of chronic brain damage syndromes with or without accompanying retardation which should be considered in the differential diagnosis of early infantile autism. While the behavioral disturbance in chronic brain syndromes includes irritability, emotional lability, hyperactivity, short attention span, and lack of impulse control, at times behavior more specifically suggestive of early infantile autism may occur. Berkson and Davenport[33] observed "hand flick-shake," "hand held before eyes," and "twirling" in severely retarded "mental defectives." As these behaviors which are probably identical with the hand-flapping, regarding, and whirling of autistic children are lumped with less specific "stereotyped movements," their incidence is unknown. Since diagnostic precision was limited to "mental defective," the number of possibly autistic individuals in the patient group is also unknown. Occasionally, in brain damage secondary to specific syndromes, we have seen whirling (tuberous sclerosis) and hand-flapping (phenylketonuria). However, it should be stressed that in all children suffering from these conditions we do not see these disturbed motor expressions which are so characteristic of autistic children. It is postulated, therefore, that in those cases with known brain damage and autistic behavior, certain specific functional systems of the central nervous system, pathology of which underlies early infantile autism, may become involved. No anatomical sites for these hypothesized functional systems are at present known. In those cases of early infantile autism which are not accompanied by evidence of brain damage, it is postulated that the same functional systems are involved on a congenital basis as suggested by twin studies.

Since early infantile autism can only be diagnosed as a behavioral syndrome,[34] it would seem that those cases of the syndrome where evidence of brain pathology, eg, phenylketonuria, encephalitis, birth trauma exists should be referred to as "early infantile autism associated with . . ., eg, PKU, encephalitis, birth trauma" rather than excluding those cases from the behavioral syndrome as is often done. Rutter[10] reports a high incidence of brain damage in a follow-up study of 63 autistic children.

The failure of speech development in both early infantile autism and aphasia creates diagnostic problems of both semantic and etiologic significance. While the autistic child without speech is by definition "aphasic" confusing cases of real differential diagnostic import are seen. The relationship between the two conditions has been thoroughly discussed by Rutter.[10,35] The fact that aphasic children may use gesture to communicate, while autistic children often do not, may help to separate the two conditions if the child is seen at an early age. If the child improves in all areas but speech, the diagnosis of aphasia is supported.

Etiologic Considerations

In the literature, the etiology of early infantile autism has been considered from several points of view: (1) hereditary tendency; (2) influence of parental personality or malignant family interaction; (3) critical or vulnerable periods in infancy; (4) possible disturbed neurophysiologic mechanism; and (5) underlying or concomitant developmental and neurologic pathology. Various investigators have stressed different symptom subclusters as expressing the fundamental and basic nature of the disorder. For example, Kanner when first describing the disease process focused on disturbed relating to the environment. The coldness, aloofness, and withdrawal of the child was described in relationship to analogous though less severe behavior observed in the parents and even the grandparents in this particular patient sample. This lent itself initially to a genetically based interpretation wherein the autistic child was seen as the final expression of an innate tendency toward intellectualism and an associated lack of emotional expression.[1] The emphasis on the disturbed relatedness, however, also lent itself to an alternative etiologic notion, namely that the children were disturbed and emotionally "refrigerated" because they were raised in an emotionally refrigerated environment.[2,36] Therefore, the etiologic emphasis was changed from faulty genes to faulty parents. A more specific emphasis on the parents' role in the development of the syndrome was postulated by Szurek[37] and by Rank[38] and has been categorically stated by Reiser.[13] The emphasis shifted from the type of environment created for the child to the parent-child interaction; a state of emotional turmoil in the parents during the critical period of infancy was postulated to compromise the essential relationship. In our own experience, however, this has not been seen in all cases; moreover, in many families where great emotional turmoil has been present during the infancy of the child, that child has not become autistic. This experience has been confirmed by others.[10]

The concept of symbiotic psychosis was introduced by Mahler[6] and emphasized the parent as the etiologic agent in the development of psychosis in the child, but for opposite reasons than those of Kanner.[2] In the development of symbiotic psychosis, the parent was described as all-enveloping and never giving the child the opportunity to differentiate himself. However, we have seen both "symbiotic" clinging and complete physical and emotional fusion alongside of, and alternating with, emotional aloofness and cold, icy withdrawal in the same child. What is basic and common to these apparently opposite disturbances is the fluctuating capacity of such a child to perceive separateness between himself and the surrounding environment. The inability to maintain a distinction between self and nonself can be expressed as readily by fusion as by lack of awareness of the other person. Thus, both behaviors, which superficially appear to be opposites, are simply different expressions of a failure in these children to delineate the boundaries between themselves and their environment.

Emphasis on the disturbances of relating has led others to pin-point the period of differentiation from the mother between 6 and 18 months of age[34,39] as the critical period of vulnerability in development of the disease. However, our clinical experience and direct observation[40] show that the onset of the illness can be manifest at birth or in the first months of life when other symptom clusters are considered.

Another subcluster of symptomatology which has received particular consideration with reference to etiology has been that of disturbance of developmental rate. Bender has emphasized this aspect of the syndrome by postulating a maturation lag at the embryonic level as being characteristic of and fundamental to the development of the entire syndrome.[41]

The disturbances of motor expression which we have described have received mention in passing, but have not been related systematically to the syndrome as a whole. Some investigators have referred to the motor behaviors as self-stimulation.[42]

Disturbances of perception have been emphasized by several authors. Bergman and Escalona[5] observed abnormal sensitivities in a small group of children, some of whom became psychotic, and postulated a low barrier to external stimulation as being of etiologic import. Goldfarb[43] has studied perception from the point of view of receptor preference in these children and has pointed up their apparent preference for the use of near receptors (tactile sensation) over far receptors (vision and audition). Schopler[44] has attempted to use near receptor preference as evidence that early sensory deprivation due to inadequate reticular arousal mechanisms is a factor in etiology. Although the linkage between near receptor preference and sensory deprivation is not made clear, an overriding consideration is that infants actually suffering known sensory deprivation exhibit an entirely different syndrome than that of early infantile autism. Contrasting with the notion of reduced arousal functions is the postulation of a chronically high level of arousal as basic to the etiology.[45] Actual observation, however, of the behavior of autistic children, either individually or as a group, reveals them at times to be in apparent states of low arousal (posturing, immobility, and unresponsiveness), and at times in apparent states of high arousal (agitation, excitation, and fearfulness). Wing[46] stressed the autistic child's inability to make meaningful patterns out of sensory stimuli, thereby linking cognitive to perceptual disturbances.

Goldfarb[12,47] has described both motility disturbances and disturbances of perception in a high percentage of schizophrenic (autistic) children whom he labels the "organic" subgroup. This subgroup is differentiated from "nonorganic" children who are relatively free of these disturbances. Goldfarb postulated a continuum of etiologic variables ranging from purely environmental to specific organic influences. These have been detailed by Sarvis and Garcia[39] who associated the illness with faulty family psychodynamics, traumatic environmental circumstances, severe physical illness, and temporal lobe and other neuropathology affecting perception. However, the absence of autistic behavior under conditions of severe environmental and organic insult, and the presence of the syndrome unassociated with such conditions suggests that a basic pathologic mechanism specific to the illness must be present. Environmental factors may determine in some cases the time at which the illness comes to clinical attention. Somatic factors may in some cases either trigger or replicate the expression of the basic pathology.

Underlying Mechanisms

Is it possible to relate the symptom clusters of early infantile autism to an underlying pathologic mechanism? All of the subclusters of symptoms can be seen as resulting from certain cardinal developmental failures occurring in the first year of life. First, many of the behaviors of an autistic infant stem from a failure to develop a distinction between himself and the outside world. Second, imitative behavior is fragmented, greatly delayed, or does not appear. Third, the autistic infant fails to develop the capacity to adequately modulate perceptual input; much of his behavior suggests that he is either getting too little or too much input from the environment. These three developmental failures can be associated and explained by assuming that autistic children do not have the ability to maintain constancy of perception. Thus, identical percepts from the environment are not experienced as the same each time. This is due, we further postulate, to an underlying failure of homeostatic regulation within the central nervous system so that environmental stimuli are either not adequately modulated or are unevenly amplified. This postulated failure to maintain perceptual constancy results in a random underloading or overloading of the central nervous system.

The autistic infant seems to get either too much or too little sensory input, and these states often alternate rapidly and without relation to the environment. Behaviors suggesting that sensory overload is being experienced include attention to inconsequential stimuli and scrutiny of tactile and visual detail. Such activities suggest that the trivial cannot be treated as trivial. More impressive is the tendency of so many of these children to respond with increased excitation, irritability, or apprehension bordering on panic to stimuli which may be either minimal or intense. Such stimuli may be in the auditory, visual, tactile, and proprioceptive modalities. Spinning objects may incite particularly intense reactions in these children. This suggests sensitivity in the vestibular modality as does the panic brought on by an elevator ride.

That these children also get too little external stimuli is inferred from their under-responsiveness.

What type of pathologic mechanism might interfere with the capacity to maintain perceptual constancy? While the failure of homeostatic regulation may represent a neurophysiologic deficiency, behaviors such as the tendency to rub surfaces, visual regarding of finger movements, hand-flapping, and whirling suggest a breaking through of a pathologic excitatory state or activating mechanism. Such a postulated state would have the characteristic of interfering with homeostatic regulation of perception.

Physiologic states can be characterized by degrees of excitation, facilitation, inhibition, or some combination thereof. In the behaviors which define early infantile autism and its allied conditions, we can discern expressions of both states of excessive excitation and inhibition. These states may occur independently in an individual child, may alternate rapidly with each other, or even appear to coexist. The hyperexcitatory state is manifested by hand-flapping, finger-fluttering, whirling, circling on tiptoes, sudden lunging and darting, accentuated startle, hypersensitivity to stimuli, and excited reactions to spinning objects. The overinhibitory state is manifested by posturing, prolonged immobility, and nonresponsiveness to external stimulation. To a considerable, though not complete extent, the symptoms indicative of the state of hyperexcitation include those behaviors which suggest that sensory input is not being adequately dampened. The symptoms indicative of the overinhibitory state, on the other hand, suggest excessive damping of sensory input whether from auditory, visual, proprioceptive or other sources.

In the Table, the symptomatology common to early infantile autism, childhood schizophrenia, atypical development, and the other related conditions is outlined for comparative purposes by chronological order of appearance, descriptive subclusters, developmental failure, and pathologic states of excitation and inhibition.

In summary, the behavior common to a group of related clinical entities, eg, early infantile autism, childhood schizophrenia, and atypical children, suggests a common underlying pathologic mechanism. This mechanism involves the presence of states of hyperexcitation and inhibition which interfere with the normal capacity to maintain perceptual constancy. The presence of these states may indicate a dissociation of a physiologic equilibrium between facilitatory and inhibitory systems which regulate sensory input.

Clinical Illustrations

How do these postulated pathologic mechanisms find expression in the multivariant clinical entities under consideration and how do they lead to the major subclusters of the symptoms?

If the dissociated excitatory and inhibitory states are not too severe, then percepts are available for imitation and self can be distinguished from nonself. In such cases, symptomatology may be confined primarily to disturbances of perception and motor behavior.

CASE 1.—This 4-year-old boy has been under psychiatric observation since 2½ years of age. His older brother was diagnosed as having early infantile autism. His parents are nonprofessional people who did not complete college. Following an uneventful pregnancy, he was born three or four weeks postterm, weighing 3,714 gm (8 lb, 3 oz). The neonatal period was not remarkable. Between 3 and 19 months of age, he had asthmatic bronchitis. Frequently, during the early months of life, his mother could not be certain when he was hungry.

226

The Symptomatology of Early Infantile Autism, Its Variants, and Certain Cases of Childhood Schizophrenia

Chronological Appearance of Symptoms	Subclusters of Symptoms	Developmental Failures Expressed by Symptoms	Excessive Excitatory & Inhibitory States Expressed by Symptoms
Postnatal Hyperirritability Failure to respond Torpor Flaccidity **First 6 mo** Failure to smile No anticipatory response Failure to vocalize Hypersensitivity to stimuli Lack of eye contact **Second 6 mo** Unwilling to chew or accept solids Flicking at objects Casting away of toys Letting toys passively drop out of hands Irregular motor development Limp or rigid when held Unaffectionate Failure to discriminate mother Failure to play "peek-a-boo," "patty-cake," or "bye-bye" Lack of words Failure to point Regarding of hands Intolerance of sensory stimulation; cupping ears May appear deaf **Second-Third Yr** Attending to self-induced sounds Ear-banging & flicking Visual & tactile scrutiny Ignoring meaningful or painful stimuli Posturing & staring Whirling Hand-flapping Darting, lunging motions Spinning of objects Deviant eye contact Use others as extension of self Early speech drops out Prolonged tooth-grinding **Fourth-Fifth Yr** Failure to speak Echolalia Pronoun reversal Atonal, arhythmic voice Severe distress in novel situations	**Disturbances of Perception** *Heightened awareness* *Auditory* Attending to self-induced sounds, ear-banging, & tooth-grinding *Visual* Regarding of hands, staring, & visual detail scrutiny *Tactile* Rubbing surfaces *Olfactory & gustatory* Bizarre food preferences, sniffing *Vestibular* Spinning objects **Heightened sensitivity** *Auditory* Fearful reactions to noise; cover ears *Visual* To change in illumination *Gustatory* Intolerance of "rough" foods *Vestibular* Fearful of roughhouse, fright in elevators **Nonresponsiveness** *Auditory* Disregard of speech, ignoring loud sounds *Visual* Disregard of surroundings *Tactile* Let objects fall out of hand *Pain* Failure to react to bumps & falls **Motor Disturbances** Hand-flapping; finger-flicking Bizarre gesticulations Whirling Toe-walking Darting & lunging Posturing **Disturbances of Relating** Deviant eye contact Absent social smile Delayed anticipatory response Limpness or stiffness when held Bizarre or stereotyped use of toys Failure to play "peek-a-boo," etc Use others as extension of self Lack of emotional responsiveness **Disturbances of Language** Lack of speech development Echolalia Pronoun reversal Atonal, arrhythmic voice **Disturbances of Developmental Rate** Retarded development Precocious development Giving up of acquired skills Scatter on developmental tests	**Failure to Distinguish Between Self and Nonself** Lack of interest in eye contact Absent social smile Failure to play "peek-a-boo" Let objects fall out of hand Use others as extension of self Pronoun reversal **Failure of Imitative Behavior** Failure to play "patty-cake" Failure to say "bye-bye" Failure to mimic sounds & expressions Lack of emotional expression **Failure to Modulate Input** *Sensory overload* Attention to trivial stimuli Visual & tactile scrutiny Irritability or apprehension to inconsequential stimuli; cover ears, etc Panic in elevator Intolerance of "rough" foods *Sensory Underload* Disregard of auditory & visual stimuli Underreactivity to painful stimuli **Dissociated Motor Excitation and Inhibition** *Excitation* Hand-flapping Whirling Circling Darting & lunging *Inhibition* Posturing Prolonged immobility	**Excitatory States** Hand-flapping Whirling Circling Darting & lunging Accentuated startle Overreactivity to stimuli in all modalities Excitation associated with spinning objects **Inhibitory State** Posturing Prolonged immobility Nonresponsiveness to stimuli in all sensory modalities

"Junior" foods were first introduced at 5 months, but were not accepted until 7 months.

Between 9 and 36 months, he was unusually aware of anything that would spin. He would go past the shower curtain, pressing his eyes very close to it, apparently preoccupied with the details in the printed pattern. At 36 months, he was particularly responsive to any change in his mother's appearance, such as a change in hair styling or make-up. From time to time, he would seem to stare as if he saw something that was not there. He was not excessively disturbed by auditory stimuli. Between 24 and 38 months he walked on his toes; when presented with a spinning top, he would flap his hands. Between 30 and 38 months he would whirl himself. The use of sounds, syllables, words, phrases, and sentences occurred on schedule. However, as he developed communicative speech, an excessive parroting of phrases and sentences also occurred. He particularly repeated questions directed to him rather than answering them. He developed a pleasant, responsive smile, an anticipatory response to being picked up, and good eye contact during the first half year of life. He was cuddly, affectionate, and always seemed to need his mother. His use of toys was limited, and he was preoccupied with any part of a toy that would spin. He played "peek-a-boo" and "patty-cake" and mimicked his parents' gestures and mannerisms. Motor development was not delayed.

He began psychotherapy at 3½ years of age. A relative paucity of fantasy was noted during the early phase of treatment. He tended to repetitively confuse the identities of persons, for example, calling his therapist "daddy" or "Dr. Smith Jones," a name combining that of his therapist and his father. He had some bizarre ideation: For example, when shown a microphone, he said, "Mommy is inside the microphone."

Such a case is often referred to as an *atypical child* or a *child with unusual sensitivities*.

In severe cases where perception is so unstable that imitation (and subsequent identification) and distinction between self and nonself is impossible, then disturbances of relatedness, language, and development are seen along with the disturbances of perception and motor expression.

CASE 2.—A 5-year, 7-month-old boy had his first psychiatric evaluation at the age of 3 years and 10 months. Since age 4 he has been an inpatient in a psychiatric hospital. He is the second child of parents whose formal education stopped at the end of high school. His father has been a truck driver and laborer. Following a normal pregnancy, he was delivered without incident at term, weighing 3,345 gm (7 lb, 6 oz). The neonatal period was not remarkable, although he was described as "irritable and oversensitive." He developed chickenpox at 12 months. The parents were first concerned at 16 months as he did not seem to respond normally. However, they had noticed that he had been preoccupied with twirling beads in his crib at 4 months and twirling ashtrays at 8 months. Furthermore, he failed to show an anticipatory response to being picked up until after 12 months. He remained on baby foods until 36 months, as he had refused to chew earlier.

He was unusually aware of visual detail and spent considerable time regarding the movements of his fingers since 15 months. He completely ignored auditory stimulation and toys presented to him. If handed objects, he let them fall out of his hand or flicked them away. From 24 months, he whirled himself, walked on his toes, and developed a repetitive, rapid oscillation of the hands. From 4 months, he rolled his head rhythmically from side to side and could only be distracted from such activity with great difficulty. Although he had spontaneously used some sounds by 6 months and some syllables by 12 months, he did not imitate either sounds or syllables. By 36 months, he had developed a 10-word vocabulary, but after that age, he ceased using words. He never combined words into phrases. He never made eye contact, and he used others as an extension of himself. The parents have said, "he pushes us to his needs." He never played "peek-a-boo" or "patty-cake." Between 18 and 24 months, he occasionally waved "bye-bye" in imitation of his father, but then abandoned this activity. He sat without support by 7 months but did not walk alone until 16 months.

In the course of extensive observation in an inpatient setting, he was noted to sustain his oscillatory hand-flapping throughout the entire day. He was never observed to use toys or other objects in any appropriate way and would only spin them.

This case demonstrates a more severe manifestation of the same basic disease than does case 1 and is usually labeled *early infantile autism*. If the development of such a child remains static, particularly when speech fails to develop, while the motor and perceptual disturbances gradually abate, he may be relabeled *pseudoretarded*.

If a child such as case 2 develops speech, particularly echolalia and pronoun reversal, he will continue to be labeled autistic.

CASE 3.—This 6-year-old boy has been under

psychiatric observation since 4 years of age. He is the third in a family of four children, and his parents are high school graduates. His father is a salesman. The pregnancy was not remarkable. He was delivered at term by breech presentation and weighed 3,970 gm (8 lb, 12 oz). His Apgar rating was 10, and the postnatal course was not remarkable.

He has been in good physical health with no illnesses other than chickenpox at age 2 years. The early feeding history revealed he was apparently unwilling to hold solid food in his mouth or to chew. He sat without support at 7 months, but did not walk until 21 months. He showed no excessive reaction to auditory, visual, tactile, or proprioceptive stimuli, but he would become excessively disturbed when given new toys or clothes. He consistently ignored people and did not respond to sounds or to painful stimuli, eg, bumps and falls. He would let toys fall out of his hands. He maintained prolonged and unusual postures and between 2 and 3 years of age, whirled himself, flapped his hands, and walked on his toes. He never showed an anticipatory response to being picked up; he seemed to look through people, stiffened when held, and ignored affection.

He spontaneously made sounds such as "coos" and "babbles" by 4 months and later used syllables. He later ceased these vocalizations. He did not use phrases until after 36 months and never used complete sentences. Prior to 24 months, he failed to imitate sounds and words, but after 36 months, he would repeatedly parrot words and phrases he had heard in the past, but which had no relationship to the present situation. His speech was characterized by a flat tonal quality without inflection.

The echolalia and pronoun reversal are sequelae of the earlier failures to imitate and to distinguish between self and nonself.[26] If, in the early arrested autistic child, the failure to distinguish between self and nonself is manifested by persistent clinging to other people, then the label *symbiotic psychosis* may be applied.

CASE 4.—This 4-year-old girl has been under psychiatric observation since 30 months of age. She is the third child in her family. The mother, a teacher, had considerable experience with school-age children and was a warm and affectionate person. Following an unremarkable pregnancy, the patient was born several days after rupture of the membranes. At delivery, the umbilical cord was looped around the neck. She was kept in an incubator during the first postnatal day because of "congestion in the lungs." The first month of life was characterized by projectile vomiting until pyloric stenosis was diagnosed and corrected surgically. Following the surgery she thrived on bottle feedings and gradually accepted strained foods. She would not, however, accept any chopped foods, and at 30 months, eating was limited to strained baby foods or puddings. Paradoxically, she chewed on crinkly cellophane.

She failed to cry to be held or fed, from birth on, and by 6 months of age, it became apparent that she did not smile at others. During the first and second years, she never indicated wanting to be held by her mother. At 27 months she first seemed to be aware of changes in her surroundings and at such times began to cling tenaciously to the mother. By 33 months, she showed persistent clinging. She would throw severe temper tantrums if the mother refused to hold her on her lap. However, she accepted being held by any other person in the same way, and then would seem unaware of the mother's absence. She would kneel for hours at a time on her mother's lap, pressing her chest against her mother, or she would stand on her mothers' lap, hanging onto her thumbs, vigorously rocking back and forth. She would press her fingers into her mother's eyes, with no apparent awareness that this caused pain. She would, on occasion, smile responsively when her hands were pushed together in the "patty-cake" game, but she did not actively imitate. By 33 months, she was saying "ring around" and "fall down" responsively to a "ring around the rosy" game, and she would also say "rock, rock the baby" while pantomiming rocking a doll in her arms. She would say "Mary, Mary" to her own image in the mirror but had no specific term for her mother. She would point to her nose and verbalize a word that sounded like a fusion between "nose" and "mouth" or mix up the words for "mouth" and "nose," and she often held her forearms flexed upward with her hands loosely waving in the air. She scratched at surfaces. In an elevator she would cry both at the beginning and at the end of the ride. From 15 months, she often engaged in peculiar posturing with her hands held in a "claw-like position." She did not sit without support until 12 months, but pulled herself to a standing position at that time and walked without support by 15 months.

Those cases in which communicative speech develops, the disturbance of relatedness is not too severe, and a thought disorder becomes manifest are usually referred to as *childhood schizophrenia*. In such cases, the perceptual inconstancy has not been so severe as to arrest the development of relatedness and language but results in distortion in these areas. This distortion is manifest in the thought disorder. The persistence of disturbances of motor behavior and perception are the pathologic sequelae of the abnormal or dissociated states of excitation and inhibition and reveal the fundamental developmental relationship between such cases of childhood schizophrenia and early infantile autism.

CASE 5.—This 11-year-old boy has been under continuous psychiatric observation since 4 years of age. His natural parents were high school graduates. Following a normal pregnancy, he was delivered at term, weighing 3,913 gm (8 lb, 10 oz). Examination at 8 days revealed good crying and color; the Moro reflex was described as "only fair." He was placed for adoption and was noted to be a quiet baby, not particularly responsive to stimulation. He entered the home of his adopting parents when 18 days old. Both adopting parents are college-educated, thoughtful, and affectionate people. The father is an engineer. A social work report at 4 months indicated a "happy and well-adjusted child." There were no early feeding problems and "junior" foods were introduced at 6 months without difficulty. He chewed well and ate everything offered until 24 months, at which time he limited his diet to liquids and soft foods. When 4 years old, he again accepted a regular diet.

From three months, he was panicked by any loud noise and startled repeatedly if one moved suddenly near him. The sensitivity to loud noises persisted until he was 6 years old. Until 15 months he became severely upset by any encounter with a strange person. He was markedly disturbed when brought into unaccustomed surroundings until 3 years old. Between 2 and 3½ years, he was panicked at any attempt to toss him in the air. He remained oblivious to any toy presented to him until he was 3 years old.

Photographs document a preoccupying interest in regarding his own writhing hand movements from 8 months and hand-flapping from 11 months. At first, he held a toy to his mouth with one hand and repetitively flapped his fingers against a part of it with the other hand. By 4 years this evolved into a stereotyped ritualistic gesticulation consisting of a rapid pushing of the fingers of the one hand against the other. At the same time, the thumb of one hand would be rhythmically pushed toward the mouth while it was pushed back by the pressure of the other hand. At 8 years of age he tried to consciously suppress this activity, but substituted a rhythmic stereotyped alternating extension and flexion of the fingers. He has always walked on his toes. When he was a baby, he would sit for hours content to be alone playing with a toy that he could spin. Later, he would say that he was inside the washing machine while he was preoccupied watching it spin.

From birth, he was described as being "very sober." When held he conformed without stiffening but did not snuggle or cuddle. He did respond to affection and to the "peek-a-boo" and "pat-a-cake" games. Although he was aware of his mother when she was present, separation evoked no response. He reacted to other children as if they were inanimate. By 4 years, he became interested in toys and began to use them functionally.

He first used syllables at 6 months and words at 9 months. He did not use speech for communication until after 4 years of age, but would parrot words and phrases up to that time. He was not able to use pronouns properly and characteristically confused and reversed the pronouns "you" and "I."

He never crawled, and while he started walking at 11 months of age, if he fell, he would not stand up again by himself. He never pulled himself up or cruised about the furniture prior to walking without support. He did not open doors or turn knobs until 3½ years old.

Once he began speaking, he revealed a preoccupation with fearful thoughts. Before the age of 6 years, he had a dream about a frightening chair and insisted on following his mother around so that he would be protected from it. He dreamed that his father or mother were in a chair costume chasing him. He became quite concrete and literal in his expressions, saying, for example, "There are so many chairs I have to be afraid of now." From 5 years to 9 years old, he thought of himself as being a car. Whenever he had to urinate, he would say that he was draining his tank. He believed that other people could control or actually think his thoughts. Between the ages of 7 and 10, he would ask his therapist, "Can you think my thoughts?" and, "Can you dream my dreams?" At 11 years, when his teacher tapped on her desk for attention he commented that her act "weakens my blood" and he often noted that everything around him seemed to grow smaller or larger.

This child experienced great difficulty in absorbing formal learning. Mastery of reading and writing was delayed and learning could only be accomplished in a special school.

The following case is presented to illustrate another clinical variant of the same basic syndrome. In this child, perceptual and motor disturbances are associated with precocious intellectual development.

CASE 6.—Case 6 is a 6-year-old boy. His parents, nonprofessional people, did not finish college. The child and a fraternal twin brother were born following a full-term pregnancy which was not remarkable except for a viral illness during the second trimester. The patient was the firstborn and was delivered by an easy breech extraction. He weighed 2,438 gm (5 lb, 6 oz). The neonatal period was not remarkable. The mother did not recall any early feeding difficulties. From the first months, he showed unusual awareness in all sensory modalities, including a tendency to stare at spinning objects such as the record player. He was easily upset by many types of stimuli. Hair clippers and vacuum cleaners were particularly disturbing to him. At 4 months, his sensitivity to noise was manifested by responding to his mother's voice with a startled reaction and scream. He flapped his hands and walked on his toes. Early motor development was not remarkable. While he smiled responsively, there were periods during his development when it was felt that he did not really look at people but rather looked through them, would stiffen when held, and seemed emotionally aloof. He would let objects fall out of his hands. His play with toys was limited, and he only became involved with toys that spin. He pointed to and gestured for what he wanted, and he communicated early with words, although his speech was described as being "a monotone with no inflection." He never confused pronouns and no echolalia was reported.

At 6 years of age, he had many fears and continued to panic at strange noises. He did not like to play with other children, apparently preferring to be alone and involved in fantasy. He became preoccupied with being able to name the capitols of all the countries of the world and with the relationship between the different species of animals in a nature book. He became fearful of things he had seen on television and reacted to them as if they were real. He learned to read early, read well, and was at the top of his class in a regular school. Such a child may be labeled *autistic, atypical, borderline psychotic,* or *schizophrenic,* depending on the clinical setting in which he is seen.

These six cases illustrate the merging of clinical entities which have been described under different diagnostic rubrics.

The following case is an example of the clinical syndrome of early infantile autism in which specific neurological abnormalities were found.

CASE 7.—Both the mother and father of this 5-year-old boy held degrees in the physical sciences and their families had a long history of intellectual achievement. During the early years of the patient's life, his mother was depressed, agitated, and emotionally labile. The pregnancy, delivery, and postnatal course were not remarkable. During the first weeks of life, he was noted to lie very quietly, and he was described as being "apathetic." The mother felt that the baby did not want to be held. He was prop-fed and was not weaned until after his third birthday. No difficulties in chewing solid food developed. Prior to 24 months of age, he responded to many types of noise by "running and screaming" and putting his hands over his ears. He responded with equal distress to change in illumination and continued to show a sensitivity to auditory and visual stimuli throughout his life. He became preoccupied with spinning tops and pot covers before 36 months, and this behavior became a persistent activity. Before 48 months, he would often ignore both people and various forms of stimuli not related to people. At 36 months, he did not respond with pain to bumps and falls. From the time he could walk, he persistently whirled himself, flapped his hands, and walked around on his toes. He failed to imitate either sounds or words during his first 24 months, and he did not use words for communication until after 5 years of age. He also failed to communicate by gesture. He never used complete sentences. He did not show an anticipatory response to being picked up until 3 or 4 years of age and earlier he would stiffen when held. He used others as an extension of himself and actively withdrew from affection. He had not played "peek-a-boo" or "pat-a-cake."

Neurological examination revealed a spreading of the biceps reflex into the finger, active finger jerks, crossed adductor reflexes, and persistent plantar grasp reflexes at 5 years, 11 months. Two EEGs showed focal slowing appearing on the right side. A pneumoencephalogram revealed asymmetry of the frontal horns of the lateral ventricles with the right appearing slightly larger than the left. A bilateral carotid angiogram revealed the right lateral ventricle to be slightly larger than the left. The findings were felt to be consistent with focal cortical atrophy on the right side.

In this case, both the development of the child and the family history are consistent with the syndrome of early infantile autism as described by Kanner. The syndrome, however, is seen to occur in association with a specific cerebral abnormality.

The following case is presented as an example of children in whom careful history and observation does not reveal evidence of the symptoms characteristic of the syndrome of perceptual inconstancy (early infantile autism, its variants, and sequelae) yet who nevertheless have severe ideational and affectual distortion of psychotic proportions.

CASE 8.—This 7-year-old boy was admitted for inpatient evaluation because he refused to eat, saying, "bad people have touched my food." History revealed that at three months' gestation, the mother had a viral illness with high fever, vaginal hemorrhaging at four months, and that the patient was delivered five weeks prior to term, weighing just 2,268 gm (5 lb). He was reported to have had intermittent difficulty breathing from birth on, and at 6 months asthma was diagnosed. All motor developmental landmarks were normal. There was a good smiling response noted by 2 months, stranger anxiety at 6 months, words and phrases by 1¼ years, and sentences were used by 2 years. No unusual sensitivities or mannerisms were noted. When the patient was 1½ years and 3½ years old, his mother was hospitalized for medical and surgical treatment. During these hospitalizations he was cared for by his grandfather. Six weeks following the mother's second hospitalization, the grandfather was killed in an automobile accident and the parents related the onset of his illness to this event. He refused to accept his grandfather's death, saying that he could see him and would speak to him. He wanted to die so that he could be with him and on one occasion released the car brake and rolled the car into the street in an attempt to get killed. He gradually withdrew interest from friends and family and evolved an elaborate fantasy world peopled by robots, devils, gods, and other powerful creatures. He became fixed in the belief that he was a mechanical robot, had switches on his body, and was impervious to pain. He was expelled from kindergarten because of unprovoked outbursts of severe hostile behavior to the other children. Psychiatric examination revealed loosening of associations, preoccupation with fantasies of being made out of steel and controlled by wires, and grossly inappropriate affect. Psychological testing revealed a psychotic ego organization with impairment of intellectual potential and no evidence of organic brain dysfunction. Prolonged observation has revealed no evidence of symptoms indicative of disturbed perceptual or motor development. Observation of his parents indicated that the mother had a severe thinking disorder; she, in fact, had frequently told her son that certain foods should not be eaten because they had been poisoned.

We consider such a case is an instance where childhood schizophrenia is not related to the syndrome of perceptual inconstancy as are other cases of childhood schizophrenia (eg, cases 5 and 6).

Comment

The basic pathologic mechanism underlying this syndrome is presumed to be on a neurophysiologic basis. A particular pathoneurophysiology will be postulated in a subsequent communication. The relationships between the basic dissociation of facilitatory and inhibitory influences, the resulting perceptual inconstancy, the major developmental failures, and the resulting symptom-complexes are illustrated schematically in Fig 2.

Early infantile autism, its clinical variants, and its sequelae can best be understood as a unitary disease with varying symptoms which are expressive of an underlying pathophysiology. With maturation the symptoms undergo certain vicissitudes. In those autistic children in whom the disease process severely limits development of intrapsychic organization, these symptoms may secondarily be utilized to modulate sensory input. For other autistic children, in whom more advanced intrapsychic organization occurs, these symptoms may secondarily serve as foci for the development of bizarre or psychotic fantasies. However, neither a "need" for self-stimulation nor the child's fantasy life explain the original development or the sustained activity level of these symptoms.

Since the symptoms of early infantile autism can be understood as expressive of a pathophysiologic mechanism related to dissociated states of excitation and inhibition, it may be possible to investigate the etiology from a neurophysiologic point of view. This seems to be hopeful since these behavioral states occur concomitantly with known brain pathology, disturbed environment, or

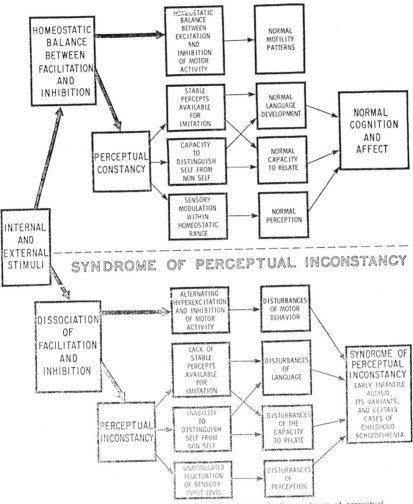

NORMAL MODULATION OF STIMULI

SYNDROME OF PERCEPTUAL INCONSTANCY

Fig 2.—Postulated pathophysiology of symptom formation in the syndrome of perceptual inconstancy compared with the regulation of sensory input in normal children.

completely independent of these factors. Therefore, such factors appear to be neither specific nor fundamental to the etiology of this disease. The overt expression of the pathologic mechanism may be triggered by some of the associated conditions. As the weight of clinical evidence suggests that a schizophrenic thought and affect disorder may be one sequela of early infantile autism, the hypothesis suggested may have applicability to certain children and adults with this major psychiatric illness.

233

Since early infantile autism, its variants —atypical development and symbiotic psychosis—and its major sequela—some cases of childhood schizophrenia—are expressions of one disease process based on faulty homeostatic regulation of perceptual input, we could refer to children within this clinical spectrum as manifesting a *syndrome of perceptual inconstancy.*

Summary

Early infantile autism and several related syndromes are described in terms of the natural history of the symptoms and their developmental relationships. Early infantile autism, atypical development, symbiotic psychosis, and certain cases of childhood schizophrenia are shown to be essentially variants of the same disease.

The symptoms of this disease have been grouped into five major subclusters: disturbances of perception, motility, relatedness, language, and developmental rate.

Disturbances of perception are shown to be fundamental to the other aspects of the disease and to be manifested by early developmental failure to distinguish between self and environment, to imitate, and to modulate sensory input.

It is suggested that these developmental failures are caused by a breakdown of homeostatic regulation of sensory input. This results in a condition of perceptual inconstancy.

The symptoms suggest that the illness is characterized by dissociated, uncoupled, and alternating states of excitation and inhibition. It is this pathophysiology which interferes with the adequate homeostatic regulation of perception and leads to a state of perceptual inconstancy.

Since the symptomatology is primarily expressive of an underlying pathophysiology, the symptoms may only secondarily in some cases come to be purposeful in the intrapsychic life of the afflicted child.

As this syndrome may be seen in children with specific organic brain dysfunction or may occur independently from birth, the pathophysiologic mechanism causing perceptual inconstancy is probably specific to the disease but may be activated in certain cases by particular neuropathologic conditions.

This work was supported by United States Public Health Service grants No. MH-12575-01 and No. MH-13517-01. Prof Henry Work and Prof George Tarjan, the Division of Child Psychiatry, UCLA School of Medicine, provided support of this study.

References

1. Kanner, L.: Autistic Disturbances of Affective Contact, *Nerv Child* 2:217-250, 1943.
2. Kanner, L.: Problems of Nosology and Psychodynamics of Early Infantile Autism, *Amer J Orthopsychiat* 19:416-426, 1949.
3. Bender, L.: Childhood Schizophrenia: Clinical Study of One Hundred Schizophrenic Children, *Amer J Orthopsychiat* 17:40-56, 1947.
4. Putnam, M.C., et al: Round Table, 1947: Case Study of an Atypical Two-and-a-Half-Year-Old, *Amer J Orthopsychiat* 18:1-30, 1948.
5. Bergman, P., and Escalona, S.K.: "Unusual Sensitivities in Very Young Children," *Psychoanal Stud Child* 3-4:333-352, 1949.
6. Mahler, M.S.: On Child Psychosis and Schizophrenia: "Autistic and Symbiotic Infantile Psychosis," *Psychoanal Stud Child* 7:286-305, 1952.
7. Despert, J.L.: Some Considerations Relating to the Genesis of Autistic Behavior in Children, *Amer J Orthopsychiat* 21:335-347, 1951.
8. Rank, B.: Adaptation of the Psychoanalytic Technique for the Treatment of Young Children With Atypical Development, *Amer J Orthopsychiat* 19:130-139, 1949.
9. Wolff, S., and Chess, S.: A Behavioural Study of Schizophrenic Children, *Acta Psychiat Scand* 40:438-466, 1964.
10. Rutter, M.: The Influence of Organic and Emotional Factors on the Origins, Nature and Outcome of Childhood Psychosis, *Develop Med Child Neurol* 7:518-528, 1965.
11. Bender, L.: Schizophrenia in Childhood—Its Recognition, Description and Treatment, *Amer J Orthopsychiat* 26:499-506, 1956.
12. Goldfarb, W.: An Investigation of Childhood Schizophrenia, *Arch Gen Psychiat* 11:620-634, 1964.
13. Reiser, D.E.: Psychosis of Infancy and Early Childhood, as Manifested by Children With Atypical Development, *New Eng J Med* 269:790-798, 844-850, 1963.
14. Brown, J.L., and Reiser, D.E.: Follow-up Study of Preschool Children of Atypical Development (Infantile Psychosis): Latter Personality Patterns in Adaption to Maturational Stress, *Amer J Orthopsychiat* 33:336-338, 1963.
15. Eisenberg, L.: The Autistic Child in Adolescence, *Amer J Psychiat* 112:607-612, 1956.
16. Darr, G.C., and Worden, F.G.: Case Report Twenty-Eight Years After an Infantile Autistic Disorder, *Amer J Orthopsychiat* 21:559-570, 1951.
17. Tolor, A., and Rafferty, W.: Incidence of Symptoms of Early Infantile Autism in Subsequently Hospitalized Psychiatric Patients, *Dis Nerv Syst* 24:1-7, 1963.
18. O'Gorman, G.: *The Nature of Childhood Autism,* London: Butterworth Co., Inc., 1967.
19. Kamp, L.N.J.: Autistic Syndrome in One of

Pair of Monozygotic Twins, *Psychiat Neurol Neurochir* 67:143-147, 1964.

20. Ornitz, E.M.; Ritvo, E.R.; and Walter, R.D.: Dreaming Sleep in Autistic and Schizophrenic Children, *Amer J Psychiat* 122:419-424, 1965.

21. Vaillant, G.E.: Twins Discordant for Early Infantile Autism, *Arch Gen Psychiat* 9:163-167, 1963.

22. Schain, R.J., and Yannet, H.: Infantile Autism, *J Pediat* 57:560-567, 1960.

23. Kanner, L.: To What Extent Is Early Infantile Autism Determined by Constitutional Inadequacies, *Proc Assoc Res Nerv Ment Dis* 33:378-385, 1954.

24. Taft, L., and Goldfarb, W.: Prenatal and Perinatal Factors in Childhood Schizophrenia, *Develop Med Child Neurol* 6:32-43, 1964.

25. Fish, B.: Longitudinal Observations of Biological Deviations in a Schizophrenic Infant, *Amer J Psychiat* 116:25-31, 1959.

26. Griffith, R., and Ritvo, E.: Echolalia; Concerning the Dynamics of the Syndrome, *J Amer Acad Child Psychiat* 6:184-193, 1967.

27. Fish, B., et al: The Prediction of Schizophrenia in Infancy: III. A Ten-Year Follow-up Report of Neurological and Psychological Development, *Amer J Psychiat* 121:768-775, 1965.

28. Creak, M.: Schizophrenic Syndrome in Childhood: Progress Report of a Working Party, *Cereb Palsy Bull* 3:501-503, 1961.

29. Ekstein, R.; Bryant, K.; and Friedman, S.W.: Childhood Schizophrenia and Allied Conditions," in Belak, L. (ed.): *Schizophrenia: A Review of the Syndrome*, New York: Logos Press, 1958.

30. Provence, S., and Lipton, R.: *Infants in Institutions*, New York: International Universities Press, 1962.

31. Coleman, R., and Provence, S.: Environmental Retardation (Hospitalism) in Infants Living in Families, *Pediatrics* 19:285-292, 1957.

32. Spitz, R.A.: "Anaclitic Depression," *Psychoanal Stud Child*, 2:313-342, 1946.

33. Berkson, G., and Davenport, R.K.: Stereotyped Movements of Mental Defectives, *Amer J Ment Defic* 66:849-852, 1962.

34. Garcia, B., and Sarvis, M.A.: Evaluation and Treatment Planning for Autistic Children, *Arch Gen Psychiat* 10:530-541, 1964.

35. Rutter, M.: "Behavioral and Cognitive Characteristics of a Series of Psychotic Children," in Wing, J.K. (ed.): *Early Childhood Autism*, New York: Pergamon Press, Ltd., 1966.

36. Eisenberg, L., and Kanner, L.: Early Infantile Autism 1943-1955, *Amer J Orthopsychiat* 26:556-566, 1956.

37. Szurek, S.A.: Psychotic Episodes and Psychotic Maldevelopment, *Amer J Orthopsychiat* 26:519-543, 1956.

38. Rank, B.: "Intensive Study and Treatment of Preschool Children Who Show Marked Personality Deviations, or 'Atypical Development,' and Their Parents," in Caplan, G. (ed.): *Emotional Problems of Early Childhood*, New York: Basic Books Co., 1955.

39. Sarvis, M.A., and Garcia, B.: Etiological Variables in Autism, *Psychiatry* 24:307-317, 1961.

40. Fish, B.: Involvement of the Central Nervous System in Infants With Schizophrenia, *Arch Neurol* 2:115-121 1960.

41. Bender, L., and Freedman, A.M.: A Study of the First Three Years in the Maturation of Schizophrenic Children, *Quart J Child Behav* 4:245-272, 1952.

42. Simmons, J.Q., et al: Modification of Autistic Behavior With LSD-25, *Amer J Psychiat* 122:1201-1211, 1966.

43. Goldfarb, W.: Receptor Preferences in Schizophrenic Children, *Arch Neurol Psychiat* 76:643-652, 1956.

44. Schopler, E.: Early Infantile Autism and Receptor Processes, *Arch Gen Psychiat* 13:327-335, 1965.

45. Hutt, S.J., et al: A Behavioural and Electroencephalographic Study of Autistic Children, *J Psychiat Res* 3:181-197, 1965.

46. Wing, J.K.: "Diagnosis, Epidemiology, Aetiology," in Wing, J.K. (ed.): *Early Childhood Autism*, New York: Pergamon Press, Ltd., 1966.

47. Goldfarb, W.: *Childhood Schizophrenia*, Cambridge, Mass: Harvard University Press, 1961.

How Far Can Autistic Children Go in Matters of Social Adaptation?

LEO KANNER, ALEJANDRO RODRIGUEZ,[1] AND BARBARA ASHENDEN

The Johns Hopkins University School of Medicine and Hospital

In a long-range follow-up study of eleven autistic children, it could be ascertained that two of them, not differing essentially from the others in their basic initial symptoms, had in their childhood attained a modus vivendi which allowed them to function gainfully in society (Kanner, 1971a, 1971b). One, Donald T., is a regularly employed bank teller who takes part in a variety of community activities and has the respect of his fellow townspeople. The other, Frederick W., has a full time job running duplicating machines; he has been described by his chief as "outstandingly dependable, reliable, thorough, and thoughful toward fellow workers."

It cannot be emphasized strongly enough that—even with the full knowledge of family background, parents' personalities, prenatal, paranatal and neonatal data, developmental milestones and complete physical and psychological assessments—it would have been impossible for anyone to predict this outcome. There was nothing in the detailed observations of the patients' childhood

[1] Requests for reprints should be sent to Dr. Alejandro Rodriguez, The Johns Hopkins Hospital, Division of Child Psychiatry, CMSC335, 601 North Broadway, Baltimore, Maryland 21205.

JOURNAL OF AUTISTIC AND CHILDHOOD SCHIZO-PHRENIA, 1972, Vol. 2, No. 1, pp. 9-33.

development and behavior, nor is there anything in the documented experiences with psychotic children generally, that would offer reasonably sure indicators of prognostic value.

It has occurred to us that an expansion of up-to-date follow-ups beyond the first eleven cases might contribute to the scope of information about the "natural history" of the autistic illness. In this investigation, we have limited ourselves to those who have by now passed the age of adolescence and we have tried to trace their destinies until the present time (January 1972). Out of the 96 patients diagnosed as autistic at the Children's Psychiatric Clinic of The Johns Hopkins Hospital before 1953, we singled out for special consideration those whom we have found to be sufficiently integrated into the texture of society to be employable, move among people without obvious behavior problems, and be acceptable to those around them at home, at work, and in other modes of interaction.

In addition to Donald T. and Frederick W., mentioned above, we came upon nine other such persons. They will be reported in the order of the age which they have now attained.[2]

Case Material

Case 1

Thomas G., born September 11, 1936, was brought to the Clinic by his maternal grandmother on April 19, 1943. The complaint story began as follows:

He acts so silly. First he kissed shoes and now it's watches and clocks. He is awful smart for his age. He is not a bad child, more of a girl, quiet. He does not play with children. He comes in the house and shuts the door when the neighborhood school is let out.

Thomas was born at term. His mother, 17 years old at the time, had "kidney trouble" during pregnancy. Delivery was normal and birth weight was 7 pounds. Thomas sat up at 6 months and walked at 18. He had measles at 2 and a T&A at 3 years of age. There was no history of severe illness.

[2] For the sake of accuracy, we must point out that we have so far been unable to trace the whereabouts of one patient since 1962, at which time he was doing exceptionally well in college; we have not given up the search but cannot include him in this report. Another patient, who excelled in mathematical physics on a scholarship at Columbia University, might well have figured in our account had he not been run over by a truck on New York's Broadway and killed several years ago.

The father, an upholsterer of Italian extraction, the son of a municipal band conductor and nephew of a composer, died in 1941 at 31 years of age in a tuberculosis sanitarium. The two parents had lived together only from January to December 1936. The mother gave Thomas little attention because "she feared he would give her tuberculosis" (which he did not have), touched him "as little as possible" and frequently went off leaving the child long periods to be cared for by the paternal grandmother who was "on relief" in New York. When the maternal grandmother finally took full charge of Thomas, who was then close to 4 years old, he still had no sphincter control and did not talk. The boy improved quickly and remained with her until he attained school age and rejoined his mother, who had remarried. He was entered in the first grade but soon had to be taken out because of his "peculiar behavior"—paying little heed to directions and insisting on kissing other children's shoes. Thomas was returned to his maternal grandmother who, sensing that he was not well, brought him to our Clinic.

He was in good physical health. At times he answered the examiner's questions and at other times stared ahead or giggled to himself. He was very preoccupied with watches, for which he had a special name: "I like to fool with *dishnishes*—they go tick-tick . . . watches get me excited. It makes me *embarranness*." He referred to his two grandmothers in terms of their ages: "One is 64 and one is 55. I like 55 best." Generally fascinated by numbers, the boy had to make sure how many pages a dictionary or a Sears Roebuck's catalog had, when he spotted them in a room.

Thomas was followed at the Clinic for several years by the social worker to whom he took a liking. For a time it was difficult to get him away from his engrossment with watches and numbers. Obsessions, after running their course, shifted consecutively to measuring cups, maps, and astronomy. He did quite a bit of drawing, was very serious-minded, never cried and became upset by sad pictures or stores. There was some slowness in the boy's response. Before giving details about what went on in school, he would say: "Wait, I have to get it in my mind first." With other children, he never took the initiative but joined in their games. Thomas took piano lessons, won a scholarship and always enjoyed playing.

At 12 years of age, he was at the top of his class in the sixth grade. The school considered him "adjusted," though he was still looked upon as a "queer fellow." Thomas' marks were excellent. He spent one term each in the school's athletic association, art club, and newspaper, and helped the librarian after school. He also took on a central part in a demonstration during a folk dance. Teachers liked him because of his good academic performance: "He works slowly but what he turns in is excellent." Schoolmates neither accepted nor entirely rejected him. He was the butt of much teasing finding it best to ignore because, if he teased back, "it got worse."

After graduation from high school, Thomas got a Johns Hopkins University Scholarship, which was discontinued after 2 years because his marks were not good enough. He then enlisted in the military service. Because of the slowness of his responses, Thomas was after 5 months directed to undergo medical examination. While at the hospital, he suddenly had a *grand mal* seizure and received a medical discharge. Thomas managed to go back to evening school and earn his college diploma. He continued to experience seizures when neglecting to take his medication regularly.

Interests in astronomy and music provided much personal satisfaction and some social contact. Thomas was a scout leader in demand to teach astronomy and also play the piano. He belongs to a swimming and athletic club and likes to read about science and astronomy, but not fiction.

Among his several jobs was that of a file clerk at a Government agency for a period of five years. He changed this position for work in a military test center focused on electronics and science.

In 1969, the grandmother, now 83 years old, had to be placed in a nursing home. Due to negligence in taking medication, Thomas had another seizure and lost his job. Rather resourceful in rapidly securing other employment, he now works for a charitable organization. Thomas owns a house which he bought several years ago, drives his own car, and plays the piano and tape recorder when at home. He is not interested in girls: "They cost too much money."

Case 2

Sally S., born May 6, 1937, was first seen at the Clinic on March 8, 1943. There were the typical pronominal reversals. An excerpt of the summary states:

> Sally is a well-developed, attractive, intelligent-looking girl. Physical examination showed no noticeable abnormalities. Her main difficulty lies in disability to relate to persons and situations. Aloneness and a marked degree of obsessiveness are the outstanding features, combined with a phenomenal memory and unusual dexterity in solving puzzles considerably beyond her age level.

Both parents were college graduates. The father, an advertising copywriter, was described by his wife as "devoted to his family, not a particularly warm person but everybody likes him; he does not put himself out for people, as I do." The mother, a librarian, spoke of herself as "extremely democratic, a high-strung person; I cross the bridge before I get there." The paternal grandfather, a "brillant lawyer, who got himself involved with women and alcohol," committed suicide; his widow ran a home for old people. The maternal grandfather, a surgeon, died of cancer; the grandmother taught school for some time. A brother, three years older than Sally, was described as rebellious and defiant.

Sally was born normally at term. Reported to be "an exceedingly healthy child," she stood up at 10 months but did not walk until 22 months. "Since a time when she was less than one year old, the girl would scream when members of the family would fail to sit down in their usual chairs, if the routine of the daily walk was changed, if the order of the dishes on the tray was altered, or when she was hindered in going through one special door leading into the garden." She was obsessively interested in all processes which had to do with body functions.

Sally went regularly to school in her home town. At 13 years of age, while in the sixth grade, she had a full scale WISC score of 110 (verbal 119 and performance 98). Among her school marks were A's in Spelling and French, B's in Geography, Mathematics, Bible, and Art, and C in English. She was reported by the school psychologist to have "difficulty with relationship aspects of adjustment."

Seen again at the Clinic on December 6, 1953, the girl was characterized by her mother as follows: "Since you saw her in 1943, Sally has learned to adjust socially. She is now in the eleventh grade. Her records show her depending too much on her memory instead of any power of reasoning." Sally spoke of herself as "a plugger," indicating that she put considerable pressure on herself in order to do well: "Up to last year, the fundamentals of learning have been easy because of my good memory but this year it is the interpretations, and this is difficult for me." Sally had the ambition to go to college but added: "I may be hitching my wagon to a star." About her relationship with schoolmates she said: "The girls are very nice and friendly. There are some points in which I am not close to them. I don't have the interest in boys that most girls of my age have." She expressed concern about her brother who was expelled from school because of drinking and misconduct and had a job at a gasoline station. Sally called him "a strong victim of adolescence—he needs real psychiatric help."

After finishing high school, Sally was successfully enrolled in a woman's college, graduating with a B average. She decided to go into nurses' training and tried to live up to the rules and regulations. Rotation through the different departments, prompted difficulties in adjustment at the beginning of a new service: "Maybe I was anxious to do too well." While on the obstetrical ward,

Sally was asked by the dean to reconsider her plans. Having been told that 20 minutes were the usual time for breastfeeding, she entered the room at the exact moment and took the babies away without saying a word; there were many complaints from the mothers.

Sally readily accepted the suggestion to take up laboratory work and has done well in this field since then. In 1968, the family moved to Chicago and the young woman secured a regular job in one of the hospitals in that city. She is appreciated "because of her excellent facility in chemistry." A psychiatrist consulted in August 1970 writes: "She struggled for a long time to expand her social life . . . . Currently she has been dating a man for the past six months but it is clear that Sally is frightened by any intimacies. She has, with some encouragement, used her interest in music to establish herself in a church-affiliated singing group."

Her father committed suicide in 1969 and her brother is an alcoholic. Sally remains interested and proficient in her work and persistent in efforts to sustain relations with friends and acquaintances. The young woman and her mother remain on good terms and are in contact with each other.

Case 3

Edward F., born October 11, 1939, was first seen on November 15, 1943. His mother said that he was a retarded child who had always appeared very withdrawn:

> He is happy in his own world. He was about 3 years old before he knew members of the family. He has certain stereotypes, has to touch telephone poles, will lay sticks against the pole and walk round and round. He talks better than he understands.

Edward was the younger of two boys and two additional brothers were born later. The father, a lawyer "of worrisome disposition," who was 34 years old at the time of Edward's birth, consulted a psychiatrist in 1939 because of "anxiety about work, fear about making mistakes, panic at night." He had always been "interested in things political, world events, hiking and mountain climbing." The mother, two years younger and also a college graduate, worked as a social worker until marriage at 26 years of age, "always interested in people, fairly well balanced, perhaps extremely logical, always has 4 or 5 reasons for or against." An older sibling was described as healthy and well adjusted.

Edward was an attractive, slender, intelligent-looking boy with vivid dark eyes. Immediately after entering the office, he went after crayons and paper and

241

became absorbed in them. At his mother's insistence, he "read" from a book which he had brought along by repeating remembered passages and interspersing them with neologisms of his own coinage. The boy then tried to jab the point of a pencil into the secretary's leg; when diverted, he attacked a paper bag. He could be engaged in games usually used with very young children.

Edward was born about three weeks before term, weighing 5 pounds and 14 ounces; his "finger nails were not quite developed." He was a planned and wanted child, "never very active." Apathetic as an infant who did not nurse vigorously, Edward did not appear to be aware of his surroundings. The difference from other children was noted when he was 4 months old: "When you picked him up, he relaxed in your arms rather supinely. Almost from the beginning he seems to have had no desire to grow up."

The child sat up at 7 months and walked at 20. "He preferred to crawl even after he learned to walk, had flat feet, wore corrective shoes, and walked like a drunken sailor." Fine muscular coordination developed better than gross motility. Speech development was "slow and unusual." When he finally started to talk, his speech consisted mainly of repetition of what he had heard. Bowel control was acquired at an early age. Wetting by day stopped when he was past the age of three.

When Edward was still an infant, his mother resumed work and he was cared for by the maternal grandmother and a maid, both described as patient with him. When seen at the Clinic, the mother had ceased to work as a result of increasing concern about her son. He was beginning to develop an attachment to her.

At five, Edward was admitted to the Henry Phipps Psychiatric Clinic where a ward had been set up for a few months to study autistic children. He seemed unaware of his environment; however, his later memory of this experience was an unhappy one as he was afraid of the other children.

At six, the boy attended a kindergarten with an understanding teacher who let him participate in group activities or keep him out depending on his readiness. The mother, pleased with his improvement, said that he talked, acted and looked like other children, but appeared different from them in his "limited social ability, restricted interests and peculiar way and rate of learning." In general, he had become "a happy and pleasant child to live with," although he "obviously had a long way to go."

At seven, Edward entered a class for the retarded where he stayed for two years. The family felt that his stay in this class under a sympathetic and interested, although not too well trained, teacher was of incisive importance for Edward's growth. Although at first difficult to control, he made much progress there. When punished by being kept home a day, the child "got the point." The principal agreed to take Edward into the second grade. He had done so well at the end of the year that advancement to fourth grade was recommended. After that accomplishment he was able to keep up with the school work, although his social difficulties continued. An attempt at participation in a scout troop proved too difficult.

Edward had always been musical. At 12 years of age, he took music lessons and seemed to have great facility in composition. The parents were unhappy when he dropped the music at the end of the year, fearing that high school work would require too much. His obsessiveness was not as bad but he continued to show "fixed ideas."

When seen at the Clinic at 13 years, Edward was doing moderately well academically in the eighth grade of a public school. He still suffered from major disabilities in his interpersonal contacts, had an idiosyncratic way of expressing himself and great difficulty in comprehending social situations.

In 1970, the mother wrote that he had gotten along so much better than they had ever expected. Edward finished high school at 19 and wanted to go to college. She attributed this to the pressure he felt to do like the others in the family. Tests were arranged which showed him high on verbal ability and mediocre in performance. It was felt, however, that he could try. Edward went to a state university and took courses in horticulture. He could not master the chemistry, shifted to history and got his B.A. degree at the end of five years. He lived at the dormitory but made no lasting friends.

After graduation, Edward obtained a good horticultural position but he could not make the grade and was asked to leave. This event was very upsetting to him. For the last few years, he has been working at a government agricultural research station in a "blue collar capacity." Edward does not like this too well preferring to associate with "educated people." He has his own apartment and entertains himself with his Hi-fi set. He has bought a car with money that he has saved. He enjoys an active social life, belonging to hiking clubs and he has led hikes. His knowledge of plants and wild life brings him respect. He has begun to date girls. He comes home on weekends when he has time, and he is very welcome.

The mother adds: "We could, of course, write volumes on all the special things we had to do for Edward and with Edward at each stage of his life—but at this time he is completely independent and self-sufficient. I do believe that he enjoys life."

Case 4

Clarence B., born June 15, 1940, was first seen on May 31, 1945. The nursery school that he had attended for two years said of him:

Clarence is an awkward, tall, thin youngster who always seems glad to come to school. His tendency to be quite tense and to repeat certain behavior patterns has been very marked. He remains an individual resisting change and appearing oblivious to his surroundings. His responses have seemed more a matter of personality pattern than a lack of intelligence. He has shown increasing interest in letters and words, the clock and pictures. Clarence rarely comes directly into the school; he had varied from stopping in the hall to look at the clock to listening to the sound of the drinking fountain. Any of these things, once started, persists day after day and week after week. Though he takes no interest in other children, he has shown real excitement over their name tags. When he entered school, he talked little or none. The few things he said, as in naming pictures in a book, were incomprehensible to most of us. Now he speaks distinctly. He repeats questions asked him rather than making a reply.

Pregnancy, birth and motor development were normal. Verbal utterances began at about two years, but were poorly enunciated. There was marked echolalia. "As a baby," the mother recalled, "he did not care much for cuddling." He had "an excellent memory for places, names, happenings, and stories."

A thorough pediatric examination proved Clarence to be in good physical health. In the Binet test, at 6 years, and 4 months, he scored at 5 and 9. He passed the third grade clinical reading test.

Clarence remained at home and went to public school. He was followed regularly by a psychologist who often informed us about developments. The parents, who also kept in touch with us, by 1951 said that he was "making a fair adjustment," that "there are times when he exhibits normal behavior," that "he is relating to people much better." Clarence read a great deal, made some progress in oral work, but did not join in conversations with his classmates. He had gone through a stage of preoccupation with "volcanoes, fires, diseases, sudden death and destruction." At one time, the parents were concerned about strong sibling rivalry.

In July, 1954, after finishing the eighth grade with A's and B's, Clarence spent the summer at the Devereux Camp, where he did well. At the Devereux Schools where he was enrolled, it was noted that he began to show concern about being accepted by his peers. He "made many continuing efforts in social relationships."

Clarence graduated from high school in June, 1958, with excellent marks and superior achievement test scores. After spending the summer with his parents, he was admitted to a college in Illinois, where he received his B.A. degree in 1962. While there, he "socialized" with a girl for a while. Going then to a college in Massachusetts on a scholarship, he felt isolated, and went home to write his thesis. After obtaining his Master's Degree in economics, he studied accounting at his home state university. Clarence got a job with the state planning office and promptly decided to study planning; he did everything required for another Master's Degree except for the thesis.

He might have done well at the job he obtained if it had not been for the fact that he was given a supervisory position. This was too much for him and he was dismissed in October, 1970. For a year he remained idle, for a time having a newspaper route. Finally, he applied for a job more in keeping with his education and is now employed as an accountant, at $7,500 a year.

Clarence gets along well now and has his own apartment. He obsessively tries to make social contacts. "He is awkward socially but can make a superficial adjustment," states a recent report. He senses embarrassing situations to the point of asking: "What am I doing wrong"? Although he dated a girl, she "broke off" after about nine months. Clarence feels that he ought to get married but that he "can't waste money on a girl who isn't serious." He likes driving a car and, as a hobby, collects time tables to maintain his interest in trains.

One sister has a Master's degree in education, the other sister in the history of art. Both are married; one has four children whom Clarence likes to play with; "he gets on the floor and they crawl all over him," the sister says.

Case 5

Henry C., born December 13, 1943, was first seen on May 26, 1947.

> He could not carry on even a simple conversation, a matter of considerable concern to his parents, even though with some coaxing he managed to say a few words. At the same time, the boy could identify every letter of the alphabet and also the punctuation marks. The child had a sizeable repertoire of tunes and exhibited considerable skill with blocks. He handled the Seguin formboard at his age level.

Both parents were college graduates. The father returned from the armed services in April 1947, having been away since Henry was 6 months old. He spoke of himself as a perfectionist ("bugs on keeping things in order"). The mother, who in her earlier years had to struggle with adjustment to her epileptic condition and to her mother's obsessive domination, was extremely tense whenever she picked up the baby for fear of dropping him during convulsion. In fact, she did so on one occasion which, though not injuring the child, increased her anxiety. She left the child alone most of the time, feeling that this was what he liked best.

On the boy's sixth birthday, he was placed by his parents in a foster home where he improved remarkably: "He does beautifully with words now" (March 1949), using good syntax, though occasionally reversing pronouns. In 1950, he was "no problem" in regular kindergarten: "He seems to be happy within himself and is slow in making overtures toward other children." There was a good relationship between Henry's foster parents and his mother. Henry's parents were considering divorce: the father was referred to as "an isolated iceberg."

In 1952, Henry decided to change his name, at first to that of his foster parents; then, retaining his first name, he gave himself a middle name after his patron saint and a last name after a movie actor. Eventually he had his name duly legalized.

When seen at the Clinic in July 1954, Henry related personal interests and incidents in a dramatic fashion but became uncomfortable when others tried to have him elaborate. He was passing into the fifth grade even though his school work was of a marginal quality; "the school recognized his difficulties and has agreed on a policy of promotion." At home, he was preoccupied with death and killing, both in his remarks and in his drawings.

In August 1956, Henry's mother was found dead (the janitor had to break into the apartment) when he and his foster mother went to visit her. The coroner's autopsy reported "natural death" (?). Henry, when informed, "cried a little but it was not difficult to distract him."

While Henry did well in school, at home he was rude and insistent, especially after visiting his father. He spent much of his time writing "horror stories, murder, science fiction." After learning to use the typewriter, "the stories became longer, more vivid, bloodier, and very often did not make much sense."

In the fall of 1958, Henry was entered in a boarding school, which he liked. Spending his weekends with the foster parents, he declined his father's invitations to stay with him.

In our usual efforts to follow the destinies of our patients, we corresponded with the father, the foster parents, and a financial guardian who for a time looked after a small sum left by Henry's mother and who, having moved to India, wrote us from there on October 4, 1971:

> . . . I first saw Henry at 2 or 3 years when my wife and I visited his parents and played bridge in their apartment. He was somewhat like a

wild animal running back and forth across the living room until he became exhausted. The next time I saw him, he was 15 and we had a very interesting conversation. I felt at that particular time that he appeared to be quite normal. His letters also indicated to me that he was being fairly well adjusted. I thought that it was quite remarkable that he was pretty much on his own since then.

We wrote to Henry himself when we learned of his address. Early in January 1972, he sent us a lengthy autobiographic letter; regretfully, we cannot reproduce it word for word but the following is an abstract:

On June 29, 1962, at 19½ years of age, he entered the armed services. Upon completion of basic training, he was assigned to one of the intelligence services, received a top security clearance, took courses until December 6, 1962 (the nature of which he could not disclose because they were of a "highly confidential nature"), and received an honorable discharge on January 18, 1963. Then follows a list of various jobs held in California and later in Pennsylvania, (six altogether) mostly as a "general office worker"; at present he is "chief inventory controller in a Motion Picture Laboratory" where he has received "several healthy pay increases." After drifting around, he feels that "perhaps at last, I have found a place worthy of my talent for settling down in." All six jobs were described in great detail, giving dates, description of responsibilities, names and telephone numbers of supervisors, and reasons for leaving the jobs. Generally speaking, "I have never been dismissed from any place of employment because of any working habits or lack of working habits."

The letter addressed "To Whom It May Concern," starts as follows:

I am writing this resume with the intention of giving any person who would wish it a lucid account of my life, educational and working background, and experiences. I am 6 feet tall, weigh 145 pounds, have medium brown hair and hazel blue eyes. I am in excellent health with no history of any severe illnesses or injuries. I have an automobile and a permanent residence. I am also draft exempt and have no criminal record of any kind.

Elsewhere he writes:

As for my future, I have absolutely no worries whatsoever. I live each day as though it were my last, and let the devil take tomorrow .... I am 28 years old and single (though several girls I know had hoped to change that) with no desire to get tied down for a good long time . . . . I neither smoke nor drink but I do have an uncontrollable urge to gamble. (We all have to have a few bad habits.)

The letter is concluded as follows:

For as long as I live, I shall always remember you, Dr. Kanner, and how you have opened many doors for me. I cannot thank you enough for the limitless kindness you have shown me while rekindling the spark of living within me that had nearly died so very long ago.

Case 6

George W., born February 27, 1944, was first seen on January 11, 1951. His mother complained:

Although he has talked clearly, using big words and sentences since he was 18 months old, he still had never spoken *with* us—that is, carry on a conversation or even answer simple yes and no questions. He lives completely in a world of his own. As an infant he had not smiled like other children. At 2 years, he knew the alphabet and numbers. He never used the first person in speaking.

George was born 5 weeks past term, weighing 8 pounds at birth. He was on a rigid schedule and was awakened for feedings. His first words were spoken at 13 months, he walked alone at 18 months, and bowel control was established at 18 months; bed wetting continued until the age of 6 years. Gross motor development was described as poor and fine motor coordination as good; he could open and close a safety pin and replace the top on a toothpaste tube.

The boy's father, of Spanish (Latin American) descent, was a civil engineer who went into the armed services when George was 6 months old; he was away for about 2 years. On his return, he "had difficulty relating to George" and "kept looking for a physical (glandular) cause of George's problems."

The boy's mother had 3 years of college. "Intellectual pursuits" were important to her and she started George very early with letters and numbers. The case history is full of her expressions of conflicts with her father—fear of his displeasure and resentment of his domination. She blamed herself for anything that went wrong with George, at the same time hoping for some quick, miraculous cure. When the child was about 4 years old, she resorted to drinking for several years until she joined Alcoholics Anonymous.

Because George was not able to get along in kindergarten, he was referred to the Clinic where he developed a tenuous relationship with his therapist. He echoed things he heard, repeated names that came over the hospital's loud speaker, and used many neologisms. Also, he was preoccupied with traffic lights and with elevators.

At the age of 9, George was admitted to a center for emotionally disturbed children where he remained for 6 years. While there, he had many consuming obsessions, mainly focused on mechanical devices (plumbing, lighting), travel, map making, and physical health (he washed many times a day because of his fear of germs). These preoccupations gradually subsided and he became more interested in group activities, regressing occasionally, usually in association with changes in personnel. However, he did fairly well with his school assignments.

At the age of 15, George returned home and entered in public school in a "slow" sixth grade where "with encouragement but not much pressure" he was able to do the work. His teacher reported:

> He conforms to rules and regulations as well as any immature sixth grade child. He plays the violin well, he appears to enjoy the company of his classmates, he is quite friendly and likes to joke. He is particularly fond of poems and plays on words.

George's mother took him out of school when he was in the eleventh grade so that he could concentrate on music. He had played violin in a number of youth orchestras and took courses at a prominent Conservatory. Concerned about not getting a high school diploma, George has, in recent years, spent much of his time subscribing to correspondence courses. He is especially interested in languages, having learned Spanish in school, teaching himself French, and having "a working knowledge" of Italian. At present George is employed as a page in a library and is also in charge of mailing books (mostly to foreign countries).

George lives with his parents. He is helpful with chores at home (to make things easier for his mother who describes him as "dependable") but has no friends and "girls are not interested in him." His major preoccupation now is an overconcern about pleasing people: "He is not relaxed and afraid of doing wrong."

Case 7

Walter P., born June 16, 1944, was first seen on July 8, 1952. He had seemed normal until he was about 3½ years old when his mother noted that his speech was not progressing, he had become unusually quiet (sitting for long periods looking aimlessly around), and finally had just about stopped talking altogether. The child became unduly interested in spinning tops and other toys, was upset when things were moved from their accustomed positions, paid little attention to the people in his environment, and was slow in responding to being called.

Walter's parents gave the impression of being sociable, well-adjusted people. The father had 2 years of college and worked as an ordinance engineer for the federal government. He was able to give more specific and accurate information about the child than his wife. The mother also had 2 years of college and worked in a bank to provide money for the child's care and treatment. Both parents emphasized the harmony of their relationship. A brother, 3 years older than Walter, was getting along well.

Walter was born at term. At 3 weeks, he developed pyloric stenosis which was relieved by an operation from which he recovered uneventfully. There were no feeding problems. The boy began to talk at 2½ years of age and was fully toilet trained by age 3 without any apparent difficulty or conflict.

When seen at the Clinic, Walter was an attractive child who cooperated in a stiff, automatic way. While he did not relate to the examiner, looking vaguely out of the window and responding only to the simplest questions, he immediately placed all the pieces in the Seguin formboard. The boy would respond to "What is your name?," "How old are you?," "Sit in the chair," but would not cooperate in any verbal tests. His behavior was repetitious, obsessive, and withdrawn.

At 9 years, Walter was still obsessive, used little speech but had progressed some in "play school," he had learned to copy and to spell some words, and was very destructive with anything chipped or broken.

At 10, the child's mother reported that he was "progressing well." Walter attended a school for retarded children, was learning to write and to do simple arithmetic, seeming to enjoy it, but reading was causing him some trouble. Also he was playing and talking better with other children and could give simple messages over the telephone (he was able to say what he wanted). The boy had a variety of rituals, first, tapping his chin until it was red, and later, rubbing his eyes. His mother found him a "lovable little boy" who behaved well when they took him out.

Arrangements were made with a psychiatric clinic near his home for follow-up consultations.

In 1971, the mother gave this follow-up report:

> Walter attended a boarding school for exceptional children from 1956 to 1962, coming home on weekends, and then lived with her (his father had died). For 2 years, he attended a day school and then worked for a short time in a sheltered workshop. "Since June 1968, he

has worked at a small restaurant as a dishwasher and bus boy, earning $1.25 an hour. He seems to enjoy his work, has pleased his employers, and has never missed a day. He is a handsome young man, takes complete care of himself and of his room, and is neat and clean at all times. There are no behavior problems. He helps with the housework and takes care of the yard, including complete care of the power mower. His main difficulty always is in communication. What he says, he says well and in a fairly clear manner, but there is no voluntary conversation. Walter talks enough to make his wishes known, will answer the phone and tell me who is calling, but when I am not home, unless I ask him, he will not tell me if someone called.

Case 8

Bernard S., born August 3, 1949, was first seen on June 7, 1952. He was referred by the nursery school which he attended. His teachers reported that he seemed "more alone than most children" and that he was "in the school but not a part of it." The child showed some bizarre behavior and echolalia. He referred to himself in the third person and often had a smile on his face which was unrelated to anything obvious to the onlooker.

Bernard's father was a pharmacist who spent long hours in his drug store. His mother had manic-depressive episodes and had been hospitalized for a few months 9 years before Bernard was born. She did not become pregnant until 14 years after her marriage, which came as a "delightful surprise."

Very soon after Bernard's birth, his mother became ill again and was hospitalized for over a year during which time Bernard was cared for by a nurse in her home. When the mother took him back, Bernard was 15 months old and was walking "but not feeding himself." The mother was a perfectionist, especially about his eating. She continued to have mood swings and was under the care of a psychiatrist.

The parents separated when Bernard was about 2½ years old. Six months later, the mother disappeared with the child to Florida. The father fetched him back, and placed Bernard with a paternal aunt. One of the nursery school teachers who visited at the time, described the boy as relaxed and happy with his aunt: "For the first time, I heard him speak quite volubly." The aunt did not return him to the nursery school as she wanted him to remain at her home "where he could get some much-needed love and attention, so that he could feel someone really cared for him." The parents came back to live together again and took Bernard home. He was reentered in the nursery school at 4 years of age. The boy had a good memory; he knew the names of all the children in the school and noted who was absent before the teacher did. However, he could be brought into group activities for only very brief times. In the neighborhood, he stayed in the house because the children would not play with him and called him "that crazy kid." Their attitude improved when he bribed them with cookies.

The father gave a follow-up report when Bernard was 20 years old:

> He had graduated from high school at 19 and was struggling with junior college in a general course. His marks had been mediocre. He is not the studying type, seeking a job and a simple uncomplicated life. He lost 2 years of school in shifting around. One year he spent in a "progressive" boarding school, but that proved to be "more of a hippie colony" and his work was poor. The mother died while he was there and then he did not want to go back. After the paternal aunt who had cared for him as a small child came to live with them following her husband's death. Bernard showed marked improvement.

The father remarried in 1968 and Bernard got along well with his stepmother. He had had "no real psychiatric treatment."

Bernard is "backward and shy but that is the way he is." He did approach a girl once for a date in a very negative manner. He hates clothes, drives a car, does best if not pressured and helped his father in the drug store (he did not wait on customers but would fill the shelves). His chief interest is the streetcar museum. He is a member of a club that goes there on Sundays, laying track, painting cars, etc. They take trips. He used to like history, is up on world politics, and reads the newspapers.

Case 9

Fred G., born December 11, 1948, was first seen on August 11, 1952. His parents gave a history of difficulties dating from colic for 6 weeks after birth. He was carried around constantly by members of the family; when the colic subsided, he continued to demand attention. A practical nurse handled this by letting him "cry it out." At 3 months, the child was taken to visit his grandmother and placed unceremoniously into her arms on arrival. He reacted with terror, screaming for the 3 weeks, and since then had a great fear of strangers.

> In spite of Fred's ability to go through some of the motions of the Binet test, it was not possible to get his full cooperation. He placed the small formboard figures. When asked to match forms, he named them

first. He ignored people in the room and repeated questions rather than answer them.

Fred was born by Ceasarean section, walked at 14 months, and began to talk at one year. His speech was good and he had a large vocabulary but would not use the first person and repeated a phrase rather than say "Yes." Weaning from the bottle was difficult and slow, and there was also conflict over bowel training.

At home, he was preoccupied with music, being able to recognize records just by looking at them when he was 3 years old. He could identify compositions after hearing them by saying: "That's the Moldau," "That's Beethoven's Fifth," etc. Six months before coming to the Clinic, he had been sent to a nursery school where he was fearful of the children. After his mother stayed with him several days, he calmed down but ignored everyone, refused to participate in any form of group activity, and "was just there." The mother said that "at home there could not be a better child." "He likes to be by himself," she added. He would go into rages over inanimate objects that would not do just as he wished.

The father, who wanted to be a physician, took up a related course of study because family finances did not allow him to go through medical school. After 3 years, he abandoned it for government work involving secret documents and assignments. The mother, a college graduate, had taught school several years and quit a year before Fred's birth. She came from "a family of pushers" and had great intellectual drive. The woman expressed a fear that she might be blamed for the child's difficulties. There seemed to be no particular domestic problems. The home atmosphere was one of emphasis on such cultural pursuits as music and intellectual discussion.

For approximately 2½ years, from 1952 to 1955, Fred regularly attended a day care center for emotionally disturbed children. He formed an attachment to the director and saw her often in the years that followed.

When tested at 16 years, he was found to have a full scale WISC IQ of 118 (verbal 126 and performance 104). His arithmetic score was at the ceiling with quick answers on the tests, and comprehension, similarities and rote memory were rated as being of high average. On the Rorschach, he showed "sharp alterations between impulsivity and repression" and "a struggle between feelings of relationship and isolation."

At 23 years of age, Fred is doing well at a university where he has a B plus average and is gifted in mathematics.

He has adjusted well in college life and his schoolmates respect his academic prowess. The young man has sloughed off his obsessive preoccupations. For instance, he dresses well but is not as compulsive about clothes as he used to be.

Though described as "awkward and intellectual," he tries, at least on the surface, to take part in the concerns which he knows should be those for his age, even "experimenting" once with a double date arrangement (not repeated). Fred drives a car skillfully, with full knowledge of all the parts, and in his spare time has done some composing and built a telescope.

Until his first year in College, Fred had always lived with his parents. After some hesitation, particularly by the father, they supported his decision to move to a dormitory.

DISCUSSION

Now that 29 years have elapsed since the identification of early infantile autism, the children so diagnosed in the first decade of its recognized existence have reached adulthood. Despite considerable mobility of some of the families, it has been possible to learn about the patients' present status. The first of an anticipated series of follow-ups appeared last year as a report of the destinies of the eleven children whose condition had suggested and crystallized the specific syndrome (Kanner, 1943, 1971). Altogether, 96 patients had been designated as autistic before 1953 at our Clinic, the "birthplace" of the syndrome. Of this number we have selected those now capable of functioning in society. Besides the two presented in 1971 (Donald T. and Frederick W.), we have sketched the biographies of nine such persons (one female and eight males), currently ranging in age between 22 and 35 years. The nosological criteria, set down in 1943, had been uniformly applied to all 96 children.

The value of catamnesis has been sensed for quite some time. As far back as the early 1940's, Cottington (1942) compared the results of shock treatment, psychotherapy and socialization of a few psychotic children, none older than 14 years. Lourie, Pacella, and Piotrowski (1943) in a review of 20 children "with schizophrenic-like psychoses," saw three types of "adjustment": (1) Apparently normal (4 cases); (2) fair to borderline (5 cases); and (3) low grade (11 cases). These reports were pioneering innovations at a time when interest was centered mainly on description and speculation about etiology. However, they dealt with categories rather than individuals, whose subsequent fate after childhood or at most the early teens has remained unknown.

Continuous curiosity about the patients' progress has always been one of the primary concerns of our Clinic (Kanner, 1937a, 1937b). Names, symptoms, diagnoses, and any other relevant items were cross-indexed for all. Since, except for our own communications, early infantile autism did not enter the public arena until about 1950, our Clinic saw itself as a quasi ex-officio archive for all that pertained to the syndrome, to be kept in flux and added to as time went on. This gave helpful information for a study (Kanner & Eisenberg, 1955) which comprised children with an average age of 14 years and yielded one finding of potential predictive value:

> The prognosis has shown to vary significantly with the presence of useful speech at the age of 5 years, taken as an index of the severity of autistic isolation.

Many are now in their 20's and 30's; all but two of them were available for "check-ups" in 1971. Their biographic profiles are—and will continue to be—a part of the "archive" and have aided us in picking out those who have gone farthest in terms of social adjustment.

Eleven autistic children (9 in this series plus Donald T. and Frederick W. reported in 1971) have emerged sufficiently to function as adults in varying degrees of nonpsychotic activity. Three have college degrees, three had a junior college education, one is now doing well in college, one graduated from high school, one passed the eleventh grade, one went to a private "boarding school for exceptional children," and one received vocational training in a sheltered workshop.

Their present occupations are bank teller, laboratory technician, duplicating machine operator, accountant, "blue collar job" at an agriculatural research station, general office worker, page in the foreign language section of a library, bus boy in a restaurant, truck loading supervisor, helper in a drug store, and college student. Two (Thomas G. and Henry C.) had enlisted and been accepted by the armed services but were "honorably discharged" within a year.

What distinguishes them from those who, remaining wholly isolated, did not make the linkage with society?

In comparing the two groups, no difference could be found with regard to ethnic origin, family characteristics, or specific intercurrent events. Nor is there anything in the features of physical health that stand out as a contrast, though Thomas G. began to experience convulsions after his twentieth year.[3]

We did, however, find a number of items which were shared by the patients who form the nucleus of this study. They have to do with a variety of maturational and environmental issues and with the patients' type of reactions to the growing awareness of their peculiarities.

---

[3] The onset of epileptic phenomena is not too uncommon in the lives of autistic persons, even when earlier EEG's had shown no abnormalities.

All of them used some speech before the age of 5 years. This in itself cannot be taken as an all-valid prognostic sign because many who had done likewise have failed to reach a similar degree of emergence. What characterizes our group is a steady succession of stages: No initiative or response—immediate parroting—delayed echolalia with pronominal reversals—utterances related to obsessive preoccupations—communicative dialogue with the proper use of personal pronouns and greater flexibility in the use of prepositions.

Not one of them had at any time been subjected to sojourn in a state hospital or institution for the feebleminded. This seems to be significant in view of our experience that such an eventuality has invariably cut short any prospect for improvement (Kanner, 1965). All of our eleven patients here considered have remained at home at least before school age and some quite a few years longer. Three still live with their families, the others—whether in foster homes or boarding schools—had regular contact with their relatives. However, many other autistic children who stayed at home did not advance as those eleven did.

One recurrent theme, though, could be noted as specific for our group in clear contrast with the non-emerging autistic children: a chronicle of gradual changes of self-concept and reactions to them along the road to social adaptation.

In the first few years of life, there was in this respect no difference between any of our 96 patients now over 20 years old. Their isolation with all its corollaries—neither chosen nor imposed from without—was a form of existence which was had, lived, experienced rather than contemplated or reacted to. It was part of an innate illness not perceived as such by the ill child who was contentedly (though pathologically) "adjusted" unless threatened by external interference with the status quo. There was a minimum of centrifugal reaching out and a minimal response to centripetal incursions. As time went on, some of the incursions began to be tolerated in varying degrees. Unless they became too overwhelming and the child was pushed back into self-incapsulation until his status was barely distinguishable from extreme mental retardation, he was making compromises to the extent of verbal interplay, demanding parental assistance with his rituals, falling in line with I-You identification, superficially going through the symbolic acts of shaking hands, hugging and kissing, and generally yielding to the rudiments of domestication. This carried over to nursery school and kindergarten, at least in terms of joining mechanically in routine activities, first on invitation and then more or less spontaneously.

Our eleven children went through the same stages. It was not until the early to middle teens when a remarkable change took place. Unlike most other autistic children, they became uneasily aware of their peculiarities and began to make a conscious effort to do something about them. This effort increased as they grew older. They "knew," for instance, that youngsters were expected to have friends. Realizing their inability to form a genuine buddy-buddy relationship, they—one is almost tempted to say, ingeniously—made use of the gains made by their obsessive preoccupations to open a door for contact.

Thomas G. joined the Boy Scouts and found recognition by teaching astronomy and playing the piano; he also joined a swimming and athletic club. Sally S. utilized her good memory, of which she was fully aware, to merit acceptance in high school and college; when she failed as a student nurse because the maintenance of a genuine relationship with the patients was beyond her capacity, she became a laboratory technician and has made a reputation for "excelling in chemistry." Edward F. enjoys an active social life belonging to hiking clubs, and his knowledge of plants and wild life brings him respect. Clarence B. "obsessively tries to make social contacts; he is awkward socially but can make a superficial adjustment." Henry C. enlisted in the Army, had several well-paying jobs and "has an uncontrollable urge to gamble." George W. is "over-concerned about pleasing people." Walter P. satisfies his social needs as bus boy in a restaurant and "pleases his employers." Bernard S. is a member of a street car museum where he lays tracks, paints cars, and goes on trips. Fred G. is respected by his schoolmates because of his academic prowess.

Again and again we note a felt need to grope for ways to compensate for the lack of inherent sociability. Out of this developed a paradoxical use of the previously self-serving, isolating obsessions which instead come to serve positively as a connecting link with groups of people.

The contacts thus established led to the discovery that the boy-meets-girl issue was paramount in the talks of the companions. Again, there was a vaguely felt obligation to "conform." Those attempts were sporadic and short-lived. The "explanations" offered indicated that there was not too much displeasure with the absence of any real involvement.

Henry C. reported that he was single, that several girls "had hoped to change that" but that he had "no desire to get tied down for a good long time." Thomas G. declared categorically that girls "cost too much money." Clarence B., who "socialized" with a girl for a short time in college, stated that he "ought to get married but can't waste money on a girl who is not serious." Bernard S. was said to have approached a girl once for a date "in a very negative way" (inviting rebuff). Fred G. "experimented" *once* with a double date arrangement (never repeated).

George W. made things easy for himself by deciding a priori that girls were not interested in him. Sally S., the only girl in our group, once asked seriously at 23 years of age what she ought to do if ever she fell in love with someone, an experience she had never had before. She said: "I have never had the interest in boys most girls my age have." At 30 years, she dated a man for a few months but gave this up because she was "frightened by any intimacy."

COMMENT

On the basis of the recorded and discussed observations, the question raised in the title of this paper can be answered with reasonable certainty. Not counting the gifted student of mathematics killed accidentally and the young man whom we have so far lost track after 1962 when he was in college, eleven of the 96 autistic children known to our Clinic since before 1953 are now in their twenties and thirties, mingling, working, and maintaining themselves in society. They have not completely shed the fundamental personality structure of early infantile autism but, with increasing self-assessment in their middle to late teens, they expended considerable effort to fit themselves—dutifully, as it were—to what they came to perceive as commonly expected obligations. They made the compromise of being, yet not appearing, alone and discovered means of interaction by joining groups in which they could make use of their preoccupations, previously immured in self-limited stereotypies, as shared "hobbies" in the company of others. In the club to which they "belonged," they received—and enjoyed—the recognition earned by the detailed knowledge they had stored up in years of obsessive rumination of specific topics (music, mathematics, history, chemistry, astronomy, wild life, foreign languages, etc.). Reward came to them also from their employers who (as confirmed in statements sent to us) remarked on their meticulousness and trustworthiness. Life among people thus lost its former menacing aspects. Nobody has shoved them forcibly through a gate which others had tried to unlock for them; it was *they* who, at first timidly and experimentally, then more resolutely, paved their way to it and walked through. Once inside, they adopted some of the values they found there. Material possession became an object of ambition. Those who are not with their families (eight of the eleven) live by themselves; one (Thomas G.) even owns a house which he bought several years ago. All drive automobiles and there is no record of accidents or traffic violations.

There have been equally duty-bound, though haphazardly pursued attempts to form personal friendships. These were far less successful. Failure apparently was not met with major frustration, self-reproach or accusation of others. There even was a sense of relief in matters of dating; ready rationalizations were: "a waste of money," "cost too much,"; Sally had a dread of "intimacy," Henry did not feel like being tied for a long time. No one in the group has seriously thought of, or is now contemplating, marriage.

This, then, is the profile of eleven autistic children, now adults, whose social adaptation does not run counter to the general run of the populace. It differs essentially from that of at least 83 of the 96 other autistic children in the series. Fascinating as it is, it does not offer a definite clue for the cause of the difference. The presence of speech before the age of 5 years and the fact of being kept out of state institutions are helpful hints but, being shared with some of the non-emerging children, they can only be viewed at best as straws in the wind pointing to prognostic probabilities.

Hence, at least for the time being, there is no alternative to the idea expressed at the close of our 1971 follow-up: "It is well known in medicine that any illness may appear in different degrees of severity, all the way from the so-called *formes frustes* to the most fulminant manifestation. Does this possibly apply also to early infantile autism"?

It must be kept in mind that our "emergers" grew up in the days before the introduction of therapeutic techniques especially intended to remedy the autistic illness, be they based on circumscribed psychotherapeutic, psycho-pharmacological, or behavioristic orientation. Would any of those have in any way altered the outlook for our 96 children? Will any of those increase the ratio of "emergers" in the future? What can we make of the fact, documented in this study, that almost 11 to 12 percent "got there" without any of those techniques? Now that a number of state hospitals have divisions for the personalized care and treatment of children, can we look upon admission of autistic patients to them with better expectations than before? Will the biochemical research now vigorously under way uncover early indications pointing to prognostically reliable assessments of the degree of severity of the autistic illness?

All these are justifiable curiosities with important practical implications. It will take time to satisfy them. Continual follow-up or even better follow-along, will—as we hope that this study does—prove in the long run to be of great importance. Our astute readers have undoubtedly noticed that this paper is being presented with a twofold purpose. One is, of course, patently announced in its title. The other, more implicit aim is an attempt to set up a sample for follow-along and follow-up studies hopefully to be conducted in clinical and research centers as the intervals between childhood and adulthood of autistic patients keep lengthening.

REFERENCES

Cottington, F. Treatment of schizophrenia in childhood. *Nervous Child,* 1942, **1,** 172-187.

Kanner, L. Problem children growing up. *American Journal of Psychiatry,* 1937, **94** 691-699. (a)

Kanner, L. Prognosis in child psychiatry. *Archives of Neurology and Psychiatry,* 1937, **37,** 922-928. (b)

Kanner, L. Autistic disturbances of affective contact. *Nervous Child,* 1943, **2,** 217-250.

Kanner, L. Children in state hospitals. *American Journal of Psychiatry,* 1965, **121,** 925-927.

Kanner, L. Follow-up study of eleven autistic children originally reported in 1943. *Journal of Autism and Childhood Schizophrenia,* 1971, **1,** 119-145.

Kanner, L., & Eisenberg, L. Notes on the follow-up studies of autistic children. In P. H. Hoch and J. Zubin (Eds.), *Psychopathology of childhood.* New York: Grune & Stratton, 1955.

Lourie, R. S., Pacella, B. L., & Piotrowski, Z. A. Studies on the prognosis in schizophrenic-like psychoses in children. *American Journal of Psychiatry,* 1943, **99,** 542-552.

CASE REPORT

THE ELIMINATION OF TANTRUM BEHAVIOR BY EXTINCTION PROCEDURES

CARL D. WILLIAMS

University of Miami

THIS paper reports the successful treatment of tyrant-like tantrum behavior in a male child by the removal of reinforcement. The subject (S) was approximately 21 months old. He had been seriously ill much of the first 18 months of his life. His health then improved considerably, and he gained weight and vigor.

S now demanded the special care and attention that had been given him over the many critical months. He enforced some of his wishes, especially at bedtime, by unleashing tantrum behavior to control the actions of his parents.

The parents and an aunt took turns in putting him to bed both at night and for S's afternoon nap. If the parent left the bedroom after putting S in his bed, S would scream and fuss until the parent returned to the room. As a result, the parent was unable to leave the bedroom until after S went to sleep. If the parent began to read while in the bedroom, S would cry until the reading material was put down. The parents felt that S enjoyed his control over them and that he fought off going to sleep as long as he could. In any event, a parent was spending from one-half to two hours each bedtime just waiting in the bedroom until S went to sleep.

Following medical reassurance regarding S's physical condition, it was decided to remove the reinforcement of this tyrant-like tantrum behavior. Consistent with the learning principle that, in general, behavior that is not reinforced will be extinguished, a parent or the aunt put S to bed in a leisurely and relaxed fashion. After bedtime pleasantries, the parent left the bedroom and closed the door. S screamed and raged, but the parent did not re-enter the room. The duration of screaming and crying was obtained from the time the door was closed.

The results are shown in Fig. 1. It can be seen that S continued screaming for 45 min. the first time he was put to bed in the first extinction series. S did not cry at all the second time he was put to bed. This is perhaps attributable to his fatigue from the crying of Occasion 1. By the tenth occasion, S no longer whimpered, fussed, or cried when the parent left the room. Rather, he smiled as they left. The parents felt that he made happy sounds until he dropped off to sleep.

About a week later, S screamed and fussed after the aunt put him to bed, probably reflecting spontaneous recovery of the tantrum behavior. The aunt then reinforced the tantrum behavior by returning to S's bedroom and remaining there until he went to sleep. It was then necessary to extinguish this behavior a second time.

Figure 1 shows that the second extinction curve is similar to the first. Both curves are generally similar to extinction curves obtained with sub-

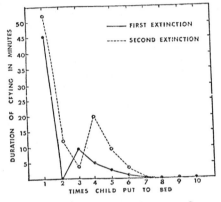

FIG. 1. LENGTH OF CRYING IN TWO EXTINCTION SERIES AS A FUNCTION OF SUCCESSIVE OCCASIONS OF BEING PUT TO BED

human subjects. The second extinction series reached zero by the ninth occasion. No further tantrums at bedtime were reported during the next two years.

It should be emphasized that the treatment in this case did not involve aversive punishment. All that was done was to remove the reinforcement. Extinction of the tyrant-like tantrum behavior then occurred.

No unfortunate side- or aftereffects of this treatment were observed. At three and three-quarters years of age, S appeared to be a friendly, expressive, outgoing child.

JOURNAL OF ABNORMAL AND SOCIAL PSYCHOLOGY, 1959, Vol. 59, p. 269.

An Experimental Approach to the Psychopathology
Of Childhood: Encopresis *

By E. J. Anthony +

There is an aphorism of Nietzche's which says, somewhat categorically,
that all prejudice can be traced back ultimately to the intestines. This statement, made in his autobiography, was clearly not intended for scientific interpretation. Nevertheless, taken as a profound insight into certain fundamental
causal connexions, it does appear to have a bearing on some present-day
beliefs in child psychology. If by 'tracing back' is implied a genetic continuity,
then this suggested association between permanent attitudes and intestinal
function can be seen as a special instance of the so-called 'Jesuitical hypothesis'
which postulates that the decisive experiences for the formation of personality
are all transacted during the first five years of life within the orbit of the
nursery world.

It is during this period that the workings of the bowel and bladder are said
to be invested with strong ideas of goodness and badness constituting a
system of 'sphincter morality'. Attitudes, such as disgust, ensuing from this
system then become inseparably linked with the alimentary tract, and are
localized, in common speech, somewhere along its course.

That, briefly, is the theme of this study. It sets out to investigate the
alleged causal relationships between bowel training, bowel functioning and the
presence of certain subsequent negative attitudes. It could therefore be quite
aptly sub-titled: An inquiry into the origins of bowel prejudice.

Problems of causality

There are many intrinsic difficulties about establishing causal connexions
in the field of the behavioural sciences, chiefly because of the longer time
intervals involved and the diffuseness and complexity of the antecedent conditions.
The problem is made no easier by the fact that the scientific worker, in common
with the unsophisticated adult and the 'prelogical' child, often seems to share in
the general human tendency to assume that the repeated juxtaposition of events
implies some form of causal relationship, or when a victim of the 'genetic
fallacy', that what comes after is necessarily associated causally with what has
gone before. He may even be misguided enough to believe that the finding of
a correlation between his two measures indicates the existence and direction
of a causal linkage.

* Based on a paper read to the Medical Section of the British Psychological
Society, on 13 April 1957.
+ Senior Lecturer in Child Psychiatry, Institute of Psychiatry, London;
Lecturer in Family Relations, London School of Economics; Consultant Physician,
Maudsley and Bethlem Royal Hospitals, London.
BRITISH JOURNAL OF MEDICAL PSYCHOLOGY, 1957, Vol. 30., pp. 146-175.

The nature of such presumed relationships also has some influence upon the judgement. Different sequences impose different degrees of taxation on our credulity. When two events are similar in kind and when one follows the other immediately in time, the case is much stronger than when there is a dissimilarity or discontinuity of experience. For example, it could be claimed, with some justification, that toilet training is a major determinant in producing a toilet-trained child. If we go a step further, we are still likely to obtain some degree of acceptance of the statement that an abnormal mode of training may, in a certain number of cases, lead to an abnormal toilet performance. When, however, the time intervals are lengthened or the subsequent event is a special attitude or 'character trait', the causal argument becomes less convincing and requires much more in the way of proof to sustain it. All these sequences may be thought of as examples of 'natural experiments'. A greater difficulty arises when a special type of experimental reaction is reported to follow a special mode of child-rearing. The experimental situation, characterized as much by its artificiality as by its rigid restrictions of time, place and purpose, exemplifies an extreme degree of dissimilarity and discontinuity of experience, and no correlational technique is sufficient in itself to bridge the causal gap between it and the original 'natural' biosocial situation.

Table 1. Some possible causal relationships in toilet training

Antecedent variables	Intermediate variables	Consequent variables
Training attitudes and behaviour of parents	Learning	Normal toilet functioning (with respect to time,
(1) The potting couple (mutuality, cue awareness)	Conditioning	place and posture)
	Imitating	Abnormal toilet functioning (encopresis,
	Introjecting	retention)
(2) Pressures used (Huschka's criteria)	Incorporating	Abnormal toilet attitudes to faeces and function
(3) Levels of aspiration		(1) Animistic attitudes towards faeces (toilet phobias)
Effects on the potting couple of:		(2) Presence or absence of shame
(1) Primitive conditions		(3) Reaction of disgust (paradoxical behaviour)
(2) Class factors		
(3) Maternal psychopathology		(4) Defiance (active or passive) prodomal syndrome, 'The Battle of the Bowel'
(4) Paternal attitudes		
(5) Traumata (physical and psychological)		(5) Anal character traits
Consistency of training. Interrelation of training systems		(6) Compulsiveness and ritualism

On the antecedent side, one can postulate a complex of child-rearing determinants of varying power and constancy. From these must be excluded the host of precipitating factors that are so readily credited with a primary causal significance but do no more than 'trigger off' the symptom. During the pilot phase of this project, when the focus was on the 'encopretic event' itself and the precipitating affect in each instance, it was only after prolonged searching had proved fruitless that it became apparent that the symptom was, in general, no more than an affectless stereotyped activity, and that the well-springs of hostile and erotic feeling from which they presumably sprang originally, no longer flowed into every act of defaecation. The abnormal toilet functioning eventually becomes as automatic as its normal counterpart. It was therefore decided to abandon this aspect of the investigation in favour of the more enduring factors listed on a hypothetical causal table (Table 1). The schema was found helpful in the analysis of each new case.

For both the precipitating and predisposing factors, the situational span seemed wider than presumed under the traumatic hypothesis as it was first formulated. The precipitating event is more frequently a 'concatenation of events'-- for example, the coincidence of the birth of a sibling, with the beginning of school and the onset of some minor illness; and the predisposing factor, often disguised as a brief traumatic incident, is shown on further analysis to constitute a 'traumatic stage' covering a period of years, so that an entire phase of rigorous toilet training may be telescoped into the remembered experience of a single enema. This is well illustrated by the case of a boy whose mother was excessively attached to the maternal grandfather and had little time for her husband and child, although she had been very solicitous during his babyhood. In the same month the grandfather had a stroke and became incontinent, the mother had a baby who was incontinent, and the little boy became encopretic. Throughout his training period he had been tied to the pot and left for hours 'until he performed'. In most of my cases, it was not at all difficult to isolate some complex of factors. The constant background, however, to these many and varied events was the abnormal training techniques used by the mother, and this ultimately became the main subject for investigation on the antecedent side.

On the consequent side, in addition to the bowel dysfunction as the outward and principal sign of failure, there occur attitudes of shame, disgust and rebelliousness. Between the antecedent and consequent variables lies an area filled by mysterious intervening variables about which there has always been, and always will be, much speculation. They form an integral part of this chain, whether causal or merely logical, and have been given both physiological and psychological connotations. When not considered as mathematical equations, they appear to have something to do with the internalization of the antecedent factors and are variously spoken of in terms of learning, conditioning, imitating, introjecting, incorporating, identifying, etc. depending upon one's psychological persuasion. I intend to leave this area severely alone.

The Antecedent Variables

The potting couple

The investigation of the antecedent variables has entailed a search for some measurable indices of maternal toilet-training behaviour. Before dealing with them I would like to say something about the less measurable, but no less important, training circumstances. In the first place, I should like to call attention to the mother-child training relationship, which I shall refer to as 'the potting couple', thus relating it to the other 'coupling' situations of childhood. It is a close mutual relationship in which both mother and child must play their parts co-operatively if the result is to be a satisfying one. In the so-called 'nursing couple', a satisfying flow of milk into the mouth of the child is evidence of a good breast relationship; the mother enjoys giving and the child receiving. In the 'potting couple', the situation is again reciprocal but the direction is reversed. It is the child who is now the main giver, and it is the mother who receives. There is the passage of faeces from the child into the mother's pot; but it still requires a good deal of give and take on both sides. Each sacrifices something for the other, and when the final bodily product reaches its proper receptacle there should normally be a feeling of gain rather than of loss. The mother loses her milk but gains a satisfied child; the child loses his faeces but gains an approving mother. He can bear to part with his product because, under normal circumstances, he has not invested them with exaggerated positive or negative feelings that may make him either want to keep them or get rid of them in a hurry.

The system of cues

The potting situation, like every other early coupling situation, is full of an unspoken language in which a system of minimal cues plays its part. The mother requires to learn the natural rhythms of her child, the rate at which food moves along his alimentary tract, the filling and emptying capacities of his visceral organs and the sensitivities of the thresholds concerned in giving signals that herald a need. The average mother learns this language without much difficulty, but in my series I found a sore deficiency in this respect.

In the normal training situation, the mother's prompt response to the child's physiological cues and her own communications during the process gradually make the child aware of his own cues, so that he is able, eventually, to take over mother's role in the potting situation and thereby become autonomous. In my sample there were two sorts of deviation from the normal. There were mothers who hopelessly muffed all the cues so that the child's learning of them appeared to become deficient. He was spoken of as passing his mothers without being aware of it. Then there were mothers who anxiously misinterpreted every physiological cue of the child, responding to each and every crisis with the production of the pot. In time, the child appeared to become hyper-sensitive to this association and would run frequently to the toilet under the merest pretext, until every disturbing situation had this effect. In one case, every time his mother got cross with a small encopretic boy he automatically pulled down his trousers. For him it seemed to be the answer to everything.

Maternal psychopathology

Another large immeasurable factor is the maternal psychopathology, especially when it is provoked by symptomatic behaviour on the part of the child. Encopresis is one of the least acceptable symptoms of childhood and seems to engender a considerable amount of hostility from the environment. No contemporary community as yet makes allowances for unconscious motivation and, therefore, once the doctor has pronounced his verdict of 'no organic cause', environmental tolerance rapidly subsides, and punitive and suppressive measures come to the forefront. I always feel that there is a special type of hatred reserved for the encopretic child which the enuretic child rarely experiences. There are systematic cruelties practised on these children which would be unbelievable in any other context; and the intensity of feeling passes from generation to generation without abatement. A little while ago a mother broke both arms of her little boy after an 'encopretic' event. (I put encopretic in inverted commas as he was only 2 1/2 years old--I have had several children referred to me for soiling under the age of 2 1/2.) She was imprisoned and the maternal grandmother took the child into her home and then promptly brought him up to the clinic, refusing to have him back until he was clean. The daughter had apparently hidden this 'terrible' fact from her. What she said to me was: 'when she hurt him I was glad she was going to be punished; but now I have found out why she did it I think they were wrong to put her away'. With this intensity of feeling involved, it would not be surprising if the effects were intense and long-lasting.

The child's task

The process of toileting is a good example of learning in the immature organism under conditions of stress. So far, we have been considering some pathologically induced stresses, but there are inherent difficulties in the situation that belong to the act and the culture irrespective of any traumatizing interference on the mother's part.

Every infant starts life with an innate physiological tendency to empty his hollow organs when they have reached a critical point of fulness. Later, he comes to regard the extruded contents with interest and even pleasure. 'The morning will arrive in every nursery when the astonished parents will observe their beloved child smearing faeces over his person, his hair, and his immediate environment, with gurgling abandon...'(Dollard & Miller, 1950).

Within a comparatively short space of time, however, the toddler must learn under pain of losing love, 'to attach anxiety to all the cues produced by excretory materials--to their sight, smell and touch...to deposit faeces and urine only in a prescribed and secret place and to clean its body. It must later learn to suppress unnecessary verbal reference to these matters...'(Dollard & Miller, 1950).

266

From the child's eye view, the toilet ritual, as practised by the adults of our compulsive communities, must sometimes appear as an exacting and complex ordeal far removed from the simple evacuations into the nursery pot. It is his business, with maternal prompting, to become aware of defaecation cues in time, to stop his play in response to this, to suppress the desire for immediate excretion to search for and find an appropriate place for the purpose, to ensure adequate privacy for himself, to unfasten his clothes, to establish himself securely on the toilet seat (no mean achievement for slender buttocks on some ancient structures), to recognize an end-point to the proceedings, to cleanse himself satisfactorily, to flush the toilet to refasten his clothes, to unbolt the door and emerge successfully to resume his interrupted play at the point where he left off.

He is often expected to learn all this at an age when his neuro-physiological apparatus is immature and he has to do without the help of words. It does seem to be the deliberate cultural intention to invest the whole process with sufficient anxiety to ensure its life-long maintenance. But what is learnt under stress may be unlearnt under stress, depending on the amount of stress undergone in the two situations.

Among the many factors that may interfere with successful learning are the level of intelligence, the presence of emotional disturbances, the occurrence of other and even unrelated traumatic experiences, the frequent shifting of environment during the training period and the incidence of frank gastro-intestinal illnesses, especially those involving diarrhoea.

Vulnerable periods during training

As far as the available evidence goes, the cortical centres governing elimination do not begin to function before the age of six months, so that, as a general rule, voluntary control is not possible before that time (McLellan, 1940). McGraw set out, in a co-twin study, to show that the sequential changes observed in the gradual achievement of bladder control tended to reflect the maturation of the neural organization. The control of bowel function usually takes place earlier, consolidates sooner and establishes itself more firmly. Nevertheless, its general pattern of development is not very different, and on the basis of McGraw's findings (McGraw, 1940) and my own data, it has been possible to construct a paradigm of a learning curve for bowel performance (Fig. 1).

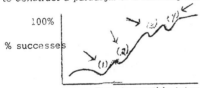

Fig. 1. Paradigm of training sequence (after McGraw). (1) First regressive phase. (2) Second regressive phase. (3) Third regressive phase. (4) Fourth regressive phase.

As with bladder training, there are four recognizable phases, each associated with a transitional episode of regression. In the first phase, potting successes can be attributed to a process of reflex conditioning. With the development of the cortex and its increasing participation in the control of bodily functions, this mechanism diminishes in sensitivity, and the infant, as it were, falls between two stool-controlling mechanisms. Following this, there is a sharp rise marking the beginnings of voluntary control when evacuations will occur into a particular pot. The capacity to undertake more complex cortical associations soon makes the child able to discriminate and generalize, so he begins to make use of a wider range of toilet facilities. Again, in the transition from the particular to the general, a mild relapse in function may occur. Before the child takes over the responsibility from the mother of demanding his pot, a period of indecision may ensue during which neither mother nor child can be said to be firmly in charge of the situation. At this point, a third regressive phase may intervene. Occasionally one may see the fourth type of regression described by McGraw, although it is much less likely to take place during the development of bowel control. The pre-school child is notoriously liable to 'accidents', and this has been ascribed to its engagement in complex mental activities that have yet to be integrated with the cortical functions controlling elimination. These transient declensions represent vulnerable periods during training when future enuretic and encopretic children are liable to be sensitized or launched into being. It is at these phases, too, that a child may first be made conscious of failure and mother's disappointment. They are invariably misinterpreted and mishandled by mothers belonging to the two extreme groups. The high-pressure ones regard them as a challenge and intensify their efforts. For them the demands of the training system are absolute and make no allowance for idiosyncracies of this sort. Their devotion to artificial norms leads them to disregard individual variations in the rate and rhythm of development. The low-pressure mothers, on the other hand, are discouraged by the child's inconsistency and tend to become more inconsistent in their own management. Since they have never been very consistent trainers, these periods may mark the beginning of complete bowel and bladder neglect. The results of over-training and under-training seem to be equally detrimental.

Maternal consistency

This study was begun with preconceptions in favour of consistent maternal practice in child-rearing. It was felt that rigidity and flexibility were responses of the personality and, as such, would not vary with the situation. I was obliged to relinquish this belief in the face of much evidence to the contrary. For example, one mother systematically overfed her child and spoke in glowing terms of his gluttony, whilst, at the same time, she oppressed and assailed his nether end with a punitive intensity matched only by the strength of his opposition. I often felt that she tried to get as much out of him at one end as she put in at the other, and only in this respect could she be called consistent. This finding is supported by both anthropological and class studies. According to Whiting & Child (1953) the intercorrelations between any one system of child-rearing and another are such that no consistency of practice, in either indulgence or severity, can be claimed. They conclude that training methods do not grow out of cultural attitudes towards children so as to produce general laxity or strictness. They appear, instead, to originate in antecedents specific to each system of behaviour. W. Davis (1946) found similar evidence of inconsistency in his social class studies. Negro middle-class mothers, for example, are lax feeders but rigid potters. Nor is there much consistency between the practice of one generation and the next, however powerful the influence of grandmothers on mothers seems to be in any individual case. Child-rearing attitudes are particularly susceptible to the oscillations of fashion. Comparing Klatskin's work (1952) with that of Davis, less than a decade earlier with respect to one criterion of coercive training--onset of potting before six months--we find that Davis has a figure of 68% to put against Klatskin's 6%, suggesting almost a Copernican revolution in the realm of child care. Most authors report a trend towards greater leniency in all areas, but despite this, 'pathological' trainers continue to attend the clinics in great numbers with their disturbed children as if they were impervious to this general influence.

Criteria for Training Pressures

The search for a measurable index on the antecedent side led inevitably to a consideration of the criteria elaborated by Huschka some fifteen years ago (Huschka, 1942) for the assessment of training pressures and adapted by me for use in the present investigation. The criteria were based on times of onset and

Table 2. The pressure of training (based on Huschka's criteria)

High Pressure or Coercive

Onset under 8 months
Completed under 18 months
Enforced by physical coercion (rigid, frequent and protracted potting, beatings, use of suppositories, purgatives, enemata)
Enforced by psychological coercion (threats, withdrawal of love, inculcation of shame, aversion, fear and guilt)

Normal Pressure

Onset between 8 months and 23 months
Completion between 18 months and 30 months
Use of co-operative techniques

Low Pressure or Pathological Deferment

Onset after 24 months
Inconsistent or neglectful techniques

269

completion of training and on the use made of physical and psychological coercion (Table 2).

Toilet inquiries of this detailed nature are not easy to conduct, especially when one is dealing with sensitive subjects. As Huschka points out, these mothers are prone to forget such data or else refashion them in keeping with their current philosophy of child-rearing. The figures they give, however, whether false or true, do seem to reflect their general tendencies in this matter, and can be interpreted as such. I have used them only in conjunction with other information obtained in the course of a lengthy fact-finding interview. The final assessment of high, average or low pressure is founded on a 'global' appreciation of the several factors involved. The ratings of two judges computing separately, correlated satisfactorily (+0.83) for the purpose of the investigation.

These training pressures have a long history and are rooted in the deeper psychopathology of the mother. There is, however, one factor that has an important bearing on the amount of coercion used on different children in the same family, and the tendency of a particular child to succumb; this is the response of the mother to success or failure in training.

Maternal 'levels of aspiration' in training

Huschka (1942) has remarked that 'competition among mothers seems to be one factor behind the frequent employment of heroic measures' in toilet training. This seems to be a cultural variant of one of the major themes in modern urban and suburban life--'keeping up with the Jones's'. It brings in a further factor in stepping up the pressure on the modern Western child and leads us to a more detailed inquiry into the sources of maternal potting aspirations.

This 'aspirant' pressure is assessed in data furnished by the mothers themselves, about which we have already made certain provisos. Only mothers giving 'confident' information repeated unchanged on a second occasion and judged to be fairly reliable were included. Only mothers with two children, the younger being the encopretic one, qualified for the analysis. Consequently, although the cases were drawn from a larger sample than the experimental one, the numbers did not exceed thirty, fifteen in the high-pressure group being compared with fifteen in the low-pressure group.

In the course of a general interview, freely conducted, the subjects were asked, but not consecutively, a series of prepared questions, viz: At what age was your first baby clean and dry? Was your second one later or earlier? What did you expect with the first? And with the second--did you think you would do as well, better, or worse? Did you mind how the training went? If you had another baby what do you think would happen? Does this business of toilet training bother you or not? How did your mother get on with her training schedules? Did you copy her ways? Were your results as good as hers, better, or worse? From where did you get your information about this?

270

The original aspiration studies carried out by Lewin (Lewin et al. 1944) took place under time-limited laboratory conditions and dealt with cognitive probability judgements. These were thought to be influenced both by the avoidance of failure and the search for success. The small aspiration study, here described, was based on 'natural' experiments taking place over protracted periods of time. The first two aspirations were retrospective estimates, and therefore prone to falsification. The last aspiration, however, was forward-looking to the training of the unborn baby. In addition, these expectations, unlike Lewin's, were rooted in deep and emotionally charged experience. Some of the mothers were much involved in their 'experiments' and highly motivated to bring them to a successful conclusion; others apparently lacked all drive in this direction, appearing to be motiveless to the point of neglect.

The results are here represented diagrammatically and not in the usual terms of difference between predicted and past scores (Fig. 2).

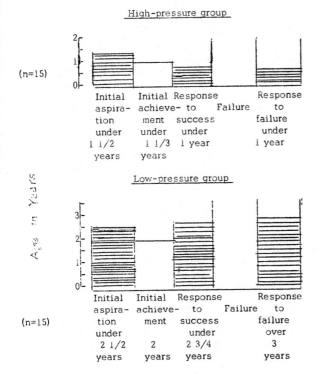

Fig. 2. Levels of aspiration and achievement in relation to toilet training.

It will be observed that the high-pressure mothers show a high initial aspiration, and that their achievements in training are even better than they themselves would have predicted. As might have been anticipated from Lewin's work, this has the effect of raising their aspirations for the next child. Failure, as judged by encopresis, leaves their level of aspiration unaffected, and in a few cases even brings about a further rise.

The low-pressure mothers start with low initial aspirations, but, even so, fall short in their first achievements. This has the effect of lowering their standards still further. The tendency to relax the pressures on subsequent children has been also observed with normal mothers of normal children. The response of the low-pressure group to failure, again as judged by encopresis, is a continued lowering of the level of aspiration, despite the fact that their regime already indicated a pathological deferment of training.

At first sight, one of these tentative findings--the maintenance or even rise of aspiration level following failure--seemed to conflict with the laboratory response, although in one particular study (Sears, 1941) child subjects responded to failure by developing 'unrealistically' high levels of aspiration. On further investigation, however, an explanation for this apparent anomaly became evident. The high-pressure mothers emerged as a group whose children generally began their soiling later on in childhood after a varying period of continence. In point of time, these children were successfully trained at a very early age, so that the mothers were, in fact reacting to the success of their training and not to the subsequent failure of the child to maintain it. For this breakdown, they unanimously blamed the soiler. He had undone their good work; he was 'lazy', 'rebellious', 'playing up', etc.

The low-aspiration group are the mothers usually of life-long encopretics, so that their failure stems directly from the period of training, and is either attributed to it or projected on to some sordid set of circumstances. It was due, they said, to 'not having the time because of work'; to 'the doodle-bugs that flew over his head whilst he "sat"--enough to upset anyone's stomach it was'; or to the absence of any proper 'facilities', etc.

The two situations of failure thus turn out to be not at all comparable. When this is recognized, the pattern of response to success and failure corresponds more closely to the laboratory model, suggesting that, at least in this case, the two situations were not antipodal. This had a supportive bearing on my intention to relate the early training procedures to more frankly experimental reactions. Whilst allowing that the two situations differed in many essentials, it seemed to me possible to exaggerate the distortions and artificialities of the contrived experiment, especially when it was carefully designed to simulate a 'miniature life situation'.

The second important finding had a bearing on so-called 'reference groups'--the social groups from whom the mother derived her 'frame of reference'. An analysis of the questionnaire data revealed two components to the 'frame'--one, that was superficial and fairly plastic, was constituted from such sources as clinics, neighbours, books, magazines, and so on; the other, deeply rooted and inflexible, had its source in the maternal grandmother and was transmitted, almost unchanged, to the mother. Sometimes the two components were in opposition, putting the mother into a state of conflict. 'When I do something new with the children, which I know mother wouldn't like, I feel very guilty. Something always seems to go wrong with it and then I go back to her way. Her way always seems to be right. I sometimes feel it's no use listening to what other people say.'

Previous research on aspiration levels had considered only the determinants resulting from individual experiences of success and failure. In their study, Chapman & Volkmann (1939) showed to what extent 'reference groups' could influence the judgement. There is no doubt that even the deep unconscious components of the frames of reference may be broken into and altered by changes in the whole climate of opinion affecting a generation. According to Chapman & Volkmann, a change in aspiration level induced by a change in the frame of reference may have 'enormous social consequences'. 'The new judgement may serve as a catalyst for major social changes in which whole groups abruptly revise their ambitions and perhaps their status.' In the context of prophylaxis, it is worth bearing this in mind.

Pressures on the primitive child

An important question, very relevant to the pressures of training, is this: Do the two types of mothers that we have so far been describing represent pathological entities or are they merely extremes of a normal cultural distribution? Have they a universal existence or are they by-products of Western life? One approach to answering this would be by an examination of the incidence, if any, in primitive societies. The anal sphincters are present in all cultures, and it is the business of mothers everywhere to give these small circular muscles a social consciousness and responsiveness. As Erikson puts it (1950): 'The sphincters, as part of the voluntary muscle system, can become the dramatic place where holding and letting go is emphasized to a degree dependent on how much the culture wants to emphasise it, and how much emphasis the individual can tolerate.' What ensues is a compromise between the individual and the cultural demand, the latter represented by the mother or her surrogate. Inasmuch as the child becomes capable of holding on to or of letting go his faeces and associated feelings at will by that amount should he develop a sense of autonomy and self-government.

The transition from maternal control to self-control of the sphincters is an important achievement in the development of the ego. Where such control remains defective or dependent on the mother's activity, the child's personality will appear unorganized and amorphous and his behaviour uncontrolled and uncontrollable. The over-trained child, on the other hand, whose sphincter later escapes from the iron control and goes its own wayward way, will show signs of over-controlled behaviour and an ego which is prematurely structured and rigid.

In general, it may be said that the mother's training behaviour, under primitive homogeneous conditions, fairly accurately reflects the accepted cultural practice, so much so that Kardiner has based his argument for the existence of a basic type of personality on the uniform conformity to primary institutions (Kardiner, 1939).

More recently, Whiting & Child (1953) have carried out a cross-cultural study of training practices in a world-wide sample of some seventy-five societies. From their data, I have extracted information on three societies in which the training pressures of the mother have been rated as severe, moderate and mild. For comparison, an American mother, according to these ratings would fall into the severe group, and I should imagine that the same applies to English culture which has also been stigmatized as 'anal'. A low rating in the Anglo-American cultural milieu would be a more pathological phenomenon than a high one. This is reflected in parental attitudes as witnessed in the clinic. The coercive ones, being in conformity with the larger group are self-righteous and assured whereas the laissez-faire types seem conscious of being out of step with their environment and are socially anxious.

In a lax primitive culture the children first learn not to defaecate near the hammocks, and are led by the mother farther and farther away from them so that by the age of 3 they are doing it outside the house and later still outside the compound; they are not held responsible for their defaecation until 6. The child passes from 'an indulgent and free excretory practice' to the culturally acceptable one, literally by a series of steps. Encopresis, in this type of culture if it occurred at all, could only be judged in terms of distance! Under such a regime training is so easy that it never becomes a conscious problem. The natives are puzzled by questions on toilet training put to them by field workers and can only reply 'Why, you just tell the child what to do and he does it' (Whiting & Child, 1953). It is as simple as that.

It seems, therefore, that our high- and low-pressure mothers can be equated with 'normal' ethnological types. The problem set by such data is as follows why do the same training techniques produce in one culture gross disturbances of functions and attitudes, whereas in another, no problem seems to exist? I can only hazard a guess that it may have something to do with uniform and accepted modes of behaviour in a homogeneous culture and with the amount of suppression of spontaneous feelings but there is clearly more to it than that.

The primitive information is given in Table 3.

In their work, Whiting & Child make use of the Freudian concept of fixation, postulating two basic types--positive and negative--the former resulting from a high degree of initial satisfaction and the latter initial frustration and punishment. Individuals with a positive fixation derive greater than normal pleasure from excretion and excretory products, whereas negatively fixated individuals show an exaggerated inhibition about these matters. According to the authors, negative fixation is stronger in establishing life-long personality traits that are less likely to be unlearned and replaced by new habits. They consider that their findings offer good support for the existence of these two fixation types. As I shall shortly show, these types are also in evidence in our experimental sample.

Table 3. Primitive data on toilet training*

	Coercive	Co-operative	Neglectful
(1) Type of training	Coercive	Co-operative	Neglectful
(2) Society	The Tanala	The Navaho	The Siriono
(3) Whiting & Child rating of training+	16	11	6
(4) Initial excretory indulgence	16	13	3
(5) Age of onset	2-3 months	About 2 years	Deferred until walking-talking stage
(6) Level of aspiration	Completion by 6 months	Between 2 and 3 years	Full defaecation responsibility not earlier than 6 years
(7) Punishment	Severely physical	'Teasing'	Little or none
(8) Inculcated disgust	Highly exaggerated	Mild	Almost absent
(9) Compulsiveness and ritualism	High	Moderate	Low
(10) Fixation type	Negative	? Some intermediate form	Positive
(11) Socialization	Early and severe	Moderate	Late and mild

* By socialization anxiety is meant the type of anxiety that develops with the imposition of inhibitory control based on punishment.
+ Rating given by Whiting & Child in their study of 20 societies.

The Consequent Variables

We have now arrived on the other side of my hypothetical causal table. I shall deal in turn with the resulting disturbances of bowel function, the disturbances of attitude and feeling, and the measurable disturbances indicated by experimental responses.

The prodromal syndrome

In many of my cases, the fully developed soiling syndrome was frequently heralded by precursory symptoms at some time during the period of 18 months to 3 years. These generally took the form of 'oppositional' behaviour--food refusals, resistances to going to sleep--which could be regarded as an amplification of the normally occurring phase of the temper tantrum. This global negativism led eventually to one of three outcomes--a shaky continence liable to break down under even minimal stress after a varying period of time; persistent soiling, or chronic

275

retention going on to 'overflow'.

Definition of a 'new' symptom

The symptom known as encopresis has a comparatively short history. It was first described thirty years ago by Weissenberg (1926) although cases of psychogenic soiling had been recognized before that (Fowler, 1882). As is usual with symptoms, once carefully defined, it was more frequently diagnosed. But this factor alone would not account for the larger numbers seen more recently in all clinics. It is possible that this increase is a false one and related to increased referrals from paediatricians. The instrumentalists of the back-passage had been accustomed to wash out the colon religiously, the rationale of which it was difficult to understand. It was like Mrs. Partington attempting to sweep out the Atlantic Ocean with her broom, which makes one inclined to think that it is a policy of despair that now sends us these children in greater numbers. It is, of course, equally possible that the increase is genuine and originates from some radical cultural shift in child-rearing methods. As previously stated, recent work would suggest that such a shift has in fact occurred. My own numbers do not represent in any way a normal intake. When I first broadcast my research intentions, the clinic trickle was rapidly converted into an appreciable stream as referring agencies rushed to rid themselves of their most unpopular customers. Clinicians on the whole, perhaps out of disgust, prefer neither to treat them nor to write about them. The literature as compared with enuresis is, surprisingly scanty, and what there is seems superficial, as if the children had been observed from a respectable distance.

For the purposes of this research, I have demanded incontrovertible evidence of the regular passage of a formed motion of normal or near-normal consistency (defined in the American literature, I am sorry to say for those who like them, as having the consistency of ripe bananas)into the clothes, bedclothes, or any receptacle not intended for the purpose. Defaecation, however successfully, into cupboards, fireplaces, the inside of pianos (one case) would, therefore, be included in this investigation as encopresis.

Clinical consideration and classifications

Although at first regarded as a monosymptomatic condition, encopresis is now recognized as a syndrome, in which the soiling acts as a nucleus around which there clusters a constellation of ancillary and related symptoms. As the child grows older, there is a tendency for these to disappear, and for the nucleus to remain tightly encapsulated for a while before its final disappearance during puberty.

Altogether about 100 cases have passed through the research clinic, of which seventy-six were set aside for the full investigation. In this experimental group, there were only thirteen girls giving a sex ratio of about 6.1 which is in excess of the usual clinic ratio. The ages ranged from 4 to 15. Three criteria were made use of in classifying the cases:

(1) The continuity or discontinuity of the encopretic symptom with the training period.

(2) The association or dissociation of the encopresis with enuresis.

(3) The presence or absence of faecal retention either as a persistent or intermittent phenomenon.

The frequencies are given in Table 4.

Table 4. Clinical types of encopresis, n=76

		No. of cases
(1)	Continuous associated	25
(2)	Continuous dissociated	5
(3)	Retentive	16
(4)	Discontinuous associated	11
(5)	Discontinuous dissociated	19
	Total no. continuous cases	30
	Total no. discontinuous cases	30

The frequencies do not in any way represent the natural distribution of the symptom in the population, but are research artefacts. The discontinuous types were easy to collect, but it took much longer to find thirty continuous cases to match with the others. Unmatched cases were excluded.

Clinical descriptions

The clinical pictures that follow are mildly exaggerated in order to accentuate the points of difference between two conditions sharing the same presenting symptom and generally regarded as similar. I will consider prototypes of 'continuous', 'discontinuous' and 'retentive' groups of children.

The 'continuous' child is a dirty child coming from a dirty family, burdened with every conceivable sort of social problem. The child's messiness forms an integral part of the general messiness and is, to some extent, camouflaged by it. Symptom tolerance in these families is surprisingly high and the parents are usually driven to the clinic, reluctantly and resentfully, by social agencies. Mother's general attitude is one of 'I couldn't care less'. She can give very little useful data on training history and is frequently unable to recall which of the children in her large family soil and wet. The child's early history is often so full of gastro-intestinal disease that it is not surprising that data on continence is difficult to elicit. The family morale is maintained by recourse to such vague somatic concepts as 'weakness' of bladder and bowel, but it is abundantly clear that the weakness lies in the maternal control. The fact that this type of case is commonly found among the lowest of the social classes would suggest the

277

operation, in part at least, of some cultural factors, although these are liable to be inundated beneath the welter of florid psychopathology. Defaecation cues are weak or absent and mother's awareness of them singularly inept. Any passing distraction seems capable of smothering it, and distractions are numerous in the life of this overactive, aggressive, dysinhibited child, who soils and smears and breaks and takes with little concern for the rights and feelings of others, and with often a complete absence of guilt, shame or disgust. As he grows older, he may tone down a lot, but the aggressive-regressive mixture is always there to distinguish him from the less rigid types of the 'discontinuous' child. According to Whiting & Child, he may be said to have a positive anal fixation. These children remain, as far as one knows, impulsive and infantile, but no one at present is at all certain what course their future psychiatric history takes. One thing is fairly sure: they undoubtedly help to breed further generations of encopretics and enuretics. The dirty mothers of these children do nothing with the dirt except live comfortably with it and teach their children to live comfortably with it. Most of them have come from 'wet and dirty' families and they seem to have stepped from one problem situation into another.

The 'discontinuous' child is the compulsive child of a compulsive family. He is over-controlled and inhibited in his emotional life and scrupulous with regard to his habits. The toilet 'leakage' is his dark secret and towards it he manifests a mixture of shame and anxiety. He is always very much on the defensive about his symptom and is therefore difficult to contact therapeutically. His reticence gradually resolves with treatment, and the words, especially dirty ones, then come pouring out. The defaecation cues are loud and clear but disregarded, so that causal explanations tend to centre on such epithets as 'lazy', 'casual', etc. As he grows older, his rigidity becomes more marked, and he may ultimately develop the rituals and compulsions of a full-blown obsessional state. A small number of older obsessional cases gives a history of soiling in childhood, although retention is the more common admission. These 'discontinuous' cases usually have normal stools, but a few are subject to episodic retention and may have had periods of constipation in early childhood.

The mothers tend to be rigid and authoritarian in their outlook, and to establish sado-masochistic relationships with their children and their husbands. They are prone to dichotomize their concepts, and the world for them is sharply divided into categories of good and bad, clean and dirty; the good being clean and the bad dirty. Their families contain two types of children, clean ones and dirty ones, and the dirty ones are made the scapegoat for all mother's ambivalent feelings towards dirt. It requires little psychological exploration to ascertain that, through their children, they vicariously gratify some of their own strongly forbidden impulses. For example, one of these meticulously clean mothers could hardly keep her punishing hands off her encopretic child when he soiled. During his remissions, however, the skin over her face would break out into an unpleasant and itchy form of rash at which she would scratch away savagely. It was 'terrible' for a woman like her to have a dirty skin or dirty child, and she was equally ashamed of both. Another woman, a typical 'encopretic mother', said to me: 'If you knew how clean I was at home, doctor, you would say I was the last person in the world to have a dirty child.' It needed only a short clinical acquaintance with her to realize that, on the contrary, she was probably destined to have other encopretic children in the future. Occasionally the husband may provide himself as an alternative scapegoat and, appropriately for the role, he is often a lavatory attendant, a coalman or a dustman, who may smell as much as the child. (The sense of smell is acute in these women.) 'One brings it from outside and the other brings it from inside and I've got to shovel it up after both of them.' If the enjoyment is not obvious, the reluctance to abandon this way of life is very much so. One encopretic mother hated the dirt of her husband—a lavatory attendant with piles. (Piles appear to be an occupational hazard with these men; they constantly indulge in lurid details about their appendages, boasting of their size in the manner of fishermen.) Nevertheless, she eschewed any thought of leaving him and of ending her dirt-shovelling, cat-and-dog, sado-masochistic existence with him. This type of mother is highly reminiscent of Bunyan's famous character in <u>The Pilgrims' Progress</u>, the muckraker, 'the person with a muck-rake in his hand who would look no way but downwards'; 'and they offered him a celestial crown for his muck-rake, but the man did neither look up, nor regard, but raked to himself the straws, the small sticks and dust of the floor.'

The 'retentive' child really belongs to a sub-grouping of both the main clinical categories, since either of them may, at times, include elements of retentiveness. He undergoes a severe toilet training and responds to it not with soiling or a precarious continence, but with stubborn constipation which later gives way to encopresis ('Obstipatio paradoxa'). For a while he may show a pseudo-bowel control largely through being constipated most of the time. Mother may later give a history of a clean period, but, on closer inquiry, this reveals itself correctly as a retentive one. The struggle between mother and child is an intense affair. It was described by one of the protagonists in the following way: 'We fight every day. He turns red and sweats, and crosses his legs together. I try and force his buttocks apart but although he's only four, his leg muscles seem stronger than my arms. But I won't give in. He's got to see who's master. Once I let him beat me, he'll always get his own way.'

The two obstinacies are evenly matched until mother brings up reinforcements in the shape of enemata, suppositories, purgatives and 'roughage'. The child's internal opposition runs parallel with its external counterpart, making an intolerable situation for the compulsive woman, who is ready to do battle on every issue and will yield no ground. It becomes the principal matter in her life. Engaged in it, she is almost immune from real disasters and tragedies which may involve her. The provocation is admittedly severe. This is the type of child who will wait for his mother to change his nappies and then immediately soil them. He will sit like Patience for hours on his pot, and then deposit his faeces on the floor beside it. He will react against the time, the place and the position. He will arch his back, cross his legs, clench his fists and redden with the effort of retention. His four abdominal quadrants are loaded with hard faeces. Periodically he passes a voluminous stool, the size of which becomes a dramatic highlight in the history of the case. One mother reiterated in every session the claim that her child had once filled 'three potfuls' in one sitting. X-rays revealed a distended colon as far as the anal sphincter, but no evidence of Hirschsprung's disease; hence the term 'psychogenic megacolon' (Richmond et al. 1954).

Three phases in the development of the condition are clinically discernible. An intense voluntary resistance emerges out of the prodromal syndrome in the toddler, which may last up to two or three years. This is followed by an apparent surrender and a period of good bowel behaviour with perhaps occasional constipation. But the 'battle of the bowel', seemingly won in the nursery, is destined to be lost on the playing fields at school. The discipline and control of the classroom, the alien toilet and the affects released in play combine to bring about a recrudescence or retention with overflow. No longer, however, is the retention associated with an active and voluntary resistance. The latter has now been internalized and opposition to the act is involuntary and effortless. As one of the children put it: 'Every time I go near the toilet, something down below seems to tighten up, and I can't make it let go however much I try. And I do try for Mummy's sake because I know how worried she gets about it, and I want to please her.' The past history in this case was of a fierce mother-child battle at the age of 4 of which the patient, at the age of 8, had no conscious recollection.

Tables 5-7 summarize the clinical characteristics of the two main categories and their relation to the type of training given.

Table 5. Differentiating factors, 'continuous' type

(1) Usually associated with enuresis
(2) Low-pressure toilet training
(3) Low levels of aspiration and achievement for mother
(4) Social and emotional regression marked
(5) Obsessional traits usually absent
(6) Anti-social behaviour
(7) 'Leakage symptoms' generally prominent
(8) 'Reaction formations' usually absent
(9) Reaction to encopresis shameless
(10) Child usually rejected and neglected
(11) Infantilizing tendency on mother's part
(12) Educational backwardness characteristic
(13) Parents frequently psychopathic
(14) Emotionally dysinhibited
(15) Weak aversion reaction

Table 6. Differentiating factors, 'discontinuous' type

(1) Usually dissociated from enuresis
(2) High-pressure toilet training
(3) High levels of aspiration and achievement for mother
(4) Social and emotional regression much less marked
(5) Obsessional traits usually present
(6) Anti-social behaviour absent
(7) 'Leakage symptoms' seldom present
(8) 'Reaction formations' usually a striking feature
(9) Reaction to encopresis--shame, guilt and anxiety
(10) Child usually over-protected
(11) Maternal tendency to hurry child through infancy
(12) Child usually doing well at school
(13) Parents generally obsessional
(14) Emotionally inhibited
(15) Strong aversion reaction

Table 7. Type of encopresis in relation to toilet training*

Type of encopresis	Coercive training (%)	Co-operative training (%)	Neglectful training (%)
Continuous (n=30)	26.7	6.6	66.7
Retentive (n=16)	75	25	0
Discontinuous (n=30)	63.3	13.3	23.4

Total n=70

* The differences for each clinical type are significant at the 1% level.

I will now turn from disturbances of function to disturbances of attitude towards the toilet function and its products.

Disturbed attitudes to function

Small children, as Freud (1910) first showed, are particularly prone to construct theories about the way in which the intimate bodily functions work. In this inquiry I found that they also theorize on the way the body, chiefly the hidden parts of it, fail to work. If cautiously approached, every child with encopresis will reveal his own idiosyncratic explanations for the dysfunction of his bowel. It is an inadequate and anxious picture to which the mother contributes her share when she attempts to force the child into conformity, with horrifying descriptions of impending intestinal catastrophes that he was building up inside him. Her own phantasies play their part in this, for, together with her frequent gastro-intestinal ailments, they furnish a conception of the hidden, inner world which is threatened or threatening. The more disturbed the child, the more frightening will this concept be. In the diagram that follows (Fig. 3), a five-year-old boy tried to explain to me what happened when he became constipated. He was a very disturbed child at the height of a bowel battle with his obsessional mother. His father suffered from chronic pulmonary tuberculosis and had been two years in a sanatorium. He was closely identified with his damaged father, who had treated his symptom much more sympathetically, and had given him a 'lecture' on his constipation before he had left him, at the age of 3, to deal with his punitive mother alone. His description was clearly an elaboration of this remembered 'lecture'. In normal defaecation, the faecal lumps queue up quietly at the point of exit. With retention, there is a damming up of the lumps which fill the stomach and then invade the lungs and the head, giving rise to shortage of breath, horrid white phlegm, occasionally blood, headaches and catarrh in the nose. If left too long, the lumps hardened to form a 'cannon-ball'. 'One day', he remarked cheerfully, 'it will come out with such a pop that it will knock Mummy right over and kill her.' The 'battle of the bowel' is not waged without ammunition on the child's side!

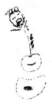

Normal   Retention of faeces

Fig. 3. Five-year-old encopretic child's concept of alimentary events.

Disturbed attitudes to faeces

Children often tend to interpret the outside world in animistic terms (Piaget, 1929). In the present investigation, I found a similar tendency with regard to intestinal events and products. In Table 8, the stages in intestinal animism are related to Piaget's stages in general animism and show an interesting correspondence.

These animistic attitudes are not difficult to elicit if one uses Piaget's method of free interrogation and follows the child passively into his magical systems of belief.

Table 8

Stages	Ages	Piaget's animistic scale	Comparable stages in intestinal animism
1	Under 5	Everything is alive	Everything inside the body is alive
2	Under 7	Everything that moves is alive	Faeces inside body are alive. Faeces outside body are not alive
3	Under 9	Everything that moves by itself is alive	Faeces that control themselves are alive. Faeces controlled by the child are not alive
4	Over 10 or 11	Clear biological concept of life	Clear biological concept of faeces

Not only, however, does the child bring his faeces to life in this striking way (Anthony, 1956), but he also endows them with special feelings, which may be roughly divided into positive, negative and neutral. Examples of each of these are given below.

Positive attitudes

L.S. 6.4 'I sometimes think my biggies fall asleep in my tummy; its so nice and warm there. Sometimes I'd like to cuddle them. They're rubber aren't they?'
P. L. 5.8 'When I do a really big job, mummy always says to me "Good girl " She should really say "Good job!" because it's jobby that does it not me.' ('But you let him out from inside, don't you?') 'No. When he grows up and becomes a big jobby, he just knocks on the door. Sometimes I say it's not time yet. Please wait till school's over. Sometimes he's nice and waits, but sometimes he just says "Oh bother school", and just comes out. And then everyone's cross with me when they should really be cross with Mr. Jobby.' (Adds rather affectionately) 'He does get me into lots of trouble, but he's not so bad really. He just doesn't think!'

Negative attitudes

M.B. 6.1 'My mum says it ends up in the sea. I think the fish might gobble it up. Then it will be a ghost and haunt me.' ('Where will it stay?') 'It might stay in the toilet and wait for me'.
A.L. 5.6 'When I drop it down in the toilet, I'm sometimes afraid it will jump back and bite me on the bottom.' ('Why would it do that?') 'Because it's cross from being sent away, I suppose.' ('Couldn't you pull the chain and send it right away?') 'That would make him much crosser. I hate pulling the chain. It only gets stuck in the pipes and can't breathe.'
N.D. 5.1 'It smells horrid. I hate it. My mummy hates it too. I could squash it. I hate it. It hurts coming out.'

Neutral attitudes

S. T. 5.10. 'You know the noise my tummy makes. Well, it's all my plops squeaking. They squeak if they're hungry.' ('Are they alive?') 'O yes. They're alive because they're inside me. But they die as soon as they come out. That's why they like to stay inside.' ('Are they ever naughty inside?') 'No. They are not naughty.' (Are they good, then?') 'No. They are not good. They are never naughty or good. They don't do anything. They just stay inside.' ('But are they alive inside?') 'O yes. They're alive inside, but they die when they come out.' ('What keeps them alive inside?') 'Because it's all alive there.' ('Why is that?') 'Because it is.'

Relation of animistic phantasies to type of toilet training

When these attitudes were correlated with the type of toilet training received by the child, a significant relationship was found between the quality of the animistic phantasies and the amount of pressure experienced (Table 9).

Table 9. Animistic feelings towards faeces in relation to the type of toilet training

Response to Piagetian 'interrogation'	Coercive training (%)	Co-operative training (%)	Neglectful training (%)
Expression of erotic, affectionate, solicitous feelings towards faeces (n=18)	11.1	33.4	55.5
Neutral feelings towards faeces (n=15)	26.6	26.6	46.8
Fearful or hateful feelings towards faeces (n=15)	73.3	6.7	20.0

Total n=48, children under 10

With regard to children trained neglectfully, the animistic phantasies are more likely to be positive than negative, the difference between the two being significant at the 5% level of confidence. With regard to children trained co-operatively the animistic phantasies are more likely to be positive than negative, the difference between the two being significant at the 10% level. With regard to coercive training, the animistic phantasies are more likely to be negative than positive, the difference between the two being significant at the 0.3% level of confidence.

The negative animistic attitudes may have a bearing on the genesis of toilet phobias. As the children outgrow their animistic concepts, they seem to lose this special fear.

Attitudes of shame and shamelessness

Attitudes of shame and disgust were closely linked together in most of the cases. When parents were questioned about the presence or absence of shame in their child, their answers frequently indicated a confusion with disgust. Among the 'continuous' cases, 76% declared the child to be shameless, 20% found that shame was present, and 4% were doubtful. Among the 'discontinuous' cases 41% were shameless, 52% were shameful, and 7% were doubtful. The difference between the 'continuous' and 'discontinuous' group with regard to shamelessness was significant at the 0.3% level. The difference between the two groups with regard to shamefulness was significant at the 1% level.

It was not found possible to measure these responses under controlled experimental conditions.

Attitudes of defiance and disobedience

On submitting questions concerning these attitudes to parents, no significant differences were found between the 'continuous' and 'discontinuous' groups, nor were any methods found to assess them in an experimental setting.

Attitudes of disgust

Having searched at the consequent end of my causal table for some form of measurable reactive behaviour in the child to set against the training activity of the parent, I concluded, after a small pilot investigation, that the reaction of disgust was one that could be most easily adapted for use in an experimental situation. Before showing how this was done, I would like to say something about the psychopathology of disgust.

The psychopathology of disgust

There is a paradoxical quality about the reaction of disgust which everyone can observe for himself. In the first place, we react to our own dirt quite differently from the way in which we react to the dirt of others; secondly, we react to the dirt inside us differently from the same dirt outside us thirdly, under the influence of strong emotion especially of the erotic kind, what is dirty for us in one situation may be less dirty in another; and finally, dirt located on one part of our bodies may be felt as 'less dirty' than its presence on some other part.

This paradoxical behaviour is not specifically a human characteristic. Kohler (1924) had noted that chimpanzees in captivity would eat their faeces. If, however, an animal stepped accidentally into a deposit of faeces, he would hobble about until he found something with which to clean his foot. During the cleansing operations his reaction seemed to be one of extreme disgust as evidenced by his gestures.

Similar behaviour can be noted in the encopretic child. One of my cases smeared the toilet room wall with his faeces and even rubbed it over his face and hands. Quite accidentally, some got on to his shoes and sent him screaming to the nurse in great distress demanding a complete change of clothing. Many encopretic children are described by their mothers as painfully fastidious. Yet they will carry faeces about in their underclothes all day with little to indicate it in their outward behaviour.

Angyal (1941) believed that the disgust reaction was made up of emotional, motor and autonomic components and was primarily directed towards one end-- the avoidance of ingesting any excremental material. He considered that the reaction was innate and universal. Had he investigated the matter from a developmental point of view, he might have been forced to agree with Freud (1910) that the basic reaction was coprophilic, and that coprophobia only developed as a result of systematic training during infancy. According to Freud, the cultural task lay in building 'psychic dams' of shame and disgust against such instinctual drives. Behind these 'psychic dams' the primary feeling and interest lay unchanged and were responsible for the paradoxical behaviour, when they did, on occasion, succeed in trickling through the dam undisguised. These primary manifestations are referred to elsewhere in the text as 'leakage' symptoms. More often, the individual's defences, chiefly his sublimations and reaction formations, desensualize and reverse the drives, and invest them with shame, anxiety, guilt and disgust. These modes of treating the original pleasurable drives bring into being certain permanent attitudes towards toilet functions, toilet products and symbolic representations of both. By such means is the 'anal character' created.

From the work of E. Jones (1948) and other analytic theorists, a check list was compiled and this was completed in each case with the help of the mother. For those unfamiliar with psycho-analytic theory, examples of expulsive and retentive types of the anal character are illustrated in Tables 10 and 11.

The 'leakage' traits allow the original drive to emerge unchanged and in the same direction. The 'sublimatory' traits have the same direction as the original drive but are altered in character through being desensualized and 'civilized'. With the 'reactive' traits the direction of the drive has been reversed.

In this investigation, the presence of 'leakage', 'sublimatory' and 'reactive' traits helped to discriminate, as will be seen later, between the main functional types of encopresis. The expulsive-retentive dimension, however, was much less useful and discriminating.

286

Table 10. Anal character traits, expulsive group

'Leakage'	Sublimatory	Reaction formation
Soiling	Generosity	Cleanliness
Smearing	Giving presents	Contamination, fear
Messiness	Sharing	Prudery
Pica	Painting	Carefulness
Swearing	Modelling	Masochism
Talking 'smut'		Modesty
Aggressiveness		'Cissiness'
Cruelty		
Activity		
Destruction		
Extravagance		
Vandalism		
Anal masturbation		
Spendthrift		
Defiling		

Table 11. Anal character traits, retentive group

'Leakage	Sublimatory	Reaction formation
Rubbish hoarding	Collecting	Orderly
Untidiness	Saving	Precise
Obstinacy	Acquisitiveness	Meticulous
Wilfulness	Possessiveness	Obedient
Disobedience	Interest in tunnels,	Submissive
Rebelliousness	caves, buried	Careful
Bossiness	treasure	Perfectionistic
Procrastination	Preoccupation	Persistent
Wooliness	with time, money,	Reliable
Unorganizing	food	Pedantic
Lack of initiative		Controlling
Giving up easily		Critical
Laziness		

Some tentative constructions

The transformation of the primary enjoyment in faeces and faecal functions into the secondary antipathetic reactions is one of the main undertakings of the 'potting couple', the training mother and the trainee child.

They are required to produce, within a certain period, a 'normal' reaction of disgust, strong enough to influence the behaviour of the individual for the rest of his life.

The following constructions can be made on the basis of this present discussion:

(1) The disgust reaction is a phenomenon relative to the culture and level of development. Its general intensity is determined by the character of the primary institutions and their application by the individual mother, with her idiosyncratic observations of cultural practice.

(2) Dependent on these factors, the mother applies strong, moderate or weak training pressures on the child, leading to the emergence of exaggerated, culturally normal, or deficient feelings of disgust. A culturally normal feeling of disgust will lead ultimately to a culturally acceptable technique for the disposal of personal excreta. Where the proper disposal of excreta is faulty, the disgust reaction will be found abnormal.

(3) One could therefore expect, on the basis of these arguments, that the disgust reaction will be abnormal in encopresis, tending towards the extreme type of response in the distribution of disgust for any particular population.

This brings us finally to the experimental reactions, which, unlike the permanent character traits we have been discussing, are limited to an artificial stimulus given in a limited period of space and time.

The Experiments

From my total sample, I excluded the 'retentive' cases who were mostly of an age between 4 and 6, and somewhat difficult to match. Of the remainder I paired off thirty 'continuous' and thirty 'discontinuous' types on the basis of age and sex. The two groups were fairly comparable in this respect, the average age for the continuous sample being 7.3 years and for the discontinuous 7.11 years.

Having carefully scrutinized the attitudes of my causal table for some form of measurable behaviour, I finally decided, after a small pilot inquiry and on empirical grounds alone, to utilize the reaction of disgust. The testing was carried out under quasi-therapeutic conditions as near to the clinic procedures of play as possible.

The following hypotheses were then made. It was predicted that the aversion reaction

(i) Would distinguish between the 'continuous', positively fixated type and the 'discontinuous', negatively fixated type of encopresis, in that the former would give a weak and the latter a strong response.

(ii) Would bear a direct relation to the length of period between training and the onset of soiling.

(iii) Would bear a direct relation to the intensity of the 'reaction formations' and an inverse relation to the 'leakage' symptoms, that constitute the anal character traits.

(iv) Would be related directly to the intensity of the training pressures.

(v) Would bear a consistent relationship to social status.

To test these hypotheses, a perceptual battery was elaborated, each sub-test of which involved one of the sensory modalities. The stimulus range was from pleasant to unpleasant, as judged by adult responses, and the subjects were rated on a seven-point scale with strong attraction and repulsion poles, and with the neutral response at point 4.

All the cases were exposed to the pleasant end of the spectrum first. In addition to verbal responses, motor and autonomic components of behaviour were noted in terms of the Angyal model (1941). In only one case was vomiting observed.

On the basis of the ratings, the subjects were classified into strong, inter-mediate, weak and unclassifiable reactors with respect to the individual sub-tests, and finally, with respect to the battery as a whole.

Attempts to assess re-test reliability, after periods of 3 and 6 months, proved impractical. Experience of this type of testing appears to provide the children with such vivid recollections of their first encounter with it, that the two situations are not at all comparable.

Smell

The first of the sub-tests took its form from the classical investigations of Henning (1938) who made use of 415 substances in constructing his 'smell prism' at the six corners of which he located putrid, fragrant, burned, ethereal spicy and resinous smells. Like most other workers, I made use of the 'smell prism' but rearranged it. No anosmic children were found in this series, but if there is such a thing as 'hyperosmia' then some of these children presented with it. On rough estimation they had extremely low thresholds to smell. Some of the mothers boasted of the child's hyper-sensitive nose which could pick up minimal smells at a considerable distance; which demonstrates how psychopathology can sharpen the faculties.

I would like to mention, in relation to my own results, a developmental investigation by Peto (1936) on about 500 normal children, in which he showed the coprophilia-coprophobia reversal with a transitional phase at the ages of 5 and 6. I have tabulated Peto's results in Table 12.

Table 12. Reaction of normal children to unpleasant odours

Sample	Ages	No disgust reaction (%)	Mixed reaction (%)	Strong disgust reaction (%)
Group I (n=92)	Under 5	96.7	1.1	2.2
Group II (n=39)	5-6	28.2	23.1	48.7
Group III (n=164)	6-16	7.9	14.6	77.5

Total n=295.
Age range 1 month-16 years.
Rural and urban populations.
Boys and girls visiting general hospital.

In comparing my seventy-six cases with Peto's norms, it became clear that my 'continuous' group behaved very much like his under 5 group, and my 'discontinuous' group very much like his over 6 group but with some exaggeration of intensities. The 'retentive' children, who clinically contain elements from both the main types, fall into line with the transitional group, but again, with a certain degree of exaggeration. The ages are not strictly comparable. Table 13, bearing Peto's in mind, demonstrates these points.

Table 13. Reaction of encopretic children to unpleasant odours

Sample	Ages	No disgust reaction (%)	Mixed reaction (%)	Strong disgust reaction. (%)	Comment
Continuous group (n=30)	4-16	83.3	10.0	6.7	Similar to normal pre-school response
Retentive group	4-6	25.0	12.5	62.5	Exaggeration of normal transitional response
Discontinuous group	5-16	3.3	6.7	90.0	Exaggeration of normal school child's response

Total n=76
Age range 4-16. Boys and girls visiting C.G.C.

Colour

Children are quite ready to admit to colour preferences, and show a strong dislike of certain colours. In general, they dislike dark colours, browns, etc. and the word 'dirty' is often applied to these even by the normal child. In this test the 'spectrum' ranged from dark brown to light yellows and reds. A colour preference is often reflected in the type of painting done by the child; for example, a preference for 'messy colours' is often associated with what clinicians have called the 'encopretic' painting--a disorganized, brownish, smudgy representation occupying the whole of a large sheet of paper. The reverse of this is a meticulous, almost colourless painting where a minimum of paint is used on a minimum of paper. A question is always included on the kind of smell any particular colour is thought to have, and, generally speaking, 'good' colours are credited with pleasant and 'bad' colours with an unpleasant smell, even though the paints are quite odourless.

Touch

In this test, an array of open vessels is placed before the child and he is asked to tell which is the warmest and which the coolest of specimens ranged before him. He is instructed to feel the contents, which range from water, through black ink, brown liquid paint, a brown cream that is quite odourless, a mixture of sand and water, to an indescribable squelchy black mess made up from several sources and which adults unanimously judged to be truly disgusting. The child is expected to move consecutively from the clean end to the dirty end. Depending on the point at which he stops, he is classified into his reaction type.

Sound

The fourth member of our perceptual battery was an auditory one--a word association test, made up of thirty words, half with a toilet reference to faeces, function and related concepts, and half neutral, given alternately. The following observations were made:

(1) The reaction time.
(2) Complete refusals.
(3) Behaviour of the subject.
(4) The galvanic skin response.

The interpretation of the test was as follows. The length of the reaction time was taken to mean a socially oriented disgust response, since it was essentially an interpersonal situation, however disguised as a stimulus-response one. The skin response, on the other hand, was an involuntary manifestation of the autonomic nervous system. It was felt, therefore, that the test provided both a voluntary and an involuntary reaction to disgust.

The reaction time results showed no significant differences between the two groups but a clear tendency in the expected direction (Table 14). The tendency for the 'discontinuous' types to have long reaction times was significant at the 1% level.

Table 14

Reaction time	Continuous	Discontinuous
Short	12	6
Intermediate	7	6
Long	11	18

n=60

The general findings with regard to the galvanic skin response were similar to Mundy-Castle & McKiever (1953) in that stable, labile and mixed skin responses to the stimulus could be isolated. The stable reactions were characterized by a tendency to adaptation, a reaction to the stimulus only, and by no fluctuation in resistance. The labile response showed no adaptation to the stimulus, a tendency to respond between stimuli, and a fluctuation in skin resistance. The mixed response contains elements of both (Table 15).

Table 15

Galvanic skin response	Continuous	Discontinuous
Stable responses	6	4
Mixed responses	7	3
Labile responses	2	8
n=30		

The figures are too small to test for significance, but it does show some interesting tendencies. The test group is of thirty of the older cases, as it was not thought wise to subject the younger ones to the procedure. The older children were carefully prepared and allowed to play with the apparatus and to subject the tester to the procedure. When it did come to their turn, they appeared fairly unruffled. They were told that they were being tested for speed of reaction, and an element of competition was brought in.

The results show that the labile galvanic skin response and long reaction times go together and are characteristic of the 'discontinuous' type, whereas the stable galvanic skin response and short reaction times go together and are characteristic of the 'continuous' type (older age group). It is understandable that the 'continuous' coprophilic cases are not put off by the anal word and, therefore, respond quickly and easily, but that they should tend to show a stable galvanic skin response is less easy to explain, since, clinically, they are a recognizably dysinhibited group. This dysinhibition is probably more external than internal. H. E. Jones (1935) has shown that children who externalize their conflicts and are outgoing have stable galvanic skin responses, whereas inhibited children may show a labile response (Figs. 4 and 5).

The reaction to toilet function

So far the work of the perceptual battery has been concerned with the response to toilet products. I made use of a well-known device to estimate the response to toilet function. The apparatus consists of a dark box, through one wall of which the subject is able to look and observe two illuminated disks on the opposite side. One of the circles is fixed, whilst the other can be made larger or smaller by means of a camera shutter device. Within the circle of the fixed disk, there is a photographed scene depicting some toilet event. The subject is asked to adjust the movable disk so as to match exactly the fixed disk, and he is rewarded for accuracy.

In the original work done with this method (Bruner & Goodman, 1947), two groups of rich and poor children estimated the size of coins. It was claimed that both groups tended to over-estimate size of the coins; that the over-estimation increased with the increasing value of the coins; and that the poor children over-estimated the size on an average more than the rich children.

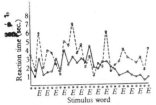

Fig. 4. Word association (reaction times). Average reaction times: ———, 'continuous type'; – – –, 'discontinuous type'; E, stress word.

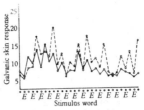

Fig. 5. Word association (galvanic skin response). Average galvanic skin response: ———, 'continuous type'; – – –, 'discontinuous type'; E, stress word.

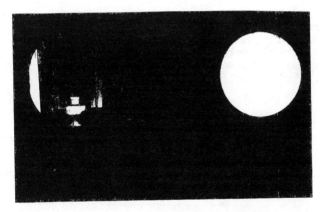

Fig. 6. What the child sees and measures in the comparometor.

293

On the basis of this and other work done, it was predicted that toilet-disturbed children would on the whole tend to over- or under-estimate a circle with a toilet content. Assuming that the 'continuous' cases were pleasure-motivated by toilet material, one would expect them to 'enlarge' on it, and over-estimate the size. By contrast, the 'discontinuous' children would be worried and repelled by the same content, and 'defend' against the percept by shutting down on it. In this context, under-estimation would be interpreted as an aversion reaction.

From the results given in Table 16 it will be noticed that the one significant tendency is for the 'discontinuous' cases to under-estimate the toilet scene (at the 10% level of confidence). No significant differences between the two functional types with respect to either over- or under-estimating is present, but again there is a consistent tendency in the expected direction.

Table 16

Estimations	Continuous	Discontinuous
Over-	12	8
Accurate	5	2
Under-	13	20

n=60

Results based on aversion reaction treated as a whole

An average figure for the aversion reactions for each sub-test of the battery was separately calculated for each individual, and plotted against the clinical variety, the length of period between training and the breakdown of training, the intensity of the training pressures as assessed by Huschka's criteria, the check list of anal character traits and finally the social class position. Tables 17 and 18 and Figs. 7-9 sum up the results.

Table 17. Strong aversion reaction for different sensory modalities

Perceptual battery	'Continuous' type (%)	'Discontinuous' type (%)	Level of confidence (%)
Smell	7	90	0.3
Colour	17	14	Not sig.
Touch	21	53	1
Sight*	43	67	10
Sound*	37	60	10

* Long reaction time in the word association sub-test and under-estimation in the comparometer test have been interpreted as aversion tendencies.

294

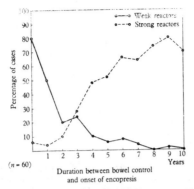

Fig. 7. Aversion reaction in relation to consolidation of training. For the purpose of clarification, the intermediate reactions have been incorporated into the strong and weak reactions.

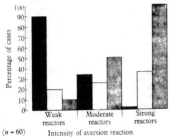

Fig. 8. Aversion reaction in relation to psycho-analytic anal character traits. ■, Erotic or 'leakage' traits; ▨, sublimations; ▦, reaction formations.

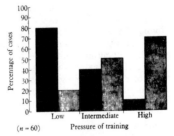

Fig. 9. Aversion reaction in relation to pressure of training. ■, Weak reactors; ▦, strong reactors. For the purpose of clarification, the intermediate reactions have been incorporated into the strong and weak reactions.

Table 18. Social class, clinical type and aversion reaction

Social Class*	I	II	III	IV	V	Totals
'Continuous'	–	–	6	13	11	30
'Discontinuous'	2	5	12	7	4	30
Strong aversion reaction	2	3	7	8	2	22
Intermediate aversion reaction	–	2	5	6	4	17
Weak aversion reaction	–	–	6	6	9	21

n=60

* According to the Registrar General's system of classification.

The 'continuous' cases are concentrated in the two bottom social groups, whereas the 'discontinuous' cases reach a peak in the third group. The weaker aversion reactions appear to be found in the lower social groups.

It will be seen that a strong aversion reaction in the experimental situation tends to be associated with a 'discontinuous' type of encopresis, a coercive toilet training, a long period of bowel continence before the onset of dysfunction, a marked development of reaction formations with respect to anal interests and drives, and, finally, a socially mobile and socially pretentious mother with high levels of aspirations in the domestic sphere.

A weak aversion reaction is more liable to be found together with a 'continuous' type of encopresis, a neglectful toilet training, a persistence of overt anally oriented interest and behaviour, and finally, a mother with a lower working class background with little or no social or intellectual aspirations, deeply inured to her way of life and without any desire to change it.

The 'overlap' between these two extreme types is related to the period of bowel continence before the loss of control, and it is this factor more than any other that adds variety to the clinical picture. From the results, however, the classificatory dichotomy appears to be justified, although the gap between the 'never-trained' and the training relapse is narrower than was first supposed.

The ability of the different sub-tests of the battery to discriminate between the two functional types is by no means the same. In this respect, they can be divided into good, moderate, and poor or absent, as follows;

> Good discrimination: smell.
> Moderate discrimination: touch.
> Poor or absent discrimination: sound, visual comparisons and colour.

The intercorrelations between smell and touch, smell and sound are fairly high, but between moderate and poor discriminators low or absent.

If any system of 'perceptual defence' (Postman, 1953) is operating in the experimental situation, it differentiates between presumably more threatening and less threatening sensory modalities. Should Angyal's theory (1941) be true, that the disgust reaction is an attempt to ward off the ingestion of excretory material, then the differential perceptual behaviour becomes more understandable, in that smell and touch can be thought of as constituting the more immediate threat. With vision and hearing there is warning of a possible threatening situation at a distance, so that withdrawal can take place in time.

Discussion and Conclusions

According to Freud (1924), the predisposition to anal fixation was determined to a large extent by the nature of the toilet training experienced by the child, and he emphasized that both a coercive and early, or a neglectful and late training could equally lead to this development. He felt unsure that this was sufficiently explanatory and therefore postulated a further 'constitutional' factor-- the so-called 'anal stamp'. Fenichel (1945) clarified the position further by classifying the fixation factors into those resulting from excessive gratification, frustration, or an alteration of either of these and those in which 'concurrence' of instinctual and security gratifications occurred.

Let us admit at once that no absolute evidence can be offered for the causal relationship between toilet training and bowel dysfunction and even less so, between toilet training and the formation of a particular character trait, but as Prugh and others have pointed out (1954) most available evidence does indicate 'a suggestive correlation'.

One has to bear in mind the following exceptions to the causal theory as simply stated:

(1) Not all children who experience an abnormal (in the sense of coercive or neglectful) type of toilet training develop bowel dysfunction or abnormal character traits.

(2) Not all children who have bowel dysfunction or abnormal traits experience an abnormal toilet training.

(3) Primitive children who have had a toilet training judged to be abnormal by the standards that are in use do not appear especially prone to develop bowel dysfunctions or abnormal character traits.

There could be two possible explanations for the insufficiency of the training hypothesis, the first being that possibly more than one cause is implicated and that the major one obscures the clear appreciation of the minor one; the second, that 'since child-rearing methods generally harmonize with other cultural influences...it is not possible to say that adult personality is related specifically to childhood experiences' (Argyle, 1957), so that other common factors may be involved.

From the findings of this research, it has emerged that toilet training is the most important and the most influential of the variables involved. The additional factors seem largely to belong to the group of 'immeasurable' variables associated with the 'potting couple' and which may help to modify the training pressure. From this point of view, it seems important that Huschka's criteria should be interpreted within the context of the total mother-child situation, and not in any simple chronological sense. The same spurious norms may be used in one instance by a pathologically motivated and anally preoccupied mother, and in another by a culturally motivated mother, anxious to keep in step with her neighbours but otherwise warm and understanding. Because of this, the same means may not bring about the same ends, and, consequently, the one-to-one relationship between means and ends is lost.

In this paper I have been mainly concerned with bowel training and its sequelae. That the same arguments may apply equally to bladder training has been shown in a paper by Bostock & Shackleton (1951) on the relationship between toilet training and enuresis. They found definite significant associations between urinary incontinence and coercive training, between coercive training and unwantedness, and between unwantedness and urinary incontinence. As a result of these findings, they elaborated a concept of enuresis as the 'end-product of a total situation...with its roots in the total personality of the child, and this includes the whole attitude of the parent to the child from the moment that breast feeding and toilet training commences'. They single out two types of mothers responsible for the enuretic outcome--the unwanting mother who compensates for her lack of love by multiplying and intensifying her ministrations, and the other, a compulsively clean and perfectionist mother, who is 'spurred to achieve early a high degree of toilet cleanliness' and who adheres to the letter rather than to the spirit of any instruction given. Nevertheless, she is a wanting mother. I would include both these as subdivisions of the high-pressure group. The prognosis is probably better with the wanting than with the unwanting mother, but no figures are available to support such a belief. The authors attempt to interpret their results in the light of learning theory. According to them the subsequent development of enuresis 'depends largely upon the degree of later frustration to which the toddler will be subjected, but the mother has created the necessary predisposition' (my italics) by means of her frustrating training techniques. The later frustrations lead to a habit disintegration and the regression to such 'stereotypies' as enuresis and encopresis. Why is the act of urination picked out before defaecation? Having reduced these complex and 'over-determined' issues to their simple formulation, the authors answer, somewhat weakly, that this is probably due to 'availability'. 'The act of defaecation is less susceptible to control by the higher centres than that of micturition' (sic). Their thinking follows closely on that of Maier. Their symptomatic stereotypies are also 'peculiarly strong and persistent', less subject to the influence of rewards and punishments, and stubborn to eradicate. Treatment consists in the removal of frustrating factors and in conditioning. They make no attempt to differentiate between continuous and discontinuous types of enuresis, which explains why they only saw the high-pressure type of mother.

The final discussion concerns the child's contribution to the formation of his symptoms. However abnormal the mother or her training behaviour, we have to remember that it is the child and not the mother who soils. There are factors in the child that respond to the mother's handling. There are Freud's 'constitutional' factors. The child may be unduly responsive to disturbed family relationships, to incidental traumata during and after the training period, to sensitization by gastro-intestinal illnesses. He may, with mother's help, mismanage his own anal phase, or react to various components in an extreme way. The developmental task is full of problems to which even a normal child may succumb temporarily. He is preoccupied with his phantasies apart from what mother is doing to him or for him. He 'appears to over-value his faeces in a magical narcissistic fashion, and at times marked anxiety over their loss "down the toilet" or in other ways may be manifest. His phantasies of omnipotence regarding this object, the stool, and its phantasied use in attacks upon others may lead to an animistic misunderstanding, related to fears or retaliation involving phantasied physical damage to his own anal region or the interior of his body' (my italics) (Prugh, Wermer & Lord, 1954). This description of the normal child passing through his anal phase is so reminiscent of the older encopretic child as he appears in this research, that it almost appears as if nothing has been added to the state of encopresis that was not already present during the anal phase of his development. As we have seen, the mother's management helps to intensify these feelings towards his faeces in a positive or negative direction.

Diagnosis, treatment and prognosis

The perceptual battery can separate two disparate groups within a mono-symptomatic clinical state. Clearly no one will want to use it simply for this purpose. Once the clinician is aware of these differences, and finds them important clinically, he will dispense with such ponderous aids. So often in child psychiatry one works on dark hunches, and if occasionally one can get along with the laboratory, so much the better. It is of some value to the clinician to know that his clinical judgements have experimental support; it subscribes to his scientific well-being. On the other hand, the diagnostic label of 'pregenital conversion' may seem unhelpful to him, although like Warson et al. (1954) he may be interested in relating encopresis to the psychosomatic disorder and the hysterical symptom and finding elements of both in it. I would agree, after a clinical experience of about a hundred cases, with Prugh et al. (1954) that these children do not appear to be using their bowels symbolically for defensive purposes, but that the symptom ensued from a 'less well-differentiated handling of tensions which could no longer be successfully dealt with in more mature fashion'.

The treatment implications are of greater importance. The 'continuous' child does not need psychotherapy, but habit training under happier conditions. He requires a warm, interested but relaxed, person operating under a more consistent régime than was ever available at home. He can be reasonably stabilized in a period of 3-5 months, although relapses are not infrequent with return to the old environment.

In the course of re-training, he needs to develop a normal degree of disgust, and he can obtain this, non-didactically, by identification with the normal adult who trains him. Failures in re-training occur when cases are severely complicated by unwantedness and backwardness. Nocturnal types of encopresis may be particularly recalcitrant.

The 'discontinuous' child is a different proposition altogether. He is generally a deeply disturbed child who needs prolonged psychotherapy and some measure of protection from his mother. Once a sado-masochistic union has been fully established, the situation may become very intractable to treatment. A disappearance of the exaggerated disgust reaction is the first hopeful therapeutic sign, but it is at this stage, when he may swing over to 'dirty' behaviour, that the mother requires expert handling if she is not to withdraw the child from therapy.

Many therapeutically heart-breaking situations in the past may be avoided by careful selection of cases for treatment. It would be illuminating to find out how many therapist-hours have been wasted doing psychotherapy with the 'continuous' group, or carrying out physical and training procedures with the 'discontinuous' group, for want of careful understanding of the treatment requirements.

The intensity of the disgust reaction may be of some prognostic value. Where it is weak, the encopretic child seems very liable to develop a passive and inadequate personality, which, if allowed to progress, can prove as difficult to influence therapeutically as the rigid character of the strong reactor. On the whole, I would agree with Whiting & Child (1953) in considering the 'continuous', positively fixated type as being more amenable to unlearning the bad habits and in reforming good ones. In a healthy environment these cases often resolve spontaneously, especially if normalizing group influences are at work. The 'discontinuous', negatively fixated types are difficult treatment problems, who may defy all attempts at psychotherapy and end, eventually as severe compulsive neurotics and with contamination phobias and washing rituals, ultimately needing a leucotomy knife to eradicate their intense disgust reactions.

It would therefore seem that the transformation of the disgust reaction in the child, from weak or strong to the normal for the environment, is one of the most important therapeutic undertakings in the treatment of these children and one with far-reaching consequences.

To return, finally, to the quotation from Nietzsche with which I started. One could say, much less categorically, much less holistically and with certain reservations, that some prejudices at least can be traced back to the primary care of the intestines in childhood.

References

Angyal, A. (1941). Disgust and related aversions. <u>J. Abnorm. (Soc.) Psychol.</u> 36, 393-412.

Anthony, E. J. (1956). The significance of Jean Piaget for child psychiatry. <u>Brit. J. Med. Psychol.</u> 29, 20-34.

Argyle, M. (1957). <u>The Scientific Study of Social Behaviour.</u> London: Methuen.

Bostock, J. & Shackleton, M. (1951). Enuresis and toilet training. <u>Med. J. Aust.</u> 2, 110-13.

Bruner, J. & Goodman, C. (1947). Value and need as organizing factors in perception. <u>J. Abnorm. (Soc.) Psychol.</u> 42, 33-44.

Chapman, D. & Volkmann, J. (1939). A social determinant of the level of aspiration. <u>J. Abnorm. (Soc.) Psychol.</u> 34, 225-38.

Davis, W. & Havighurst, R. (1946). Social class and colour differences in child rearing. <u>Amer. Sociol. Rev.</u> 11, 698-710.

Dollard, J. & Miller, N. (1950). <u>Personality and Psychotherapy.</u> New York: McGraw-Hill.

Erikson, E. (1950). <u>Childhood and Society.</u> New York: Norton.

Fenichel, O. (1945). <u>The Psychoanalytic Theory of Neurosis.</u> New York. Norton.

Fowler, G. B. (1882). Incontinence of faeces in children. <u>Amer. J. Obstet.</u> 15, 985.

Freud, S. (1910). <u>Three Contributions to the Theory of Sex.</u> New York. Nervous and Mental Disease Pub. Co.

_____(1924). The predisposition to obsessional neurosis. In <u>Collected Papers.</u>

Henning (1938). Quoted in Woodworth, R. S., <u>Experimental Psychology.</u> New York: Holt.

Huschka, M. (1942). The child's response to coercive bowel training. <u>Psychosom.</u> <u>Med.</u> 4, 301.

Jones, E. (1948). Anal-erotic character traits. Chap. 24 in <u>Papers on Psycho-analysis</u>, 5th ed. New York Wood and Co.

Jones, H. E. (1935). The galvanic skin reflex as related to overt emotional expression. <u>Amer. J. Psychol.</u> 47, 241-51.

Kardiner, A. (1939). <u>The Individual and his Society.</u> New York: Columbia University Press.

Klatskin, E. H. (1952). Shifts in child care practices in three social classes. <u>Amer. J. Orthopsychiat.</u> 22, 52-61.

Kohler, W. (1924). <u>The Mentality of Apes.</u> London: Kegan Paul.

Lewin, K. et al. (1944). Level of aspiration. Chap. x in Hunt, J. McV., <u>Personality and the Behaviour Disorders.</u> New York: Ronald.

McGraw, M. B. (1940). Neural maturation as exemplified in achievement of bladder control. <u>J. Pediat.</u> 16, 580-90.

McLellan. Quoted by McGraw, M. B. above.

Mundy-Castle, A. C. & McKiever, B. L. (1953). The psycho-physiological significance of the galvanic skin response. J. Exp. Psychol. 46, no. 1.

Peto, E. (1936). Contributions to the development of smell feeling. <u>Brit. J. Med. Psychol.</u> 15, 314.

Piaget, J. (1929). The Child's Conception of the World. New York: Harcourt, Brace.

Postman, L. (1953). On the problem of perceptual defense. Psychol. Rev. 60, 298-306.

Prugh, G. P. et al. (1954). On the significance of the anal phase in pediatrics and child psychiatry. Workshop, 1954. Amer. Orthopsychiat. Ass. in Case Studies in Childhood Emotional Disabilities, vol. 11. Ed. Gardiner, G. E.

Richmond, J. B. et al. (1954). The syndrome of fecal soiling and megacolon. Amer. J. Orthopsychiat. 24, 391-401.

Sears, P. S. (1941). Level of aspiration in relation to some variables of personality: clinical studies. J. Soc. Psychol. 14, 311-36.

Warson, S. R. et al. (1954). The dynamics of encopresis. Amer. J. Orthopsychiat. 24, 402-15.

Weissenberg, S. (1926). Über Enkopresis. Z. Kinderpsychiat. 1, 69.

Whiting, J. W. & Child, I. L. (1953). Child Training and Personality. New Haven: Yale University Press.

Continuities and Discontinuities in Childhood and Adult Moral Development[1]

L. KOHLBERG and R. KRAMER

Harvard University, Cambridge, Mass.

It may be useful to begin a discussion of the central issue of this symposium, continuity and discontinuity in the study of child and adult development, with a history of the origins of our interest in it. As a graduate student planning a study of moral development, the first author knew superego formation was pretty well completed by age 6. As an enthusiastic reader of PIAGET, however, he knew that the development of autonomous morality was not completed until the advanced age of 12 or 13. To allow for the laggards, he decided to include children as old as 16 in a study of the development of moral autonomy. When he actually looked at his interviews, it dawned on him that children had a long way to go beyond PIAGET's autonomous stage to reach moral maturity. Accordingly, he constructed a six-stage scheme of moral development, a schema in which superego morality was only stage 1 and what PIAGET termed autonomous morality was only Stage 2. His thesis data left him uncertain as to when Stage 6, the stage of mature morality, was finally reached; but at least he knew that it was fully reached by age 25, his age at the time of the study.

For reasons having nothing to do with an interest in adult development as such, he decided to follow his thesis subjects along longitudinally. The second author continued the study and developed hypotheses about moral judgment in late adolescence which he applied to the data for his dissertation [KRAMER 1968, 1969]. The findings we shall discuss today are these findings on longitudinal subjects as they progressed from age 16 to 25, and on their middle-aged fathers.

HUMAN DEVELOPMENT, 1969, Vol. 12 pp. 93–120.

Eventually we want to take these findings as a spring board for some speculations on adult development rather than to focus upon the more central and obvious conclusions to be derived from them. As we shall discuss shortly, their obvious import is that our cocky graduate student view was correct and moral development is all nailed up by 25. Put more elegantly, the two questions centrally answered by KRAMER's data are those which child psychologists typically ask when their longitudinal subjects start to grow up and when they don't know how to get disengaged from studying them. The first is whether there is age increase in a trait like 'moral maturity' after adolescence. The second related question is whether a trait is stabilized by adolescence, in the sense that an individual's score on the trait in adolescence correlates well with his score on the trait in later life.

Essentially, KRAMER found that there was no further age increase in moral maturity after age 25, and that high school scores on moral judgment maturity were highly predictive of adult scores on moral maturity. As child psychologists, our response to these findings is relief. We can finally pack up and go home without another wave of longitudinal interviewing three years hence. The story of moral development is complete. The response of the student of adult development to these results is quite different. As BERNICE NEUGARTEN's paper clearly points out, the child psychologist's triumph in nailing down a terminus of development is the child psychologist's failure in offering anything useful to the student of adult development. To the extent that moral development is nailed down by late adolescence, concepts of moral development tell us nothing about what goes on in adulthood, what goes on in adulthood tells us nothing about moral development, and the studies of adult development and of child development have nothing to offer one another in the moral domain.

To clarify NEUGARTEN's point, let's take the example of general intelligence, of general cognitive or mental maturity, which is pretty completely developed by the early twenties. The fact that cognitive development increases throughout childhood is a central key to understanding childhood personality development, as the cognitive developmental personality theories of J. M. BALDWIN, PIAGET, G. H. MEAD and WERNER have stressed [KOHLBERG 1968].

The structural transformations in conceptions of the physical world discussed as cognitive stages by PIAGET are paralleled by cognitive transformations in the child's conception of his social world and of himself as a social being. Because of this, empirical research has demonstrated that the timing of onset of new stages of social development (psychosexual and moral) is heavily influenced by such cognitive factors as general mental age or general intellectual maturity [KOHLBERG 1968].

The role of intelligence in the understanding of adult development is quite a different matter. While individual differences in adult intelligence tell us something about an adult's functioning and interests, they do not explain much about the way the individual develops or changes in adulthood, just because such differences are a constant. Adult psychosexual or moral development could certainly not result from cognitive tranformations or growth, as can childhood development, because there appears to be no such adult cognitive transformations. Accordingly, adult functioning in the area of general intelligence can hardly be the key to understanding adult development.

It may be that writing off general intelligence as a key to understanding adult development is premature, in light of our child centered psychometric concepts and measures of intellectual development. But something is more obviously amiss if we write off moral judgment or ideology as a key to understanding adult development.

Morality and moral change is clearly a focal point for adult life in a way cognitive change is not. We do not need ERIKSON's studies of MARTIN LUTHER and MAHATMA GHANDI to know that the crises and turning points of adult identity are often moral. From ST. PAUL to TOLSTOY, the classic autobiographies tell us the dramas of maturity are the transformations of the moral ideologies of men. Clearly, then, morality cannot be studied with a polite agreement between child psychologists and adult psychologists to go their separate ways in studying development.

If morality is clearly a focus for adult personality change, does this mean that moral development goes on after biological maturity? The question appears to be an exercise in making refined semantic distinctions between the words personality 'change' and personality 'development', semantic issues raised by the question: 'Is there development past biological "maturity"?' The question, however, is not merely semantic, it is critical for the relations between child and adult psychology. As ALBERTA SIEGEL's paper points out, the concept of stage has been critical to the distinctive theories of child development, the theories of FREUD, GESELL, ERIKSON, and PIAGET. As SIEGEL's paper also points out, this stage conception has roots in the biological-maturational tradition to which all the child-psychologists have been strongly exposed. In one form, then, the question of 'Is there adult development?' is the question of whether the child psychologist's general conception of stage with its biological roots, is useable to describe or understand personality change after biological maturity has been reached. As our phrasing suggests, the issue of adult development is also closely linked to the issues of whether the general concept of maturity, a biologically rooted word for ideal endpoint of development, has any meaning for the study of adult personality change.

It may not appear to you, as it does to us, that it would be of great value to determine whether child psychology's conceptual apparatus of 'stage' and 'maturity' could be used for the study of adult personality change. This value lies first in the implications of the answer for child development theory. While all stage conceptions have relied on biological metaphor, some theories, like GESELL's, treat stages as direct products of maturation, while others, like PIAGET's, treat stages as the result of organism—environment interaction, as primarily the result of psychological experience. As long as the study of stage-development is limited to childhood, it is almost impossible to empirically separate the roles of maturation and experience in stage-development in a way which would bear upon these theoretical differences. The study of adult stage-development could open this door.

There is a second reason for searching for continuity between the conceptions of development used by child and adult psychologists which is of special importance in the moral domain. This reason may be termed either philosophical or practical.

For aeons of history, it was assumed that the middleaged and the aged had a wisdom denied to the youth. In modern society, formal education and the written word has made the full knowledge of the culture symbolically accessible to the youth and the criteria of wisdom have become more public, more defined by the methods of science and logic. Value questions have come to be viewed as historically relative, as out of the domain of rational discourse. All youth know that values change rapidly, that their elder's values are different from their own and that their children's will differ from their own. Their elders protest that the generational differences are due to the fact that the values of the young are based on the immediate intellectual or emotional appeals of images and ideas, not on their meaning as integrating the experience of living. If there is any germ of truth in the elder's view, it rests on the assumption of adult development.

The assumption that the adult possesses some wisdom which the youth cannot appreciate by the usual criteria of rational discourse is the assumption that the adult has developed a higher mode of thought, is at a higher stage. If adult developmental psycholgy can define such higher modes of thought, it will have a use quite different from the uses of child psychology in contributing to communication between the generations. Child psychology has assumed it knows what maturity is. While using biological metaphors for maturity, in operational practice, child psychology has assumed that maturity is conventional adult knowledge, success, and social conformity (otherwise termed socialization, adjustment, ego strength, or 'the reality principle'). Deviation from the conventional is then labelled infantile; at best, as creative regression in the service of the ego. From such a framework, child psychology teaches the adult how to speak 'childrenese,' how to speak down to the child. The young, however, refuses to accept socialization into the current society as representing maturity. The failure of communication is not because adults can't talk childrenese, it is because the young believe that the adults can't talk real 'adultese,' that the adults don't have any deeper notion of maturity than that instilled in them when they were children. If developmental psychology is to take the maturity concept seriously, it must find it, not in the cliches of the conventional culture, but in the findings of universal patterns of adult change, and communicate these findings about a 'true adultese' which is more mature than the conventional culture to both the young and the middle aged.

As we read conceptualizations of adult development, they slide over the issues we have just raised. It is fairly common to talk loosely of adult development and stages in terms of developmental tasks. Such discussion assumes that there are age-typical changes in personality, linked to focal tasks, and that successful resolution of these tasks leads to characteristic attitudinal outcomes. Even if 'stages' in this sense can be clearly documented empirically, they would not deal with the basic issues I have mentioned. Before explaining why 'developmental tasks' will not deal with these issues, let me first clarify what child psychology in the PIAGET-WERNER tradition has meant by 'development' and 'stage' [WERNER, 1948; PIAGET, 1964; KOHLBERG, 1968]. There are three criteria used by the tradition to distinguish psychological development from behavior change in general.

The first criterion is that development involves change in the general shape, pattern, or organization of response, rather than change in the frequency or intensity of emission of an already patterned response. Under reinforcement, bar-pressing increases in frequency; such increase is not development. Under food deprivation, hunger behaviors increase in frequency and intensity; such behavior is not development. With age, sexual impulses wax or wane in intensity. Such changes are not development.

A second criterion, closely related to the first, is that developmental change involves newness, a qualitative difference in response. Developmental change does not have to be sudden or saltatory but it does entail the emergence of a novel structure of response. Novelty involves the quality-quantity distinction, which in turn involves the distinction between form and content. In a sense, any change in content is new. A really new kind of experience, a really new mode of response, however, is one that is different in its form or organization, not simply in the element or the information it contains.

The third criteria implied by the word development is irreversibility. Once a developmental change has occurred, it cannot be reversed by the conditions and experiences which gave rise to it. Learned bar pressing can be reversed or extinguished by withdrawing the reinforcement which conditioned it. A developmental change cannot. SMEDSLUND [1961] has used this criterion to distinguish cognitive development from associationistic learning. He reports that if a PIAGET conservation was taught to a preconserver by instruction and reinforcement, it could be reversed by use of the same mechanisms. Naturally developing conservation could not be reversed by the same procedures. The concept of developmental irreversibility does not rule out the existence of behavior change backward to a previous pattern. As an example, seniles and schizophrenics seem to lose the PIAGET conservations. Such backward changes are labelled regression; however, it is important to point out that they are rare and their conditions or causes are markedly different from the conditions or causes of forward development.

The three criteria of development just mentioned, plus three others, are involved in the concept of developmental stage. The stage concept not only postulates irreversible qualitative structural change, but in addition postulates a fourth condition that this change occurs in a pattern of universal stepwise invariant sequences. Fifth, the stage concept postulates that the stages form a hierarchy of functioning within the individual. This implies, sixth, that each stage is a differentiation and integration of a set of functional contents present at the prior stage.

On the face of it, developmental task conceptions meet none of the criteria we have mentioned. Sexual intimacy and marriage, vocational identity and achievement, parenthood, acceptance of life's completion and conclusion are matters of content, not form. According to ERIKSON, [1950] the *content* of parenthood forms the focus of development of a generalized or *formal* attitude of generativity toward the world and toward the self which is *new* in development. It is just the question of whether such a novel formal attitude develops apart from parental content which lies at the heart of any investigation of ERIKSON's adult ego stages.

Related to the ambiguity of the formal aspects of stages defined as resolutions of developmental tasks is the ambiguity of their irreversibility and invariance of sequence. Developmental tasks of content in themselves have no order, i.e., individuals can face vocational commitment or identity before or after sexual intimacy and parenthood. Psychologically it is even possible to develop competent parental attitudes before developing capacity for sexual intimacy. Finally, the irreversibility of development defined in terms of developmental tasks is much in question. There are certainly many older adults, apparently mature and ready to face the tasks of integrity vs. despair, who suddenly seem to prefer regression to the tasks of establishing heterosexual intimacy.

My sketch of the developmental task approach does justice neither to its usefulness for personality study nor to its theoretical richness as elaborated by ERIKSON [1950]. My caricature does, however, point to the inability of the developmental task approach to speak to the two problems mentioned. A study of adult developmental tasks will tell us little about the general role of experience in childhood structural change. It will also do little to establish communication between the generations. The older may indeed have wisdom in the sense of awareness of the problems that the young have not faced and will inevitably face. That does not, however, prove that it is wise for the young to face their problems in terms of the problems of their elders. The old may have developed a style of coping with the immanence of death which is effective and admirable. This does not mean that the young should cope with the problem or use a similar style. Only if there is a form of thought or a form of coping more mature or integrated in its application to a problem that is also the youth's problem, can the development of the older help the younger.

We have talked of the potential value for adult psychology of the rigorous conception of stage used in Piagetian child psychology. Before considering its application to adulthood, let me first quickly sketch how the criteria implied by this rigorous conception have been met in child psychology. For obvious reasons, our example will come from our work on stages of moral judgment [KOHLBERG, 1958, 1963, 1968, 1969]. Table I presents a summary characterization of six stages of moral judgment.

Table I. Definition of moral stages

I. Preconventional Level

At this level the child is responsive to cultural rules and labels of good and bad, right or wrong, but interprets these labels in terms of either the physical or the hedonistic consequences of action (punishment, reward, exchange of favors) or in terms of the physical power of those who enunciate the rules and labels. The level is divided into the following two stages:

Stage 1: *The punishment and obedience orientation.* The physical consequences of action determine its goodness or badness regardless of the human meaning or value of these consequences. Avoidance of punishment and unquestioning deference to power are valued in their own right, not in terms of respect for an underlying moral order supported by punishment and authority (the latter being Stage 4).

Stage 2: *The instrumental relativist orientation.* Right action consists of that which instrumentally satisfies one's own needs and occasionally the needs of others. Human relations are viewed in terms like those of the market place. Elements of fairness, of reciprocity and equal sharing are present, but they are always interpreted in a physical pragmatic way. Reciprocity is a matter of 'you scratch my back and I'll scratch yours', not of loyalty, gratitude or justice.

II. Conventional Level

At this level, maintaining the expectations of the individual's family, group, or nation is perceived as valuable in its own right, regardless of immediate and obvious consequences. The attitude is not only one of *conformity* to personal expectations and social order, but of loyalty to it, of actively *maintaining*, supporting, and justifying the order and of identifying with the persons or group involved in it. At this level, there are the following two stages:

Stage 3: *The interpersonal concordance or 'good boy—nice girl' orientation.* Good behavior is that which pleases or helps others and is approved by them. There is much conformity to stereotypical images of what is majority or 'natural' behavior. Behavior is frequently judged by intention—'he means well' becomes important for the first time. One earns approval by being 'nice'.

Stage 4: *The 'law and order' orientation.* There is orientation toward authority, fixed rules, and the maintenance of the social order. Right behavior consists of doing one's duty, showing respect for authority and maintaining the given social order for it's own sake.

III. Post-Conventional, Autonomous, or Principled Level

At this level, there is a clear effort to define moral values and principles which have validity and application apart from the authority of the groups or persons holding these principles and apart from the individual's own identification with these groups. This level again has two stages:

Stage 5: *The social-contract legalistic orientation* enerally with utilitarian overtones. Right action tends to be defined in terms of general individual rights and in terms of standards which have been critically examined and agreed upon by the whole society. There is a clear awareness of the relativism of personal values and opinions and a corresponding emphasis upon procedural rules for reaching consensus. Aside from what is constitutionally and democratically agreed upon, the right is a matter of personal 'values' and 'opinion'. The result is an emphasis upon the 'legal point of view', but with an emphasis upon the possibility of changing law in terms of rational considerations of social utility, (rather than freezing it in terms of Stage 4 'law and order'). Outside the legal realm, free agreement, and contract is the binding element of obligation. This is the 'official' morality of the American government and Constitution.

Stage 6: *The universal ethical principle orientation.* Right is defined by the decision of conscience in accord with self-chosen *ethical principles* appealing to logical comprehensiveness, universality, and consistency. These principles are abstract and ethical, (the Golden Rule, the categorical imperative) they are not concrete moral rules like the Ten Commandments. At heart, these are universal principles of *justice* of the *reciprocity* and *equality* of the human *rights* and of respect for the dignity of human beings as *individual persons*.

The operational meaning of these stages is suggested by table II with regard to one moral concept, the worth of human life.

Table II. Six stages in conceptions of the moral worth of human life

Stage 1: No differentiation between moral value of life and its physical or social-status value.

Tommy, age ten (III, Why should the druggist give the drug to the dying woman when her husband couldn't pay for it?): 'If someone important is in a plane and is allergic to heights and the stewardess won't give him medicine because she's only got enough for one and she's got a sick one, a friend, in back, they'd probably put the stewardess in a lady's jail because she didn't help the important one'.

(Is it better to save the life of one important person or a lot of unimportant people?): 'All the people that aren't important because one man just has one house, maybe a lot of furniture, but a whole bunch of people have an awful lot of furniture and some of these poor people might have a lot of money and it doesn't look it.'

Stage 2: The value of a human life is seen as instrumental to the satisfaction of the needs of its possessor or of other persons. Decision to save life is relative to, or to be made by, its possessor. (Differentiation of physical and interest value of life, differentiation of its value to self and to other.)

Tommy, age thirteen (IV, Should the doctor 'mercy kill' a fatally ill woman requesting death because of her pain?): 'Maybe it would be good to put her out of her pain, she'd be better off that way. But the husband wouldn't want it, it's not like an animal. If a pet dies you can get along without it—it isn't something you really need. Well, you can get a new wife, but it's not really the same.'

Jim, age thirteen (same question): 'If she requests it, it's really up to her. She is in such terrible pain, just the same as people are always putting animals out of their pain.'

Stage 3: The value of a human life is based on the empathy and affection of family members and others toward its possessor. (The value of human life, as based on social sharing, community and love, is differentiated from the instrumental and hedonistic value of life applicable also to animals.)

Tommy, age sixteen (same question): 'It might be best for her, but her husband—it's a human life—not like an animal, it just doesn't have the same relationship that a human being does to a family. You can become attached to a dog, but nothing like a human you know.'

Stage 4: Life is conceived as sacred in terms of it's place in a categorical moral or religious order of rights and duties. (The value of human life, as a categorical member of a moral order, is differentiated from it's value to specific other people in the family, etc. Value of life is still partly dependent upon serving the group, the state, God, however.)

Jim, age sixteen (same question): 'I don't know. In one way, it's murder, it's not a right or privilege of man to decide who shall live and who should die. God put life into everybody on earth and you're taking away something from that person that came directly from God, and you're destroying something that is very sacred, it's in a way part of God and it's almost destroying a part of God when you kill a person. There's something of God in everyone.'

Stage 5: Life is valued both in terms of it's relation to community welfare and in terms of being a universal human right. (Obligation to respect the basic right to life is differentiated from generalized respect for the socio-moral order. The general value of the independent human life is a primary autonomous value not dependent upon other values.)

Jim, age twenty (same question): 'Given the ethics of the doctor who has taken on responsibility to save human life—from that point of view he probably shouldn't but there is another side, there are more and more people in the medical profession who are thinking it is a hardship on everyone, the person, the family, when you know they are going to die. When a person is kept alive by an artificial lung or kidney it's more like being a vegetable than being a human who is alive. If it's her own choice I think there are certain rights and privileges that go along with being a human being. I am a human being and have certain desires for life and I think everybody else does too. You have a world of which you are the center, and everybody else does too and in that sense we're all equal.'

Stage 6: Belief in the sacredness of human life as representing a universal human value of respect for the individual. (The moral value of a human being, as an object of moral principle, is differentiated from a formal recognition of his rights.)

Jim, age twenty-four (III, Should the husband steal the drug to save his wife? How about for someone he just knows?): Yes. A human life takes precedence over any other moral or legal value, whoever it is. A human life has inherent value whether or not it is valued by a particular individual.'

(Why is that?): 'The inherent worth of the individual human being is the central value in a set of values where the principles of justice and love are normative for all human relationships.'

The concept of human life is valued at each stage. The way in which this value is conceived differs, however, at each stage. In parentheses we indicate the sense in which each higher stage involves a differentiation in thinking about life's values not made at the immediately preceding stage of thought. The sense in which each stage is a new integration is more difficult to define, but will be intuitively evident to you in reading the examples. The table illustrates this one aspect of moral development with responses from two boys in the 10-year longitudinal study. Tommy was first interviewed at 10, and then again at 13, and 16. At 10 he is Stage 1, at 13 Stage 2, at 16 Stage 3. To represent more mature stages we have used Jim.

Jim, when first interviewed at 13, is primarily Stage 2. At 16 he is Stage 4, at 20 Stage 5, at 25 Stage 6 on this aspect. These two boys, then, suggest a sequential pattern holding for each individual. While Tommy is slower in development than Jim and likely will never get as far, both go through the same steps insofar as they move at all. While various statistical qualifications are required in making the generalization, it is true that the pattern of most of our longitudinal data is a pattern of directed irreversible onestep progressions.

We have said that our sequence is invariant for individuals in the United States. Our evidence also suggests that this sequence is culturally universal.

Figure 1a presents age trends for middle class urban boys in the United States, Taiwan and Mexico. At age 10 in each country, the order of use of each stage is the same as the order of its difficulty or maturity. In the United States, by age 16 the order is the reverse, from the highest to the lowest, except that Stage 6 is still little-used. At age 13, the middle Stage (Stage 3) is most used. The results in Mexico and Taiwan are the same, except that development is a little slower. Figure 1b presents similar trends for two isolated villages in Turkey and Yucatan. Here development is slower, but the trends for these far distant villages are very similar to one another.

Let us now turn to the facts of adult development of moral thought. Some of these are contained in the graphs of figure 2. Figure 2 shows the percentage usage of each type of thought by our middle class and slower class longitudinal sample at ages 16, 20 and 25. While not all boys were seen at every age, the trends shown fairly represent both longitudinal and cross-sectional trends. The middle-aged group were the fathers of the longitudinal subjects and so comparable to them in all the usual ways.

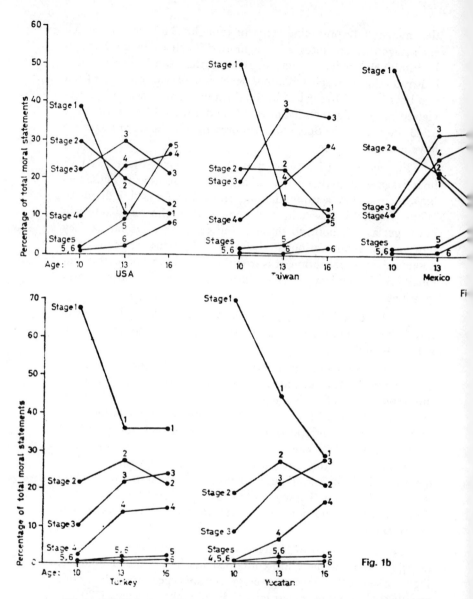

Fig. 1a. Middle-class urban boys in the U.S., Taiwan and Mexico. At age 10 the stages are used according to difficulty. At age 13, Stage 3 is most used by all three groups. At age 16. U.S. boys have reversed the order of age 10 stages (with the exception of 6). In Taiwan and Mexico, conventional (3–4) stages prevail at age 16, with Stage 5 also little used.

Fig. 1b. Two isolated villages, one in Turkey, the other in Yucatan, show similar patterns in moral thinking. There is no reversal of order, and preconventional (1–2) does not gain a clear ascendancy over conventional stages at age 16.

314

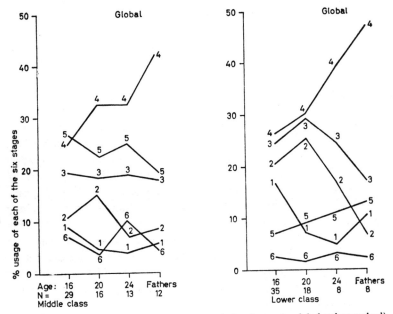

Fig. 2. Moral judgment profiles (percentage usage of each stage by global rating method) for middle and lower class males at four ages. [From RICHARD KRAMER 'Changes in Moral Judgment Response Pattern During Late Adolescence and Young Adulthood' Ph. D. dissertation, University of Chicago, 1968].

The first question to be asked is answered by the fact that there is no Stage 7 on the graph. In other words there was no way of thinking about our moral situations found in adulthood and not found in adolescence. While no new modes of moral thought are born in adulthood, there is a not quite significant (p. < 15) increase in Stage 6 thinking from 16 to 25. The figure indicates about twice as much Stage 6 thinking at 25 as at 16. To a certain extent, some of this Stage 6 thinking is new at age 25. 80 % of the middle-class high school students who showed no use of Stage 6 thought showed at least a little such thought (5 %) by age 25. It is difficult to speak very definitely about the development of Stage 6 in our small longitudinal sample because clear Stage 6 types are so rare in every population. HAAN, SMITH and BLOCK [1968] found 4 % of their Bay area college students to be predominately Stage 6. HOL-STEIN [1968] gets about the same percentage in 106 suburban college-educated parents. In our longitudinal sample, we get about the same percentage, amounting to one of our 14 middle class 25 year-

315

olds. He was predominantly Stage 5 in late high school and early college.

While there is some evidence that Stage 6 thinking can be born or at least stabilized in the post-high school years, principled thought of the stage 5 variety is pretty completely developed by the end of high school. Figure 2 indicates no clear increase in Stage 5 thinking from high school to age 25. All young adults showing appreciable amounts of Stage 5 thinking (over 15%) also showed appreciable (over 15%) amounts of Stage 5 thinking in high school. The 25% of Stage 5 thinking in our college educated young adults sample is also about that found in the other studies mentioned. We can summarize our results by saying that principled thought, especially Stage 5, is born in adolescence, but that Stage 6 principled thought tends not to become crystalized until the early 20's. Figure 2 also indicates that little development occurs after the early 20's. Our middle class college educated fathers are slightly, but not quite significantly (p. <20) *lower* on Stage 5 and 6 thought than their sons. Like the young, we put the advantage of the younger generation to social or cultural evolution.[2]

Regardless of the ambiguity of the cross-sectional differences graphed in figure 2, it is evident that adult development is primarily a matter of dropping out of childish modes of thought rather than the formation of new or higher modes of thought. Figure 2 indicates that the major change in moral thought past high school is a significant increase or stabilization of conventional morality of a Stage 4 variety, at the expenses of preconventional stages of thought. This stabilization of moral thought is not only reflected in the trends of stage usage for the group as a whole, it is also reflected in the trends of variability of stage usage within individuals. Figure 3, presents these trends, as analyzed by TURIEL [1969] using KRAMER's [1968] raw data.

Figure 3 presents the amount of spread (usage of stages of thought other than the individual's modal or preferred stage of

[2] The case for historical or cultural evolution of moral thought, as made by HOB-HOUSE [1906] is well thought through. Its appeal at the moment is enhanced by the relative position of the generations about the universal moral issues of war. The writer finds no reason to find generational increase in moral level more surprising than the documented generational increases in general intelligence. Recent longitudinal findings [BAYLEY, 1955] indicate historical or cohort increases in intelligence in adulthood masked by cross-sectional estimates. We would not be surprised to find a similar masking in our cross sectional comparison of our subjects and their fathers.

thought) found among higher (Stages 4, 5, 6) and lower stages (Stages 1, 2, 3). The age trend for higher stage is toward a reduction of usage of stages other than their preferred stage, a trend which is significant (p. <.05). In other words, young men at higher stages are stabilizing at their higher stage with age in young adulthood, although lower stage men are not.

Another word for the adult stabilization which represents the major trends of figure 2 and 3 is consistency. While our data do not present direct evidence for it, there is reason to believe that adult age change is not only toward greater consistency of moral judgment but toward greater consistency between moral judgment and moral action. HARTSHORNE and MAY [1928–30] found that in the period 11 to 14, there was no decline in cheating behavior but there was a decline in the inconsistency of cheating behavior. With age some children became more consistently honest, some more consistently dishonest, leaving a net mean amount of cheating that was constant. Comparison of cheating studies in preadolescence and in college suggests that not only is cheating behavior more consistent in college

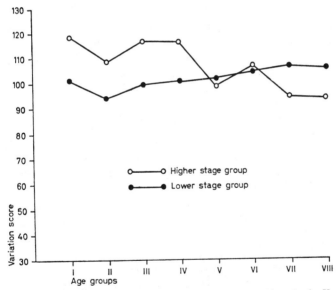

Fig. 3. Mean variation scores for higher stage and lower stage subjects in the KRAMER group at the following 8 age ranges: 14.0–15.11 (I); 16.0–16.11 (II); 17.0–17.11 (III); 18.0–18.11 (IV); 19.0–20.11 (V); 21.0–22.11 (VI); 23.0–23.11 (VII); and 24.0–26.11 (VIII).

but it is more consistently related to level of moral judgment in college than in preadolescence [KOHLBERG, 1969]. These fragments of data on consistency suggest support for the folk wisdom which proclaims that the middle aged are more reliable or trustworthy than the young, even if they seem less given to expressing lofty moral ideals in either words or heroic action.

Adult stabilization is not adult development. We could dignify an increase in the consistency of moral ideology with itself and with moral action under the name of integration, the integration of moral thought with itself and with one's self-concept. One reason we hesitate to do so is because much adult moral stabilization seems to be not development but socialization or internalization of the conventional code. This is suggested by the fact that conventional (Stage 4), as well as post-conventional, moral ideologies stabilize in adulthood. There is no Babbitt like an old Babbitt.

While the Babbitts become even more conventional with age, to some extent so do the deviants and the rebels. One of the best predictors for parole is chronological age. Old criminals get burnt out and learn that you can't beat the system. The interpretation that adult moral stabilization is 'socialization' not 'development' is further suggested by the fact that the breed of conventional morality which stabilizes in adulthood depends upon one's adult social sex role. Only 6% of our Stage 3 boys in high school remained Stage 3 in young adulthood, the rest having moved to Stage 4. In contrast, Stage 3 appears to be a stable adult stage for women. At high school there are about the same percentage of Stage 3 boys and girls [TURIEL, 1968]. In the Bay area college population of HAAN, SMITH and BLOCK [1968] there are about twice as large a percentage of Stage 3 girls as boys. Among the parent samples of HOLSTEIN [1969], the difference is even more marked, about four times as many Stage 3 women as men. In other words, while girls are moving from high school or college to motherhood, sizeable proportions of them are remaining at Stage 3, while their male age mates are dropping Stage 3 in favor of the stages above it. Stage 3 personal concordance morality is a functional morality for housewives and mothers; it is not for businessmen and professionals.

Adult moral stabilization, then, appears to be more a matter of increased congruence between belief and social role than of novel integration of experience. As such, it appears to be more like 'socialization' or 'social learning' than development. As we have dis-

318

cussed at length elsewhere [KOHLBERG, 1968], there is plenty of evidence that while the ordinary mechanisms of social learning (repetition, reinforcement, observational learning) or of attitude change (dissonance reduction) cannot cause or explain structural development, they can cause or explain the strengthening or weakening of 'naturally' or 'structurally' developing systems of response, a strengthening or weakening that seems to be what we have discussed as 'stabilization.'

Before dismissing adult functional stabilization as 'socialization,' however, it will pay to examine the most dramatic finding of the KRAMER study. This finding seems to fit neither our generalization that adult change is functional stabilization nor our earlier generalization that developmental change is forward and sequential. These generalizations hold true for our longitudinal subjects at every age and social class with one exception, the college sophomore. That paradigm of the psychological study of the normal, the college sophomore, turns out to be the oddest and most interesting moral fish of all. Between late high school and the second or third year of college, 20 % of our middle class sample dropped or retrogressed in moral maturity scores. Retrogression was defined as a drop in maturity scores greater than any found in a two-month-test-retest sample. This drop had a definite pattern. In high school 20 % who dropped were among the most advanced in high school, all having a mixture of conventional (Stage 4) and principled (Stage 5) thought. In their college sophomore phase, they kicked both their conventional and their Stage 5 morality and replaced it with good old Stage 2 hedonistic relativism, jazzed up with some philosophic and sociopolitical jargon. An example of a college Stage 2 response is given in table III along with Stage 2 responses by children and delinquents which are structurally similar to it.

Table III. Examples of sophisticated and unsophisticated Stage 2 responses to one story

Story III American

In Europe, a woman was near death from a very bad disease, a special kind of cancer. There was one drug that the doctors thought might save her. It was a form of radium that a druggist in the same town had recently discovered. The drug was expensive to make, but the druggist was charging ten times what the drug cost him to make. He paid $200 for the radium and charged $2,000 for a small dose of the drug. The sick woman's husband, Heinz, went to everyone he knew to borrow the money, but he could only get together about $1,000 which is half of what it cost. He told the druggist that his wife was dying, and asked him to sell it cheaper or let him pay later. But the druggist said, 'No, I discovered the drug and I'm going to make money from it.' So Heinz got desperate and broke into the man's store to steal the drug for his wife.

Should the husband have done that? Why?

Guide for Scoring Story III at Stage 2—as oriented to instrumental necessity of stealing:

1. *Value.* 'The ends justify the means.' Says has to, is best to, or is right to steal, to prevent wife from dying. (Without implication that saving the wife is a good deed.)
2. *Choice.* Little conflict in *decision to steal.* Implies decision is based on instrumental reasoning or impulse.
3. *Sanction.* Little concern about punishment, or punishment may be avoided by repayment, etc.
4. *Rule.* Little concern about stealing in this situation. May see stealing in this situation as not hurting the druggist.
5. *Husband role.* Orientation to a family member or a relative whom one needs and is identified with. May be an act of exchange, but not of sacrifice or duty.
6. *Injustice.* Druggist's 'cheating' makes it natural to steal. However, not actually indignant at the druggist, who may be seen as within his rights to charge whatever he wants.

Roger (age 20, a Berkeley Free Speech Movement student).

He was a victim of circumstances and can only be judged by other men whose varying value and interest frameworks produce subjective decisions which are neither permanent nor absolute. The same is true of the druggist. I'd do it. As far as duty, a husband's duty is up to the husband to decide, and anybody can judge him, and he can judge anybody's judgment. If he values her life over the consequences of theft, he should do it.

(Did the druggist have a right?) One can talk about rights until doomsday and never say anything. Does the lion have a right to the zebra's life when he starves? When he wants sport? Or when he will take it at will? Does he consider rights? Is man so different?

(Should he be punished by the judge?) All this could be avoided if the people would organize a planned economy. I think the judge should let him go, but if he does, it will provide less incentive for the poorer people to organize.

John (age 17, reform school inmate).

Should the husband steal the drug for his wife? I would eliminate that into whether he wanted to or not. If he wants to marry someone else, someone young and good-looking, he may not want to keep her alive.

(How about the law, he is asked): He replies, The laws are made by the rich, by cowards to protect themselves. Here we have a law against killing people but we think it's all right to kill animals. In India you can't. Why should it be right to kill people but not animals? You can make anything right or wrong. To me what is right is to follow your own natural instincts.

Hamza (Turkish village, age 12).

Yes, because nobody would give him the drug and he had no money, because his wife was dying it was right.

(Is it a husband's duty to steal the drug?) Yes—when his wife is dying and he cannot do anything he is obliged to steal. If he doesn't steal his wife will die.

(Does the druggist have the right to charge that much for the drug?) Yes, because he is the only store in the village it is right to sell.

(Should he steal the drug if he doesn't love his wife?) If he doesn't love his wife he should not steal because he doesn't care for her, doesn't care for what she says.

(How about if it is a good friend?) Yes—because he loves his friend and one day when he is hungry his friend will help him.

(Should the judge punish him?) They should put him in jail because he stole.

320

Jimmy (American city, age 10).

It depends on how much he loved his wife. He should if he does.
(If he doesn't love her much?) If he wanted her to die, I don't think he should.
(Would it be right to steal it?) In a way it's right because he knew his wife would die if he didn't and it would be right to save her.
(Does the druggist have the right to charge that much if no law?) Yes, it's his drug, look at all he's got invested in it.
(Should the judge punish?) He should put him in jail for stealing and he should put the druggist in because he charged so much and the drug didn't work.

The college response is that of a new left Bay area student, from the HAAN, SMITH and BLOCK [1968] study. Very similar statements are made by new right Ayn Rand objectivist students. Our Stage 2 longitudinal college subjects had similar ideologies but without extremist sociopolitical affiliations, except for one self-defined Nietzschean racist, a Chicagoan who went to a Southern all-white college.

In terms of behavior, everyone of our retrogressed subjects had high moral character ratings in high school, as defined by both teachers and peers. In college at least half had engaged in anti-conventional acts of a more or less delinquent sort. As an example, our Nietzschean racist had been the most respected high school student council president in years. In his college sophomore interview, however, he told how two days before he had stolen a gold watch from a friend at work. He had done so, he said, because his friend was just too good, too Christ-like, too trusting, and he wanted to teach him what the world was like. He felt no guilt about the stealing, he said, but he did feel frustrated. His act had failed, he said, because his trusting friend insisted he lost or mislaid the watch and simply refused to believe it had been stolen. This personal moral rebellion in the behavior of college Stage 2 men must be added to the picture of political protest behavior of Stage 2 college men provided by the HAAN, SMITH and BLOCK [1968] study.

Now if the mysterious forces of development have led our 20% from upstanding conventional morality to RASKOLNIKOV moral defiance, these same mysterious forces set them all to right. Every single one of our retrogressors had returned to a mixed Stage 4 and 5 morality by age 25, with a little more 5 or social contract principle, a little less 4 or convention, than at high school. All too are conventionally conforming in behavior, at least as far as we can observe them. In sum, this 20% was among the highest group at high school, was the lowest in college and again among the highest at 25. The correlation of moral maturity from age 16 to age 25 is .89, the correlations from high school to college and of college to 25 are only .41[3].

In what sense is the story just told, the story of rebellious use of lower stages followed by a return to the suburbs of conventional-principled moral stabilization, a story of development? Our interpretation of this story allows us to consider the sense in which the universal stabilization of morality in adulthood may be a form of adult development, even if it is not the structural transformation of moral thought itself. By focussing upon the dramatic cases of stabilization involving retrogression, rather than the placid cases of stabilization which look like ordinary socialization and social learning, we may perhaps arrive at an answer to the question. The first point in our argument is that the retrogression of our subjects it more like a functional regression than it is like a structural regression. While our retrogressors choose to use Stage 2 relativistic egoism, they have not lost their earlier capacity to use Stage 4 and Stage 5 thinking. This is evidenced by three facts. First, the retrogressors continue to use a little Stage 4 and 5 thinking. Second, when asked to give what the world would consider a high moral response to our stories, the retrogressors tend to give straight Stage 4 responses. Third, the fact that the retrogressors eventually return to Stage 4 and 5 strongly suggests that these stages were never lost. In contrast to this group there do appear to be some groups in which cases of genuine structural regression in adulthood can be found. We have found adults who were pure Stage 1, pure Stage 2, or combinations of Stage 1 and 2 among schizophrenics, among people over 65, and among incarcerated criminals. The schizophrenics were college educated, currently functioning well on psychometric tests of intelligence and preparing to leave the hospital. The criminals were in our longitudinal sample and had shown some Stage 3 and 4 thinking earlier. The elderly were college educated, and intact in intelligence according to norms for their age. While interviews of these cases did not use the methods of testing the limits for structural capacity or understanding of higher stages we have recently developed [REST, 1968] they give an overwhelming impres-

[3] The pattern of correlations I have just discussed is pointed to in MARJORIE HONZIK's paper in this symposium as the adolescent sleeper effect, an effect not unique to the moral area.

sion of unawareness of alternative or higher points of view which contrast with our college retrogressors.

If the regression of our college sophomores is functional, not structural, does it fit formulations of ego-psychology about 'regression in the service (function) of the ego'? One way of stating this question is provided by a graduate student, who proclaimed in a seminar that Stage 7 is reached when you can use all six stages for whatever you want. This student formulates regression in the service of the ego 'as a way of life', and ends up advocating plain old regression to Stage 2. Surely, when we cut through the cloudy lofty aura of such words as 'identity', 'self-realization', 'authenticity' which hover around the ego, we must recognize that an ego which uses moral values for whatever it pleases is just our good old instrumentally egoistic, manipulating Stage 2 ego.[4] Moral 'regression in the service of the ego' is not the usual law of life. It is true that everyone seems to share our retrogressors capacity to fall back upon lower stages. REST [1968] has demonstrated that the capacity to comprehend and (less clearly) to use lower stages of thinking remains, even where these lower stages are never used spontaneously in response to moral problems. He has also demonstrated, however, that the polymorphous-perverse flexibility of stage usage called Stage 7 by the graduate student, the use of various stages for whatever you want, is extremely uncharacteristic of adolescents. In spontaneous usage, people are quite consistent from situation to situation in use of a modal stage and the stages immediately adjacent to them [KOHLBERG, 1969]. In confronting the moral judgments of others, people prefer the highest level they can comprehend [REST, 1969; REST, TURIEL and KOHLBERG, 1968]. In a sense, the kind of adult change we called stabilization is exactly a further increase in consistency of response, a further decline in moral regression in the service of the ego.

In summary, while there is nothing unusual in our retrogressor's capacity to use lower stages of thought, their actual usage of such thinking is not evidence of a general human tendency to-

---

[4] There is a sense in which there is morally 'legitimate' regression of moral thought in the service of the ego. The hierarchy of moral stages is only a hierarchy in moral situations. No one uses Stage 6 thinking in bargaining in an Oriental marketplace, anymore than does anyone use PIAGET formal operations to drive a car or paint a picture. The capacity to write a compelling novel or to tell a good off-color joke depends upon using lower stages of moral thinking; the inability to think lowerstage thoughts is the mark of the prig.

ward regression in the service of the ego. It is not an adaptive bending to particular social situational presses in the service of some general ego needs.

The fact that awareness of relativism constitutes a universal developmental challenge or task for men attending a college with some claims to intellectual standing is clearly documented by the work of PERRY [1968]. In the case of our retrogressors, there is considerable use of relativism and of anti-moral protest to free themselves from familialy induced guilt. At least half of our regressors gave conscious and clear statements of strong sensitivity to and preoccupation with guilt feelings in preadolescence and adolescence. In this preregression period, the guilt was completely accepted as the voice of higher morality, as something self-accepted and internal. At the same time, the capacity of the boy's parents to inflict this sense of guilt was also noted by the boys. After they left home, they started to test out their capacity to be guilt-free. The most striking example was the Nietzschean who stole the watch from his friend (Raskolnikov). We labelled him 'Raskolnikov' with good reason. Like Raskolnikov's crime, his crime was an effort to prove that the strong need not be moral, and that the good were good only out of stupidity and weakness. Like Raskolnikov's crime, his crime too was an effort to prove that he need never feel (or fear) guilt [KOHLBERG, 1963]. After the theft he kept remarking that it was strange, but he felt no guilt. Four years later, after his return to the fold, he spontaneously announced that he had later felt guilt about it. The use of relativism by young men, then, is similar to that noted by PERRY [1968, p. 137]. 'The reactive students, in becoming aware of intellectual and moral relativism, see authorities as imperialistically extending their prejudices over the underdog's rightful freedom, and engage in a fight against the constraint of (unwarranted) guilt. Consider the conventional misuse of cultural relativism "Since it's all right for the Trobriand islanders to do thus and so, you have no right to make me feel guilty about it. It's purely a matter of individual decision". Far from being amoral, such pronouncements are made in a tone of moralistic absolutism, which reveals its emotional continuity with the earlier absolutistic structures' (which we term Stage 4).

While using relativism to free themselves from guilt, our retrogressors are equally upset at relativism and deviance, i.e. at the disappearance of the moral world they believed in in childhood. Our regressors are acutely aware of the breakdown of their expectations of a conventional moral world in the college environment. When they left high school, they thought that people lived by conventional morality and that their rewards in life depended on living that way, too. In college, they tell us, they learned that people did not live in terms of morality, and that if they did, they weren't rewarded for it. As one college Stage 2 said in explaining his 'regressive' shift. 'College accounts for the change. You see what a dog-eat-dog world it is. Everyone seems to be out for himself. When you live at home you're always trying to please your parents. You don't notice it, but in some way you are. Now I hang around with guys I don't try to please'.

Related to this theme is the theme that morality doesn't get you ahead. This boy says, 'I'd try to get as far as I can without becoming totally dishonest'.

The 'oppositional' quality of our regressor's moral ideology is, then, as much to be understood as being as a protest against the immorality of the world as it is a protest against the authoritarian morality of parental figures.

There are, then, two developmental challenges to conventional morality to which our regressors are unhappily responding. The first is the relativity of moral expectations and opinion, the second is the gap between conventional moral expectations and actual moral behavior. Now it is clear that these developmental challenges are universal general challenges. The integration of one's moral ideology with the facts of moral diversity and inconsistency is a general 'developmental task' of youth in an open society. So, too, are the more 'psychodynamic' problems faced by our regressors, the problems of freeing themselves from childhood moral expectations and childhood moral guilt. While 'psychodynamic', these conflicts are neither unusual nor pathological. Who has not desired to free himself from parentally induced guilt, who has not faced the shocks of finding there are no rewards for being a good boy or girl? The conflicts of our regressors differ only in quantity, not in quality, from our own.

If the challenges which our retrogressors face are universal, in what sense can their responses to them be said to be 'development'? We shall contend that our retrogressors are in a sense taking a developmental step forward, even though this step is reflected in a lower stage. We shall further contend that in 'returning' to their high school pattern of Stage 4 and Stage 5 thought, they are not simply reverting to an earlier pattern, retreating to the suburbs after the failure of rebellion; but are taking a still further developmental step forward.

In discussing these changes as development, we shall first cast them in ERIKSON's [1950] familiar terms. In such terms, our retrogressors are living in a late adolescent psychosocial moratorium, in which new and non-conforming patterns of thought and behavior are tried out. Their return to the high school pattern of moral thought is the eventual confirmation of an earlier identification as one's own 'identity'. To find a socio-moral identity requires a rebellious moratorium, because it requires liberation of initiative from the guilt which our retrogressors suffer from. At the 'stage' of identity the adult conforms to his standards because he wants to, not because he anticipates crippling guilt if he does not.

In introducing such terminology, we are indicating that late adolescent or adult moral changes reflect ego development rather than representing the development of morality or moral stage structures itself. Our moral stages are hierarchical structures for fulfilling the function of moral judgment. Ego development in the moral sphere is learning how to use the moral structures one has for one's personal integration. From this point of view, modes of moral thought are structures developed in childhood, but the uses of these modes of thought, their significance for the individual self are matters for late adolescent development. Until late adolescence, the child lives within a world he did not make and in which the choices he must make are circumscribed. His moral ideology is not a direct reflection of his home-school-class-nation environment; it is his own construction designed to make sense of it. However, use of his moral ideology in childhood is primarily to fit and make sense of his given world, not to guide him in autonomous choice. It gives him a rationale for accepting and conforming to the bulk of the patterns of his home, his peer group, his school. This rationale also allows him to reject some patterns in his environment, his world. It does not lead him to question or reject his entire world, however.

The early adolescent's characteristic pattern is either to protest or to secretly deviate from the particular rejected pattern, but to place it in the context of a world he must accept. Sometimes in the back of the conventionally moral high school boy's mind is the notion that he is 'putting in time' in the family and the high school until he can live a free life in terms of his own values and desires. While the adolescent may see a free life as a living out of hedonistic values, he may at the same time look forward to the opportunity to live or act in terms of sacrifice to higher moral principles, to give a moral meaning to his life in a way he cannot within the conventional structures of family and school.

ERIKSON has made us familiar with the fact that Western society provides the post-high-school student with a psychosocial moratorium which allows him to live out either hedonistic or morally idealistic impulses (reflected in anything from life in protest groups to life in the Peace Corps) with a freedom he has neither earlier or later in life. This moratorium comes to an end when inner establishment of an identity or outer pressure to take responsibility in a role of work and parenthood lead the individual to a commitment to a pattern of values which 'works' within a definite social world. The restraint which results from adult role-commitment differs vastly from the childhood restraint which comes from a dependent acceptance of such a world. They share in common, however, the acceptance of a core set of rules required to keep a social group or system going.

Neither the egoism of Stage 2 relativism of our retrogressors, nor its pretentious world-changing 'idealism' will keep a social world of responsibility for other people going. It is not, of course, that our retrogressors' moral code does not work at all, it can work to the extent of creating social movements, but it does not work if these movements are to become worlds of life-long responsibility and commitment. When the communist movement became an enduring one, it lost its orientation toward the pursuit of happiness and human equality and hardened into a Stage 4 morality of party loyalty as an absolute value. Our retrogressors 'return to the suburbs' of contractual (Stage 5) and conventional (Stage 4) rules is not, then, a defeat. It is not so much that Stage 2 Yippie or Hippie or objectivism is tried and found not to work, as it is that our late adolescent retrogressors were in a moratorium in which they didn't care about having an ideology that 'worked', that formed a foundation for life-long responsibility or commitment.

Not only is the retrogressors' return not a defeat, but it clearly brings something to conventional contractual morality which is in some sense a developmental advance. When the retrogressors return to a morality of contract and rules, they do so with less distortive idealization of their own group and authority system, and with greater tolerance and realism about those who deviate from it or are outside of it.

The formulation we have just made is inadequate. We have superimposed developmental task 'stages' of ego function in adulthood upon childhood stages of moral structure and claimed structural regression was functional advance. Obviously, such an attempt to have one's cake and eat it too is inadequate. A sequel to the paper attempts to correct this inadequacy by defining ego 'stages' in terms of metaethical theories and world views, in contrast to moral stages which are normative ethical theories for making moral judgments in specific moral conflict situations. For the moment, however, our formulation allows us to approximate some conclusions about the relations between childhood and adult moral development.

Moral development involves a continual process of matching a moral view to one's experience of life in a social world. Experiences of conflict in this process generate movement from structural stage to structural stage. Even after attainment of the highest stage an individual will reach, there is continued experience of conflict. The developmental product of such conflict is stabilization, i.e. a greater consistency of structure with itself (greater stage 'purity') and a greater consistency between thought structure and action. The evidence that adult stabilization is the integration of conflict rather than 'social learning' or socialization, is indicated by our finding one pattern of adult stabilization that involves temporary retrogression. The integration of conflict in adult development may be conceived in terms of functional 'stages' of ego development which are quite different from structural stages. While I have discussed only moral change at the 'ego stage' of late adolescent identity, the moral changes in late adulthood of the Tolstoys or the Saint Paul presumably could be discussed in the same general terms.

There is, then, a sense in which there is adult moral development. There is an adult movement toward integration in the use of moral structures, in the integration of moral thought in its application to life. There may even be typical phases in this integrative process. There are, however, no adult stages in the structural sense, and accordingly no clear solution to the two problems of adult development which we initially posed. We cannot integrate childhood and adult moral development into a single theoretical series or sequence of stages. Nor can we claim that adulthood has a moral wisdom denied to the youth. While structural stages involve a logic of responsiveness to the next stage up, this is not true of ego functional stages.

We may conclude with a concrete example of the discrepancy of implication between ego functional stages and moral structural stages for communication between the generations. The HAAN, SMITH, and BLOCK Berkeley studies indicated [1968] that those most likely to engage in social protest were students at Stage 2 and Stage 6 in moral judgment. The official stance of the University administration was variously Stage 5 and Stage 4, depending upon whom one considers the spokesman. On the face of it, this and other administrations were in a bad way as far as generational communication goes. Some dissidents were Stage 6, one step above the administration Stage 5 position, whereas others were Stage 2, so far below the administration position as to be indifferent to it. Short of moving up to an adult equivalent of the Stage 6 dissident view, the administration's appeal to the police seemed the inevitable alternative. Limiting ourselves to the Stage 2 'retrogressed' dissidents, however, our findings suggest that the Stage 5 administrator could be structurally understood by the dissident even though it was typed and rejected as Stage 4 'law and order' authoritarianism. In fact, many of the Stage 2 dissidents might end up as Stage 5 'administrators' in the course of adult development.

Aside from the concrete dividing political issues, the administrators and the Stage 2 dissidents are divided by the fact that the administrators have made peace with the problems of relativism and moral inconsistency in the world. Such peace is perceived as a sense of balance and moderation by the administrator, as 'sellout' and 'machine-likeness' by the dissident. The impasse in communication, then, are due less to the fact that lower stages do not understand higher stages than it is to a discrepancy in developmental task. This is shown by the fact that there are a number of middle-aged adults who speak vital and authentic 'childrenese' to the youth, because as they publicly proclaim, they are still pursuing the developmental task of seeking identity and commitment in a society which is not ideal.

If the Stage 5 and 6 'administrators' of our society are to speak effective 'adultese' to the young, they must give up talk about responsibility and moderation as well as talk of law and order. Instead they must try to express whatever sense of commitment they have found genuinely meaningful. As we suggest in the sequel, if developmental psychology is to aid in such communication between the generations, it must learn the language of philosophy.

References

BAYLEY, N.: On the growth of intelligence. Amer. J. Psychol. *10:* 805–815 (1953).

ERIKSON, E.: Childhood and society (Norton, New York 1950).

HAAN, N.; SMITH, M.B. and BLOCK, J.: The moral reasoning of young adults: Political-social behavior, family background, and personality correlates (in press);

HOBHOUSE, L.T.: Morals in evolution (Chapman and Hall, London 1906).

HOLSTEIN, C.: The relation of children's moral judgment to that of their parents and to communication patterns in the family. Unpublished dissertation, University of California, Berkeley 1969.

KOHLBERG, L.: Psychological analysis and literary forms. A study of the doubles in Dostoevsky. Daedalus *92:* 345–363 (1963).

KOHLBERG, L.: Stage and sequence: the cognitive-developmental approach to socialization, in GOSLIN Handbook of socialization theory (Rand McNally, Chicago 1968).

KOHLBERG, L.: Stages in the development of moral thought and action (Holt, Rinehart and Winston, New York 1969).

KRAMER, R.: Moral development in young adulthood; unpublished doctoral dissertation, Univ. of Chicago (1968).

KRAMER, R.: Progression and regression in adolescent moral development. Soc. Res. Child Development, Santa Monica, March 26, 1969.

PERRY, W.: Forms of intellectual and ethical development in the college years. Mimeo monograph. Bureau at Study Counsel, Harvard University.

PIAGET, J.: The general problems of the psychobiological development of the child; in TANNER and INHELDER, Discussions on child development: Proceedings of the World Health Organization study group on the psychobiological development of the child, vol. IV, pp. 3–27 (International Univ. Press, New York 1960).

PIAGET, J.: Cognitive development in children; in RIPPLE and ROCKCASTLE Piaget rediscovered: A report on cognitive studies in curriculum development (Cornell Univ. School of Education, Ithaca, N.Y. 1964).

REST, J.: Developmental hierarchy in preference and comprehension of moral judgment; unpublished doctoral dissertation, Univ. of Chicago (1968).

REST, J.; TURIEL, E. and KOHLBERG, L.: Relations between level of moral judgment and preference and comprehension of the moral judgment of others. Journal of Personality (1969).

SMEDSLUND, J.: The acquisition of conservation of substance and weight in children. Scand. J. Psychol. *2:* 85–87, 156–160, 203–210 (1961).

TURIEL, E.: Developmental processes in the child's moral thinking; in MUSSEN, LANGER and COVINGTON New directions in developmental psychology (Rhinehart, New York 1969).

WERNER, H.: The comparative psychology of mental development (Wilcox and Follett, Chicago 1948).